The New Consumer Drug Digest

Revised and Updated

Staff
American Society of Hospital Pharmacists

Mary Jo Reilly
Senior Vice President

James P. Caro
Director, Special Projects Division

Susan R. Dombrowski
Assistant Editor

Shelly Elliott
Production Manager

Luan Corrigan
Consultant

The New Consumer Drug Digest

Revised and Updated

American Society of
Hospital Pharmacists

FACTS
ON FILE

The New Consumer Drug Digest

The nature of drug information is that it is constantly evolving and often subject to interpretation. Therefore, while the American Society of Hospital Pharmacists has made every effort to ensure the accuracy and completeness of the information presented, the reader is advised that no claim can be made that all possible adverse reactions or interactions are contained in this book. Additionally, the reader is reminded that the CONSUMER DRUG DIGEST is not to be considered a substitute for the professional judgment of a physician or pharmacist.

Library of Congress Cataloging in Publication Data
Main entry under title:
Consumer drug digest.
  Includes index.
  1. Drugs—Popular works. I. American Society of Hospital
Pharmacists.
RM301.15.C66 615'.1 81-12499
ISBN 0-8160-1254-7   AACR2
ISBN 0-8160-1255-5 (pbk.)

Printed in the United States of America
10 9 8 7 6 5 4 3 2 1

Contents

Introduction

Many people want—and need—more information about medicines. The CON-SUMER DRUG DIGEST is an authoritative handbook on drugs, written in language that is readily understood by lay readers. The purpose of this book is to help consumers, as patients, understand the medications they take and learn what they can do to help their doctors prescribe the most beneficial drug therapy. It should help patients become responsible participants in their own health care.

This book is both a general source for information about drugs and a quick reference handbook for patients who want to supplement the information provided by doctors and others involved in the care of their health. It is *not*, however, intended as a do-it-yourself handbook or as a substitute for doctors' recommendations. Nor is it intended to help patients "second-guess" their doctors. The guiding assumptions of this book are that its readers have faith in their doctors and the others who are participating in their health care, and that they want to help assure that their drug therapy contributes to their overall good health.

The CONSUMER DRUG DIGEST concentrates on the rational use of legitimate drugs in the treatment of properly diagnosed medical problems. It does not discuss the abuse of prescription drugs, illegally obtained drugs or "street drugs." It includes entries on over 250 of the most frequently prescribed prescription drugs, comprising over 1,000 brand-name products. Selected non-prescription drugs are also included. The index includes the generic and brand names of all of the drugs covered in the book. *You must know either the generic or brand name of the drug you are taking to look it up in this book.* Simply find the name in the index and turn to the entry on the page to which you are directed. Only some of the many brand names of drug products are included. The brand names included here were selected according to the frequency with which they are prescribed. If you know the generic name of the drug you are taking, but can't find the brand name, the information in the entry on that generic drug will still apply.

Similarly, only a few of the many products that contain more than one drug (called combination products) are included here. If you know the names of the individual drugs in your combination, you can read about those drugs by looking them up in the index.

The information provided here is intended to help consumers take commonly prescribed medicines in a responsible manner. No attempt has been made to provide *complete* information on any drug or to cover all drug products. This book will provide answers to some of your general questions about the drugs you are taking and offer suggestions concerning their proper use. It is not intended as a substitute for your doctor's judgment about your particular medical condition. Always tell your doctor everything you know about your general health and medical problems.

It will help your doctor direct your health care. Drugs act differently in different people, and only your doctor can prescribe and direct your drug therapy effectively. Frequent suggestions are made to "contact your doctor for more information." Always follow your doctor's advice and the instructions on your prescription label, even if they are different from what you read here.

As indicated above, drugs act differently in different people. This is especially true in children and in old or debilitated patients. Many drugs have not been tested or used extensively in children. Generally speaking, someone younger than 12 is considered a "child"; however, depending on physical maturity, a "child" could be up to 16 years old. Sometimes a drug's effects on children may be very different from its effects on adults; some drugs should not be given to children under any circumstances. These precautions are noted in the entries on those drugs. No general precautions are made concerning the use of drugs in children, but it is always a good idea to discuss thoroughly with your doctor the use of any drug to treat your child.

Similarly, changes that occur as part of the aging process can affect the way one responds to drugs. Drugs may act quite differently in elderly patients than in younger ones. It is not possible to pinpoint a specific age at which this may begin to occur, but you should be aware that more frequent adjustments of dosages—and more frequent undesired effects—can be expected as the aging process advances. This precaution is not noted in the entries on individual drugs; in general, it applies to all drugs.

While medicne—and drug therapy—are precise sciences, they are also arts. "Always" or "never" situations rarely occur. It must be emphasized again that this book is a guide for you as a patient, and that your doctor must remain the one primarily in charge of your drug therapy. In an entry on a specific drug here you may be advised, for example, that "large doses" of that drug may produce a particular undesirable effect or that the drug may have such an effect "when taken over a long period of time." There are, however, no absolute answers to the questions "how large" or "for how long." Only your doctor, who knows your individual medical condition, can make that judgment. The information in this book can help you to help your doctor in monitoring your therapy and can bring to your attention questions you may wish to discuss with him.

While, in general, the language in this book can be understood by the average reader, some medical and technical terms are used. This occurs primarily in the section of each entry entitled "Precautions," where it is suggested that you tell your doctor if you have certain medical conditions—diabetes, porphyria or lupus erythematosus, for example—before you begin taking the medication in question. These terms describe chronic or inherited diseases; if you suffer from them, you have almost certainly undergone extensive diagnostic investigation or treatment for them in the past, perhaps by doctors other than the one you are now seeing. Thus, while these are technical medical terms, it is assumed that if you have any of these conditions, you know it. "Translations" of these terms into ones more readily understood by other users of this book have consequently been avoided. The important point is that you must always give your doctor a complete medical history, including any major illnesses you have suffered in the past and any chronic or inherited diseases you may have.

Drugs are grouped in this book according to the major body systems whose ailments they are designed to combat. It is of course impossible to include here every disease. Many drugs are used to treat many different diseases or conditions. To make this book less cumbersome, drugs are described under only one medical condition. For example, prednisone is a "steroid" or cortisone-like drug used to treat many illnesses. It is described in this book under arthritis. If you are taking prednisone for asthma, however, you can use the index to find the entry on prednisone under arthritis; the information in that entry will apply equally to your prescription.

Brief descriptions of some diseases are also included in this book. These descriptions are intended to offer some background information that will help you understand your drug therapy. Again, your physician should be your main source of information about your disease or medical problem.

HOW DRUGS ACT

Drugs are chemical compounds that modify the body's characteristic natural chemical reactions. In many cases, drugs do not cure the disease they have been prescribed to treat—they merely ensure that the body's chemical processes take place normally for as long as they are used. Drugs alone are often insufficient to restore normal function. The body's natural ability to recuperate is often at least equally important. For example, many antibiotics do not actually kill bacteria; they merely retard their growth so that the body's normal defense mechanisms can eliminate the infection. Most drugs are not naturally occurring substances. After they have been at work in the body for a certain period of time, they are gradually eliminated, just like waste products. The exact path that specific drugs follow varies a great deal. Some drugs are broken down into other compounds by the liver before they are eliminated, while others remain unchanged. Ultimately, most drugs (or their by-products) are excreted in the urine, feces, sweat or tears. Some drugs are even eliminated through the lungs—alcohol, for example.

The length of time that it takes for different drugs to be absorbed, exert their intended effect and be eliminated varies considerably. This is why dosage schedules are different for each drug.

DOSAGE FORMS AND ROUTES OF ADMINISTRATION

Oral dosage is the most common and convenient route of drug administration. Tablets, capsules and liquids are common forms in which drugs may be administered orally. Some medications are available in the form of chewable tablets, particularly those that are commonly prescribed for children; certain medications are available as long-acting tablets or capsules. It is important that long-acting tablets and capsules be swallowed whole. If they are chewed, the medication may be released all at once rather than over an extended time.

Syrups, suspensions, solutions and tinctures are various liquid forms in which drugs may be administered. *Syrups* are liquids that contain sugar; they are usually thick. Many cough medications are available as syrups. *Suspensions* are liquids that contain large amounts of solid material that is suspended rather than dissolved. The medication in a suspension will settle to the bottom rather quickly, so it is important to shake a suspension thoroughly before pouring each dose. Most liquid antacid preparations are suspensions. *Solutions* and *tinctures* are clear liquids containing dissolved medication. Some special oral dosage forms are powders, granules or effervescent tablets that are mixed with or dissolved in water before use.

A special form in which some drugs are taken orally is the sublingual tablet. These tablets are *not* swallowed—they are placed under the tongue and allowed to dissolve slowly. The medication is absorbed directly into the bloodstream through the blood vessels under the tongue. This route of administration is useful when a rapid effect is desired, as is often the case in heart patients.

Inflammations or infections of the skin, eyes or ears are frequently treated by means of topical dosage—that is, the application of ointments, creams, solutions, lotions or dusting powders directly to the site of the problem. In some cases—when the skin is severely infected, for example—an antibiotic ointment may be used in conjunction with an oral antibiotic.

Injectable medications may be used when a very rapid effect is required, when a drug is ineffective if taken orally or when the presence or likelihood of nausea or vomiting precludes oral administration. Usually injectable medications are administered by nurses or physicians, unless the patient or a member of his or her family has been specially trained to administer injections.

Some drugs are administered by rectal suppository or enema, particularly in patients who are unable to take oral medication. For example, some anti-nausea medications are available as suppositories. Enemas are commonly used to treat constipation, but may also be used to treat bowel inflammations such as colitis.

Skin patches contain a premeasured supply of drug (e.g., nitroglycerin) in a specially designed material that releases the drug for absorption through the skin over a period of time (usually 24 hours).

TOXICITY

Most drugs are relatively free from toxic effects, but any drug can produce unwanted effects under certain circumstances.

Undesirable drug effects can be classified as follows:

Pharmacologic Effects.   Unwanted effects due to a drug's pharmacologic actions (side effects) are predictable and, therefore, somewhat controllable. The action of most drugs depends on the size of each dose. If too much of a drug is taken, the drug's action may be stronger than necessary and unwanted effects may occur. In addition, most drugs exert more than one kind of action. Those actions that are unrelated to the intended effect may also cause undesirable symptoms. In some cases, these symptoms can be eliminated or minimized by adjusting the dose; in other cases, the unwanted symptoms may decrease or disappear after the patient's body adjusts to the medication.

Undesirable drug effects are more likely to occur in those whose bodily functions are impaired. Age is an important factor, since the function of certain organ systems may be impaired in the very young and the very old. For example, kidney and liver functions are not well developed in the newborn; these same functions tend to deteriorate in the elderly. As a result, young or old patients may metabolize and excrete certain drugs at a relatively slow rate, causing the drug in question to build up in the bloodstream and, perhaps, to produce undesirable effects.

Other medical conditions can also increase the chances of adverse drug effects. Be sure to tell your doctor about any medical condition you may have, even if it seems unrelated to your current problem.

Allergic Reactions. Allergic reactions are unrelated to the pharmacologic action of a drug or to dosage. Such reactions are unpredictable. Practically any drug has the potential to cause an allergic reaction if it is given to a susceptible individual. It is difficult to predict whether a person will be allergic to a particular drug, although, in general, people with hay fever or other allergies are more likely to develop allergies to drugs.

Drugs that are chemically related to a drug to which a person is allergic may also produce an allergic reaction. For example, a patient who develops an allergy to one particular sulfa drug will probably also be allergic to many other sulfas.

Allergic reactions may involve many different types of symptoms; such symptoms may appear immediately, or not until several weeks after the patient has begun to take a drug. Skin disturbances are the most common symptom. These range from mild redness and itching to severe swelling and skin destruction. Other, less common symptoms of allergic reactions include fever, jaundice and blood reactions, such as certain types of anemia.

The most dangerous type of allergic reaction is anaphylaxis. This life-threatening condition involves a decrease in blood pressure and spasm of the breathing passages. This reaction occurs, if at all, immediately after the administration of a drug and is most common when the drug is given by injection.

Any type of allergic reaction is treated by discontinuing the use of the medication immediately. If symptoms are severe, antihistamines or steroids may be used to help relieve them. Anaphylactic reactions require immediate treatment at a hospital.

To minimize the chance of developing an allergic reaction, it is important to tell your doctor if you have a history of any type of allergy, including hay fever or asthma. This information may provide useful clues to drugs that you should avoid. It is also important that you tell your doctor about any unusual symtoms that develop after you begin to take a medication.

Drug Interactions. A drug interaction results when two or more drugs that are used concurrently affect each other's actions in some way. One or both drugs may become more or less effective, or undesirable effects may occur. Drug interactions are not necessarily bad; in fact, some are brought about intentionally to increase the therapeutic effect of certain drugs. The mechanisms through which drugs can interact are complex and involve changes in the ways that each is absorbed, metabolized and excreted.

Alcohol, because of its widespread use, is probably responsible for more interactions than any other drug. The drowsiness caused by many common medications (antihistamines, tranquilizers, sedatives, pain relievers) may be increased by even small amounts of alcohol.

It is important to note that many liquid medications such as cough syrups contain enough alcohol to produce this effect. If you have questions about the alcohol content of any medications you are taking, ask your pharmacist or check the label.

The important point about drug interactions is that they may occur any time you are taking more than one drug, including nonprescription drugs. Be sure to tell your doctor about all the medications you are taking before beginning to take a new medication, and always check with your doctor or pharmacist before using nonprescription medications.

TERATOGENICITY

The abnormal development of a fetus as a result of events that take place in the mother's body during pregnancy is known as teratogenesis. Known teratogens include X rays, certain diseases (for example, rubella or German measles) and some drugs. The first trimester of pregnancy (from conception to 90 days after conception) is the period during which malformations are most likely to occur.

A few drugs are known to cause teratogenic effects, but the vast majority have not been adequately evaluated for possible teratogenic effects. As a result, the safest course is to avoid taking any unnecessary medication during pregnancy, particularly during the first trimester. Be sure to tell your doctor if you are pregnant or if you are planning to become pregnant while taking medication.

HOW DRUGS REACH THE MARKET

Federal regulations require that a new drug cannot be marketed—that is, made available for general use by physicians throughout the country—unless it has been shown to be both safe and effective. In other words, a company that wishes to sell a drug must prove that it is safe for use in humans and, further, that it actually produces the intended effect. (You should realize that "safe" is a relative term; no drug is totally safe, and a physician must decide whether the benefits of a specific drug outweigh the dangers it may pose to the patient.)

To show that a drug is safe and effective, its manufacturer must carry out proper scientific studies, first in animals and then in humans. The drug will be given to animals, usually mice, rats and dogs, and information on its activity, potential usefulness in people, dosage and toxicity will be collected. If, after considering the results of these studies, the company feels the drug is promising, it will cautiously (starting with very low doses) give the drug to a small number of healthy human volunteers. These studies are aimed primarily at finding out how the drug acts in humans; that is, how long a dose remains effective, whether it can be taken by mouth, what side effects can be expected and so on.

If the drug is found to be safe, the question "Is it effective?" must be answered. A large number of patients (up to several thousand) are thus carefully treated with the drug. These patients are closely watched for signs of improvement in their illness and for the appearance of side effects. Over time, a complete picture of how well the drug works and how it is best used will develop.

If at this stage (usually several years, at least, after the drug's development) its manufacturers believe it is safe and effective, they will ask that they be allowed to market it. The Food and Drug Administration (FDA) is the branch of the federal government that makes this decision. The FDA will review the results of all research on the drug (actually, it will already have reviewed the research at several points as it was taking place) and decide whether the drug can be placed in general use or whether more study is necessary.

Patients who receive an experimental drug (referred to as an "investigational drug") are given complete information about its intended use, its expected side effects and how it compares with other treatments already in general use. These patients must voluntarily agree to have an investigational drug prescribed for them. Once patients have been informed about such drugs, their voluntary consent to receive them is known as "informed consent". It is required in all research studies involving human subjects.

Sometimes, a severe side effect may be observed only after the drug has been marketed and used to treat many thousands of patients. Such a side effect may occur in only one out of every 10,000 patients; therefore, it may not have occurred in the comparatively few patients who were given the drug before it was marketed. If the side effect is excessively severe in comparison with the benefits of the drug (or with the side effects of other, similar drugs), the drug will be *recalled*—removed from the market. Drug recalls are rare, but they do happen. If you hear that a drug you are taking has been recalled, ask your doctor or pharmacist what to do. Sometimes only a particular batch of drug or form of the drug is recalled; therefore, don't stop taking it until you have contacted your doctor or pharmacist.

OVER-THE-COUNTER VS PRESCRIPTION DRUGS

A wide variety of medications are available without a doctor's prescription. These so-called "over-the-counter" drugs can be safely used to treat minor illnesses that do not require medical supervision. The primary distinction between prescription and "over-the-counter" drugs is that the latter have a wider margin of safety. They have fewer and milder side effects and little or no potential for addiction. In many cases, a drug will be available only as a prescription drug until experience shows that it is suitable for use by the general public.

This does not mean that "over-the-counter" drugs are harmless. They can and do cause problems if they are not used according to instructions on the labels or when they are used to treat conditions that should be evaluated by a physician. "Over-the-counter" drugs may also affect the way your body responds to other medicines you may be taking. For this reason, you should always check with your pharmacist before beginning to use an "over-the-counter" product if you are already taking medication for another conditon.

In contrast to "over-the-counter" drugs, prescription drugs are potent drugs that should only be used after thorough evaluation of a medical problem. They are more likely to cause unwanted effects and, therefore, can only be used safely under the supervision of your physician.

UNDERSTANDING THE PRESCRIPTION
Prescriptions are usually written in a format similar to the one illustrated below.

John Jones, M.D.
125 Main Street
Cornstalk, NB 10123

Name: Joe Smith
Address: 41 S First Street

℞

   Ampicillin 250 mg
    #20
   Sig: 1 tid

Do not refill   _____
Refill 1 times

       Date _____

Although the exact placement of information may vary, the following information should appear:

1. The patient's name and address.
2. The superscription—The "℞" symbol is the heading for the prescribed medication. The origin of this symbol is uncertain. It may have developed either from an abbreviation of the Latin word for recipe or from the sign of Jupiter, which was included on ancient prescriptions in order to invoke the god's blessing. In any case, the symbol has become a standard notation.
3. The name and strength of the drug.
4. Quantity.
5. Directions for use—the notation "sig." precedes the directions for the use of the medication. The actual directions are usually abbreviated in Latin notation. The most commonly used abbreviations are:

qd—every day	q __ h—every __ hours
BID—twice a day	ac—before meals
TID—three times a day	pc—after meals
QID—four times a day	prn—when needed

6. Refill information.
7. Date.
8. The prescriber's name, address and registry (DEA) number.
9. The prescriber's signature.

In many cases, a physician will transmit the prescription to the pharmacist via telephone. This cannot be done, however, with prescriptions for controlled substances (narcotics, stimulants, etc.). The law requires that pharmacists dispense these medications only upon receipt of a written prescription signed by the physician.

Refill Laws.   Regulations on refilling prescriptions vary from state to state. Federal law, however, stipulates that prescriptions for Class II controlled drugs may not be refilled and that prescriptions for Class III, IV, and V drugs are valid for only six months. A maximum of five refills are allowed during the six-month period.

Pharmacists exercise considerable judgment in determining whether or not to contact a physician regarding refills. Any time that there is a question about the advisability of refilling a prescription, the pharmacist will check with your physician to be sure that he wants you to continue taking that medication. In the event that the pharmacist is unable to reach your doctor for a refill authorization, he may dispense a small quantity to tide you over until he can reach your doctor.

EXPENDITURES FOR DRUGS

The prices of drugs, like those of almost all consumer products, are affected by our general economy. In recent years, these prices have climbed, and many consumers now shop for the "best buy" in their prescriptions, just as they shop for the best buy in a TV set. Prices for identical medications can vary greatly; the reasons for this are numerous.

The price of a prescription must obviously cover the cost of the ingredients, the container used, labor, professional services, overhead and a reasonable level of profit. Different pharmacies have different expenses, which are reflected in the prices you pay. Moreover, some pharmacists calculate their fees and profits in relation to the cost of the ingredients in each prescription, while others set standard fees that they apply to all of their prescriptions.

But when you think of the prices you pay, more than the prescription itself should be considered. A discount pharmacy may offer a cost savings, but it is unlikely that the pharmacist there will inform you about how to take your prescription, warn you about side effects, keep a patient profile on all of the medications you are taking and answer your questions. This type of care and expenditure of time are built into the price charged for the same drug at another pharmacy. In addition to price, such factors as the convenience of the location, the hours the store is open and the availability of delivery service will obviously affect your selection of a pharamcy.

Generic vs. Brand-Name Prescriptions.   The generic name is the official name given to a drug, while the brand name is the registered trade name given to a drug by its manufacturer. Generic drugs are often less expensive than brand-name products. Since the manufacturer of a specific drug has a large investment in research and advertising, the cost of brand-name products must cover these expenses. For example, a brand-name anti-anxiety agent might cost twice as much as its generic equivalent, chlordiazepoxide. Consumers concerned about costs should discuss this question with their doctors so that prescriptions are written for the least expensive form of a specific drug. And they should ask their pharmacists for help in selecting generic "over-the-counter" drugs, as opposed to more expensive brand-name products. Some drugs, however, are not available under generic labels because the patents obtained by their original manufacturers have not yet expired. Furthermore, some brand-name items are priced so low that they don't cost much more than the generics.

Drug Prices in Hospitals.   Among hospitals, the charges made to patients for drugs also vary widely. Some hosptials simply add a specific percentage to the cost of acquiring the medication. Others charge a dispensing fee, which is calculated according to the cost of acquiring the medication, operating expenses, a profit margin and the number of units that are dispensed. Still other hospitals price their drugs by a markup fee system, which combines features of each of the other two systems. The most recent pricing method tried by hospitals is the per diem system; a uniform drug charge is made per day to each type of patient.

Heart Diseases and Diseases of the Circulatory System

DRUGS USED TO TREAT HEART DISEASES AND DISEASES OF THE CIRCULATORY SYSTEM

Heart Attack and Stroke

HEART ATTACK

Typically, a person who suffers a heart attack has a history of heart pain (angina), but many heart victims have never experienced any symptoms of heart problems.

"Myocardial infarction," "coronary occlusion" and "coronary thrombosis" are other terms used to describe a heart attack.

A heart attack is usually caused by a sudden blockage in blood flow through the coronary blood vessels that supply oxygen and nutrients to the heart. The blockage is usually caused by atherosclerosis, the buildup of fatty substances on the inner walls of the blood vessels, but may also be caused by a blood clot. The sudden reduction in blood flow deprives the heart muscle of oxygen and nutrients and may result in extensive damage.

Once a heart attack has occurred, immediate treatment is required. The goal of treatment is to relieve pain, limit the extent of damage to the heart muscle and allow the damaged heart muscle to heal. The victim of a heart attack must rest. Drugs and other measures, including surgery, are used to help restore normal blood flow through the heart and heart function.

Drug therapy and proper exercise and diet are important for recovery from a heart attack.

STROKE

The damage to a portion of the brain due to bleeding from a ruptured blood vessel is known as a stroke. Strokes can also occur when blood flow to the brain is severely reduced because of the presence of blood clots within the vessels in the brain. Other terms used to describe a stroke include "cerebral vascular accident (CVA)," "intracranial hemorrhage," "cerebral thrombosis," "cerebral embolism" and "apoplexy."

Recovery from a stroke generally requires a long time; sometimes permanent brain damage occurs, and full recovery is impossible. A stroke victim may suffer paralysis on one or both sides of the body, speech impairment or the loss or impairment of other body functions. A rehabilitation program which includes exercise, physical therapy and speech training is often necessary.

The goal of drug therapy is to control blood pressure and prevent blood clots.

Congestive Heart Failure

The medical term congestive heart failure refers to a condition in which the weakened heart does not work as efficiently as it should. To say that the heart is "failing" does not mean that it will stop beating. The term "congestive" refers to a backup or slowdown in the movement of blood and fluids through the circulatory system.

Congestive heart failure occurs when the heart's ability to pump blood has been reduced by congenital heart disease, rheumatic heart disease, high blood pressure, narrowing of the arteries by atherosclerosis, coronary artery disease or heart attack. The heart muscle lacks sufficient strength to keep the blood circulating normally throughout the body. As a result, the flow of blood is inadequate to meet all the body's needs. The heart goes on working, but not as strongly as it should to maintain good health.

To understand what happens when heart failure occurs, it is necessary to know something about how the heart works as a pump. The heart is a hollow, muscular organ that pumps blood to the lungs and through the body. An adult's heart is about the size of a man's clenched fist and is shaped like an egg. It is located slightly to the left of the center of the chest and is protected by the breastbone and the rib cage.

In an adult, the heart normally beats between 60 and 90 times per minute, or about 100,000 times a day. It pumps blood, which carries nourishment and oxygen through the arteries to billions of body cells. The veins then carry blood back to the heart.

The amount of blood pumped by the heart varies with the body's activity and oxygen requirements. The heart and blood vessels can adjust the flow of blood to meet the body's needs. Most of the time the heart does not work at full capacity. Sitting, standing, walking and other moderate activities place only slight demands upon the heart. During strenuous activity the heart must pump faster than while resting to supply the required oxygen. Also, during some illnesses and when a fever is present, the heart must work harder.

When the heart is weakened by a heart attack, rheumatic fever, high blood pressure or gradual narrowing of the body's arteries, the heart does not pump efficiently. Blood which is returning to the heart tends to back up and pool in the veins. Fluid is forced out through the thin blood vessel walls into surrounding tissue resulting in swelling or "edema," especially in the legs and ankles. Sometimes fluid collects in the lungs, causing shortness of breath.

Heart failure also affects the ability of the kidneys to eliminate salt and water, further aggravating the edema.

Treating the underlying cause of congestive heart failure is often an important part of therapy for congestive heart failure. For instance, if high blood pressure is placing strain on the heart, it can often be reduced or controlled by drugs and a restricted diet. Or when defective heart valves are causing heart failure, they can often be corrected by surgery.

The successful treatment of congestive heart failure requires a clear understanding of the importance of rest, drugs, diet and physical activity.

Many people need rest. Physical activity should usually increase only gradually. To avoid strain on the heart, some patients may have to adjust to a slower pace and take things a bit easier. A sodium-restricted diet is almost always necessary in the treatment of congestive heart failure to prevent or reduce edema or fluid accumulation. Sodium is a mineral essential to life, but ordinarily we get more than we need from the food we eat. Because table salt contains a large amount of sodium, a diet designed to reduce the amount of sodium and fluid in the body restricts the use of table salt and may also require abstaining from certain foods that contain a high amount of sodium. Salt substitutes are available, which makes this task much easier.

Several medications may be prescribed for the treatment of fluid accumulation. One may be a drug called a diuretic or "water pill," which increases the amount and frequency of urination. A diuretic helps the kidneys get rid of excess water and sodium. This not only relieves edema but may also help in controlling high blood pressure.

The most common drugs given orally to patients with congestive heart failure are digitalis glycosides (digitoxin, digoxin, lanatoside C and gitalin). These drugs can also be used to treat other heart disorders, including atrial fibrillation, an irregular heart rhythm (arrhythmia).

Digitalis Drugs
(di ji tal' is)

PRODUCT INFORMATION
Brand names for digitoxin (di ji tox' in): Crystodigin, Purodigin
Brand names for digoxin (di jox' in): Lanoxin, Lanoxicaps
Brand name for gitalin (ji' tal in): Gitaligin
Brand name for lanatoside C (lan at' oh side): Cedilanid
Brand names for a mixture of chemicals from the digitalis plant: Digifortis, Digiglusin, Pil-Digis

USES
All drugs in the digitalis group act on the body to produce the same effects, both beneficial and harmful. They are prescribed for people suffering from congestive heart failure and other heart diseases.

Digitalis helps an injured or weakened heart to work more efficiently and send more blood through the body. Digitalis acts directly on the heart muscle to strengthen the force of the heart muscle's contractions. By improving the circulation of blood, digitalis helps remove excess water from the tissues and relieves symptoms of heart failure such as edema (swelling, usually of the lower legs or ankles) and shortness of breath. Digitalis is usually used with a diuretic (water pill) such as hydrochloro-thiazide or furosemide. See the general statement titled Thiazide Diuretics for more information.

A low-salt diet is usually recommended, because salt holds water in the body and makes diuretics less effective in removing excess water.

Digitalis also slows the heart rate and helps restore a normal, steady rhythm. It can be used alone or in combination with other medications that help regulate the heartbeat.

UNDESIRED EFFECTS

Digitalis is a potent drug. Keep in close contact with your doctor to find the dosage that works best without producing side effects. You will probably have to take digitalis for a long time—possibly for the rest of your life.

When you first start to take digitalis, your doctor will probably prescribe a large (loading) dose; the dosage will be reduced later. It is important that you cooperate with your doctor by always taking the amount prescribed and by reporting any bad effects.

Contact your doctor immediately if you experience loss of appetite, excessive salivation, nausea, vomiting or diarrhea; changes in vision such as blurring, color changes (usually in yellow-green vision) or seeing spots or halos; headache, confusion or depression; irregular heartbeat or changes (slow) in heart rate (pulse). These could be signs that you are taking too much digitalis; your doctor needs to know about them to adjust the dosage or change the drug.

It is possible to have more digitalis in the body than is needed, but having too little can also be a problem. Difficulty breathing and swelling in the legs and ankles are the most common signs that your dose is too low. If normal activity causes shortness of breath, or if you awaken frequently during the night due to shortness of breath, tell your doctor.

Once you and your doctor have determined the dosage that is right for you, you will not usually experience side effects as long as you take digitalis exactly as prescribed.

PRECAUTIONS

Digitalis can cause you to lose potassium, an important mineral or electrolyte, especially if you are also taking a diuretic (water pill). Your doctor may prescribe a potassium supplement. You should also ask for a list of foods that are high in potassium and emphasize them in a well-balanced diet. (See the monograph titled Potassium Supplements for more information.)

Before you start to take digitalis, tell your doctor what prescription and nonpre-scription drugs you are taking, including antacids, cholestyramine, cimetidine, colestipol, corticosteroids, diltiazem, diuretics (water pills), kaolin-pectin (diarrhea medicine), laxatives, magnesium trisilicate, medicine for coughs, colds or allergies, nifedipine, phenobarbital, phenylbutazone, phenytoin, procainamide, propranolol, quinidine, reserpine, rifampin, sulfasalazine, verapamil and other drugs for your heart condition. These medications can decrease the effect of digitalis or increase it to a potentially dangerous level. If you do not know the names of the drugs you are taking or what they were prescribed for, take the labeled containers to your doctor or pharmacist.

Tell your doctor if you have ever taken digitalis and what reaction you had to this medication. Allergies can occur, although they are uncommon. Your general state of health can affect the way digitalis acts on you. Tell your doctor everything about your health and medical history especially thyroid, kidney or liver problems.

If you develop an illness (other than your heart disease) with vomiting and diarrhea, the amount of digitalis absorbed into your bloodstream and reaching your heart can be affected. If you go to another doctor for such an illness, be sure to state that you are taking digitalis. You may wish to carry a card indicating you are taking digitalis so that doctors will know this information in the event of an accident that renders you unconscious.

Your doctor may perform certain tests including blood counts, tests to determine your blood level of certain electrolytes (especially sodium and potassium) and electrocardiograms (EKGs) to determine the effect of digitalis on your body. *Keep all appointments with your doctor and the laboratory.*

If you are pregnant, plan to become pregnant or are nursing a baby, tell your doctor before you start to take digitalis.

Do not stop taking digitalis unless you have your doctor's permission. Do not take any new drugs without checking first with your doctor.

DOSAGE

The digitalis drugs are similar but not interchangeable. The body metabolizes them differently and, therefore, different dosages are required. If you switch to a different digitalis drug, follow the directions on the prescription label for dosage.

The digitalis drugs come in tablets, capsules and liquid form and should be used only under the close supervision of a doctor. *It is very important that digitalis be taken on a regular schedule.*

You may be instructed to take a large (loading) dose at first and reduce it to your maintenance (continuing) dose after a few days. Your doctor may change your maintenance dosage later depending on your response to the drug. Carefully follow the instructions on your prescription label, and ask your doctor or pharmacist to explain any part you do not understand.

If your doctor tells you to take digitalis once a day, take it at the same time you do something else every day, such as brushing your teeth in the morning or going to bed at night, to help you remember to take it.

If you are taking antacids, cholestyramine, colestipol, kaolin-pectin, magnesium trisilicate, neomycin or sulfasalazine, take it at least two hours after digitalis to prevent interference with the absorption of digitalis.

If you forget a dose, do not take the missed dose when you remember it. Omit that dose and take only the scheduled dose at the next scheduled time. *Do not take a double dose.* If you forget to take two or more doses in a row, contact your doctor or pharmacist for instructions.

Your doctor may recommend a low-salt or low-sodium diet. Follow this recommendation, because it will help your medication work as it should. Your doctor may also suggest that you stop smoking cigarettes, because they can make the heart muscle more sensitive to digitalis. Ask your doctor about the use of alcohol and caffeine. They are usually safe when used in moderation.

While you are taking digitalis, your doctor may ask you to check your pulse every day. Your doctor or pharmacist can show you how to do this; your doctor will tell you how rapid your pulse should be. If your pulse is slower than it should be, contact your doctor to find out whether you should continue taking digitalis.

STORAGE
It is important to keep digitalis out of the reach of children. It is a frequent cause of accidental poisoning in children. Keep digitalis in the container it came in and do not allow anyone else to take it.

Diuretics

Diuretics are also used in the treatment of congestive heart failure. See the sections on Diuretics and Thiazide Diuretics (page 9) and discussion of individual diuretic drugs under High Blood Pressure or Hypertension.

High Blood Pressure or Hypertension

You may have high blood pressure (hypertension) for many years without experiencing any symptoms other than tiredness, nervousness, dizziness or headaches. Your blood pressure should be checked every time you visit a doctor, for whatever reason, so that high blood pressure can be detected as early as possible. You should have your blood pressure checked annually, even if you have no symptoms of high blood pressure and have not visited a doctor for any other reason.

High blood pressure can be treated easily with a proper diet, moderate lifestyle and drug therapy. If high blood pressure remains untreated, it can lead to serious health problems, including congestive heart failure, heart attacks, strokes and kidney disease.

High blood pressure occurs when the blood vessels constrict or narrow, causing resistance to the flow of blood. The causes of high blood pressure include abnormalities in the heart, kidneys or nervous control of the blood vessels.

The drugs used to treat high blood pressure may act on the heart, the nervous system or the kidneys. Frequently, more than one drug is used.

Thiazide diuretics are considered the most useful drugs in the initial treatment of high blood pressure. If a diuretic alone does not effectively control blood pressure, other drugs (generally referred to as antihypertensive drugs) are added.

DIURETICS

Diuretics are commonly referred to as "water pills." They act on the kidneys, causing them to eliminate excess water and salt from the body in the urine. Diuretics are the mainstay of treatment for high blood pressure. They help control high blood pressure with minimal side effects. Diuretics can help control high blood pressure, but do not cure it. They are also used to treat the fluid retention caused by heart, liver and kidney disease. Certain drugs, such as steroids or estrogens, can cause your body to retain water; diuretics can be used to relieve this side effect.

Thiazide Diuretics

USES

Thiazide diuretics are a "family" of drugs that are closely related in chemical structure and action in the body. Their blood pressure-lowering effects and undesired effects are very similar, but they may differ in the duration of their diuretic action. Your doctor will choose the one best-suited for you and for your lifestyle. Included in the ''family'' of thiazide diuretics are chlorothiazide, hydrochlorothiazide, methyclothiazide and chlorthalidone. Metolazone is a diuretic that is similar to the thiazides in chemical structure, uses, undesired effects and precautions.

Thiazide diuretics reduce blood pressure by acting on both the kidneys and the blood vessels. In the kidneys, these drugs eliminate salt and water. Urine production and the frequency of urination are increased. Thus the volume of fluid in the body and the amount of salt (whose most important component is sodium) in body tissues are reduced.

Thiazides also act on the small blood vessels, causing the walls of the vessels to relax—the blood vessels consequently expand, and the space available for the circulation of blood is increased. The combined effect of reduced volume of fluid and expanded space is a reduction in blood pressure. Thiazide diuretics, given alone for mild high blood pressure, often reduce the pressure to a normal range. They are usually considered the drugs of choice for the initial treatment of high blood pressure when there is no underlying kidney disease. *Unless your doctor tells you to stop, you should continue to take your diuretic even if you feel good.* If you have edema (swelling caused by fluid retention) or high blood pressure, you will usually have to take a diuretic, and possibly other drugs, for the rest of your life.

UNDESIRED EFFECTS

Side effects may occur during the first week you take a thiazide diuretic, but often go away within the second week. While you are taking a thiazide diuretic, the levels of minerals or electrolytes such as potassium in your body can get too low. If you suffer from muscle cramps, nausea or weakness, excessive thirst, drowsiness or restlessness or a rapid pulse, call your doctor right away. You may need to eat foods rich in potassium (e.g., bananas, oranges and other fruits) or take a potassium supplement. (See the monograph titled Potassium Supplements for more information.) Sometimes you can take a thiazide diuretic in combination with certain other diuretic drugs to avoid excessive loss of potassium.

PRECAUTIONS

Before starting to take any diuretic, discuss your general health and medical history with your doctor. Tell your doctor if you ever had liver disease, since the loss of salts and water caused by diuretics can worsen liver disease. Similarly, diuretics can increase blood sugar, so if you are diabetic or have a tendency toward diabetes, a change in diet or medication for diabetes may be needed. Diuretics can cause a gout attack in people with a history of gout. Rarely, diuretics can worsen or activate lupus erythematosus. Since these drugs act on the kidneys, tell your doctor if you ever had kidney disease or problems. If your kidneys are not working properly, the drug or your dosage may need to be changed.

Most diuretics are chemically similar to the ''sulfa drugs'' (anti-infectives) and to some of the drugs taken orally for the treatment of diabetes. If you have ever had an allergic reaction to sulfas, oral medication for diabetes or any diuretic, be sure to tell your doctor before you begin to take a thiazide or other diuretic.

Also, tell your doctor about any other drugs you are taking, especially cholestyramine, cortisone-type drugs or steroids, digitalis heart medicines, lithium or medicine for diabetes. The effects of these drugs may change when you begin taking a diuretic, or they may increase or decrease the action of the diuretic.

While taking a diuretic, avoid excessive heat; sweating can cause the loss of too much water and salt from your body.

DOSAGE
Taking a diuretic may make you urinate more often—these drugs are designed to remove excess water from your body. Unless your doctor tells you otherwise, take your diuretic in the morning. If you have to take the drug more than once a day, take the second dose before 6:00 p.m. to avoid having to urinate after you have gone to bed.

If you are taking cholestyramine, take it at least one hour after this medication to prevent interference with absorption.

Chlorothiazide
(klor oh thye' a zide)

PRODUCT INFORMATION
Brand names: Diuril, SK-Chlorothiazide

USES
Refer to the general statement titled Thiazide Diuretics.
Chlorothiazide begins to act as a diuretic, increasing excretion of water and salt, about two hours after it is taken and goes on working for six to 12 hours. No effect on blood pressure may be seen for two or three weeks.

UNDESIRED EFFECTS
Chlorothiazide causes frequent urination; this effect should decrease after a few weeks. Because chlorothiazide removes potassium from the body, you may experience muscle weakness, cramps, dizziness or lightheadedness, especially when you stand up or arise from a lying position. If your doctor has prescribed a potassium supplement for you, take it as prescribed. Allergic reactions such as skin rash or hives, nausea, vomiting, reduced appetite, stomach cramps, diarrhea, headache or blurred vision may also occur.

While you are taking chlorothiazide, you run an increased risk of sunburn. Limit the amount of time you spend in the sun or under a sunlamp. Wear sunglasses and be sure your body is covered by clothing or protected by a sunscreen preparation when you go out in the sun.

If you experience a sore throat or easy bruising, contact your doctor. If you have an illness that causes vomiting or diarrhea, the fluid balance in your body may be upset, so discontinue taking chlorothiazide and contact your doctor.

PRECAUTIONS

Laboratory tests for kidney and liver function, blood counts and tests to determine the levels of sodium, potassium, sugar and uric acid in your blood will probably be done periodically while you are taking chlorothiazide. *Be sure to keep all appointments with your doctor and at the laboratory.* Before taking chlorothiazide, inform the doctor of other prescription and nonprescription drugs you are taking. If you do not know the names of the drugs or what they were prescribed for, take the labeled containers to your doctor or pharmacist. Alcoholic beverages may exaggerate the degree to which chlorothiazide lowers blood pressure, causing lightheadedness and dizziness.

If you become pregnant while taking chlorothiazide, stop taking it and contact your doctor.

DOSAGE

Chlorothiazide comes in tablets and liquid to be taken orally. Your prescription label tells you how much to take at each dose and how often to take it. Follow the instructions carefully and contact your doctor or pharmacist if you have any questions. *Do not take more of this drug than your doctor prescribes* because excessive loss of water and salt from your body can cause unpleasant side effects.

If you are to take this medication twice a day, it is best to take it once in the morning and again in the middle of the afternoon so that you will not have to urinate during the night.

Chlorothiazide should be taken right after meals or with a snack. The liquid should first be thoroughly shaken.

If you forget to take a dose, do not take the missed dose when you remember it. Omit that dose and take your regular dose at the next scheduled time. Your doctor may recommend that you eat a low-salt or low-sodium diet, take a potassium supplement or increase the amount of potassium-rich foods in your diet (such as bananas and orange juice). Follow these recommendations; the medication will work better and you will feel better.

STORAGE

Keep this medication in the container it came in and out of the reach of children. Do not allow anyone else to take it.

Chlorthalidone
(klor thal′ i doan)

PRODUCT INFORMATION

Brand names: Hygroton, Thalitone

USES
Refer to the general statement titled Thiazide Diuretics.

Chlorthalidone is a long-acting diuretic. It begins to work as a diuretic, increasing elimination of water and salt, about two hours after it is taken and goes on working for 24 to 72 hours. You will have to take chlorthalidone for two or three weeks before you will know if it is effective in lowering your blood pressure.

UNDESIRED EFFECTS
Common effects of chlorthalidone are frequent urination and dry mouth. These effects tend to disappear after a few weeks. Dry mouth can be relieved by chewing gum, sucking on hard candy or drinking fluids.

Because this drug removes potassium as well as salt from the body, you may experience muscle weakness or cramps, dizziness or lightheadedness, especially on arising from a sitting or lying position. Contact your doctor if you experience these effects. If your doctor prescribes a potassium supplement, be sure to take it as instructed.

While taking chlorthalidone you run an increased risk of sunburn. Limit the amount of time you spend in sunlight or under a sunlamp. When you go out in the sun, wear sunglasses and be sure your body is covered with clothing or protected by a sunscreen preparation.

If you experience a sore throat or easy bruising, contact your doctor. Stomach upsets can be relieved by taking chlorthalidone with meals or a snack. If you have an illness that causes vomiting or diarrhea, the fluid balance in your body may be upset. Stop taking chlorthalidone and contact your doctor.

PRECAUTIONS
Laboratory tests of kidney and liver function and blood levels of sodium, potassium, sugar and uric acid and blood counts will probably be done periodically while you are taking chlorthalidone. *Be sure to keep all appointments with your doctor and at the laboratory.*

Inform your doctor of all the prescription and nonprescription drugs you are taking. If you do not know the names of the drugs or what they were prescribed for, take the labeled containers to your doctor or pharmacist.

Alcoholic beverages may exaggerate the effect of chlorthalidone in lowering your blood pressure and cause lightheadedness or dizziness.

If you become pregnant while taking chlorthalidone, stop taking it and contact your doctor.

DOSAGE
Chlorthalidone tablets are usually taken once a day or once every other day. Your prescription label specifies how much to take at each dose and when to take each dose. Follow the instructions carefully and contact your doctor or pharmacist if you have any questions. *Do not take more of this drug than your doctor prescribes* because excessive loss of water and salt from your body can cause unpleasant side effects.

It is a good idea to take this medication in the morning with your breakfast so that you will not have to urinate during the night.

If you forget to take a dose, take it when you remember if this is at least 12 hours before your next dose. If it is less than 12 hours before the next scheduled dose, skip the missed dose and take only your next scheduled dose at the regularly scheduled time.

Your doctor may recommend that you follow a low-salt or low- sodium diet, take a potassium supplement or increase the amount of potassium- rich foods (such as bananas and orange juice) in your diet. Follow these recommendations; the medication will work better and you will feel better.

STORAGE
Keep chlorthalidone in the container it came in, and out of the reach of children. Do not allow anyone else to take this medication.

Hydrochlorothiazide
(hye droe klor oh thye′ a zide)

PRODUCT INFORMATION
Brand names: Esidrix, HydroDiuril, Oretic, Thiuretic and others

USES
Refer to the general statement titled Thiazide Diuretics.

Hydrochlorothiazide begins to work as a diuretic, increasing elimination of water and salt, about two hours after it is taken and goes on working for six to 12 hours. You will have to take this drug for two or three weeks before you will know if it is effective in lowering blood pressure.

UNDESIRED EFFECTS
Frequent urination is a common effect of hydrochlorothiazide but should disappear after you have taken it for a few weeks.

Because hydrochlorothiazide removes potassium from the body, you may experience muscle weakness or cramps or lightheadedness on standing or arising from a lying position. If your doctor prescribes a potassium supplement, be sure to take it as instructed. Allergic reactions such as skin rash or hives, nausea and vomiting, reduced appetite, stomach cramps, diarrhea, headache or blurred vision may also occur.

You run an increased risk of sunburn while you are taking hydrochlorothiazide. Limit the amount of time you spend in the sun or under a sunlamp. When you go out in the sun, wear sunglasses and be sure your body is covered with clothing or protected by a sunscreen preparation.

Contact your doctor if you experience a sore throat or easy bruising. If you have an illness that causes vomiting or diarrhea, the fluid balance in your body may be upset, so stop taking hydrochlorothiazide and contact your doctor.

PRECAUTIONS

Laboratory tests for kidney and liver function, tests of the levels of sodium, potassium, sugar and uric acid in your blood and blood counts will probably be done periodically while you are taking this drug. *Keep all appointments with your doctor and the laboratory.*

Inform your doctor of all prescription and nonprescription drugs you are taking. If you do not know the names of the drugs or what they were prescribed for, take the labeled containers to your doctor or pharmacist.

Alcoholic beverages may exaggerate the effect of hydrochlorothiazide in lowering your blood pressure and cause lightheadedness or dizziness.

If you become pregnant while taking hydrochlorothiazide, stop taking it and contact your doctor.

DOSAGE

Hydrochlorothiazide comes in tablets to be taken orally. Your prescription label tells you how much to take at each dose and how often to take it. Follow the instructions carefully and contact your doctor or pharmacist if you have any questions. *Do not take more of this drug than your doctor prescribes* because excessive loss of water and salt from your body can cause unpleasant side effects.

If you are taking this medication twice a day, it is a good idea to take it once in the morning and once in the middle of the afternoon so that you will not have to urinate during the night. Hydrochlorothiazide should be taken right after meals or with a snack.

If you forget to take a dose, do not take the missed dose when you remember it. Omit the missed dose and take only the scheduled dose at the next scheduled time.

Follow your doctor's dietary recommendations. These may include a low-salt or low-sodium diet, taking a potassium supplement or increasing the amount of potassium-rich foods (such as bananas and orange juice) in your diet. The medication will work better and you will feel better.

STORAGE

Keep this medication in the container it came in and out of the reach of children. Do not allow anyone else to take this medication.

Methyclothiazide
(meth i kloe thye' a zide)

PRODUCT INFORMATION
Brand names: Aquatensen, Enduron

USES

Refer to the general statement titled Thiazide Diuretics.

Methyclothiazide is the most potent thiazide diuretic. Methyclothiazide begins to work as a diuretic, increasing excretion of water and salt, about two hours after it is taken and goes on working for about 24 hours. It may take two to three weeks for methyclothiazide to lower your blood pressure.

UNDESIRED EFFECTS

Frequent urination, a common effect of methyclothiazide, should decrease after a few weeks. Another effect is dry mouth; this effect will disappear after a few weeks. Dry mouth can be relieved by chewing gum, sucking on hard candy or drinking fluids.

You may experience muscle weakness, cramps or dizziness because this drug removes potassium as well as sodium. Contact your doctor if these side effects persist. Be sure to take your potassium supplement as instructed if one has been prescribed for you. Allergic reactions such as skin rash or hives, nausea and vomiting, reduced appetite, stomach cramps, diarrhea, headache or blurred vision may also occur.

While taking methyclothiazide you run an increased risk of sunburn. Limit the amount of time you spend in sunlight or under a sunlamp. When you are in sunlight, wear sunglasses and be sure your body is covered with clothing or protected by a sunscreen preparation.

Contact your doctor if you experience a sore throat, easy bruising or a skin rash. If you have an illness that causes vomiting or diarrhea, the fluid balance in your body may be upset. Stop taking methyclothiazide and contact your doctor.

PRECAUTIONS

Laboratory tests for kidney and liver function, blood counts and tests to determine the levels of sodium, potassium, sugar and uric acid in your blood will probably be done periodically while you are taking this drug. *Keep all appointments with your doctor and at the laboratory.*

Inform your doctor of all prescription and nonprescription drugs you are taking. If you do not know the names of the drugs or what they were prescribed for, take the labeled containers to your doctor or pharmacist.

Alcoholic beverages may exaggerate the degree to which methyclothiazide lowers blood pressure, causing lightheadedness or dizziness.

If you become pregnant while taking methyclothiazide, stop taking it and contact your doctor.

DOSAGE

Methyclothiazide comes as tablets. Your prescription label specifies how much methyclothiazide to take at each dose and how often to take it. Follow the instructions carefully and contact your doctor or pharmacist if you have any questions. *Do not take more than your doctor has prescribed.* Excessive loss of water and salt can cause unpleasant side effects.

If you are to take this medication once a day, take it in the morning so you will not have to urinate during the night. Methyclothiazide may be taken after breakfast or lunch or with a midmorning snack.

If you forget to take a dose, take it as soon as you remember. If you do not remember until the next day, omit the missed dose and take only the scheduled dose.

Follow your doctor's dietary recommendations. These may include eating a low-salt or low-sodium diet, taking a potassium supplement or increasing the amount of potassium-rich foods (such as bananas and orange juice) in your diet. If you follow your doctor's dietary recommendations, the medication will work better and you will feel better.

STORAGE
Keep this medication in the container it came in, and keep it out of the reach of children. Do not allow anyone else to take it.

Other Diuretics

Amiloride
(a mill' oh ride)

PRODUCT INFORMATION
Brand name: Midamor
Brand name of a combination product containing amiloride and hydrochlorothiazide: Moduretic

USES
Amiloride acts as a diuretic to increase excretion of salt and water by the kidneys and reduce blood pressure. It is usually used with another diuretic (water pill) such as hydrochlorothiazide (see the monograph titled Thiazide Diuretics for more information) to treat high blood pressure or congestive heart failure. Amiloride is known as a potassium-sparing diuretic because it does not cause the potassium loss produced by other diuretics.

UNDESIRED EFFECTS
Frequent urination is a common effect of amiloride but should decrease after a few weeks. Amiloride may cause nausea, abdominal pain, gas, loss of appetite or a mild skin rash. Take amiloride with food to decrease stomach problems. If these symptoms persist or are severe, contact your doctor.

Amiloride may cause you to retain too much potassium in your body. Signs of high blood level of potassium are muscle weakness, irregular heartbeat, fatigue and a "pins and needles" or tingling feeling (usually in the hands and feet). Stop taking amiloride and contact your doctor immediately if any of these symptoms occur.

PRECAUTIONS
Amiloride can make certain medical conditions worse. Tell your doctor if you have diabetes or kidney or liver disease.

If you have an illness that causes nausea and vomiting, the fluid balance in your body can be upset; stop taking amiloride and contact your doctor.

Certain foods should be avoided by people who are taking amiloride. Do not use salt substitutes unless your doctor has given you specific instructions for their use. Do not consume grapefruit juice, orange juice, tomato juice, bananas, apricots, coconut, dates, figs, peaches or prunes. These fruits and juices are high in potassium and could give you more potassium than you need. Consume these foods only with your doctor's permission.

Tell your doctor what prescription and nonprescription medications you are taking, particularly captopril, digoxin, lithium, medicine for high blood pressure, other diuretics (water pills) and potassium supplements. Do not take amiloride if you are taking spironolactone or triamterene (other potassium-sparing diuretics). If you do not know the names of the drugs you are taking or what they were prescribed for, take them in their labeled containers to your doctor or pharmacist.

Tell your doctor if you are pregnant or breast-feeding a baby. It is not known if it is safe to take amiloride during pregnancy or while breast-feeding.

Keep all appointments with your doctor and the laboratory. Your doctor will probably want to monitor your blood level of potassium regularly with blood tests to be sure it is not too high.

Alcoholic beverages may exaggerate the blood pressure lowering effect of amiloride, causing lightheadedness or dizziness.

DOSAGE

Amiloride comes in tablets. Your doctor will determine how much you should take at each dose and when you should take it. Follow the instructions on your prescription label carefully and ask your doctor or pharmacist to explain any part you do not understand.

Amiloride is usually taken once a day. Take it at the same time you do something else every day, such as brushing your teeth in the morning, to help you remember to take it. Amiloride should be taken with food to prevent stomach upset. It may be taken at the same time as another diuretic. It is a good idea to take this medication in the morning so that you will not have to urinate during the night.

Do not take more medication than your doctor has prescribed because excessive loss of water and salt from your body can cause unpleasant side effects and your potassium level may rise to a dangerously high level.

If you forget to take a dose, take it as soon as you remember. If you do not remember until the next day, omit the missed dose and take only the scheduled dose. *Do not take a double dose to make up for a missed dose.*

STORAGE

Keep this medication in the container it came in and keep it out of the reach of children. Do not allow anyone else to take your amiloride.

Ethacrynic Acid
(eth a krin' ik ass id)

PRODUCT INFORMATION
Brand name: Edecrin

USES
Ethacrynic acid causes the kidneys to excrete salt and water in the urine. Ethacrynic acid is one of the "loop" diuretics because it acts on the loops of the tiny filtering tubes in the kidneys. It is a strong and effective diuretic used to treat high blood pressure and the swelling and water retention caused by a number of medical problems including heart disease and certain diseases of the kidney and liver.

This medication begins to work as a diuretic about 30 minutes after it is taken, and it keeps on working for six to eight hours. Ethacrynic acid may be useful in treating conditions that have not responded to other diuretics or when kidney function is decreased. You may have to take ethacrynic acid for one or two weeks before you know if it lowers your blood pressure.

UNDESIRED EFFECTS
Frequent urination occurs commonly but usually decreases after a few weeks.

Ethacrynic acid can cause nausea or loss of appetite. These effects should be lessened if you take this medication with meals or immediately after eating. Contact your doctor if these problems continue. If you have any illness that causes vomiting or diarrhea, the fluid balance in your body may be upset; stop taking ethacrynic acid and contact your doctor.

If your doctor prescribes a potassium supplement for you, be sure to take it exactly as instructed. Because this drug causes potassium loss, you may experience muscle weakness or cramps. Contact your doctor if these symptoms occur.

Report any unusual bleeding or bruising, sore throat, fever, skin rash or yellow skin discoloration to your doctor. If you experience ringing in the ears or decreased hearing, contact your doctor.

PRECAUTIONS
Because ethacrynic acid is a powerful medication, your doctor will want to monitor your response to it carefully. Among the laboratory tests that will probably be performed while you are taking ethacrynic acid are tests for liver and kidney function, complete blood counts and tests to determine the levels of sodium, potassium, sugar and uric acid in your blood. Keep in touch with your doctor while you are taking ethacrynic acid, and *keep all appointments for checkups and laboratory tests.*

Before you take ethacrynic acid, tell your doctor what other prescription and nonprescription drugs you are taking, particularly corticosteroids, digitalis drugs (e.g., digoxin), diabetes medication, lithium, probenecid and sulfinpyrazone (gout medication) and warfarin (a blood thinner). If you do not know the names of the drugs or what they were prescribed for, take the labeled containers to your doctor or pharmacist.

Alcoholic beverages may exaggerate the degree to which ethacrynic acid lowers blood pressure, causing lightheadedness or dizziness.

Pregnant women and nursing mothers should not take ethacrynic acid.

DOSAGE

Ethacrynic acid tablets are usually taken once or twice a day. Carefully follow the instructions on your prescription label. Ask your doctor or pharmacist to explain any part you do not understand. *Do not take more of this drug than your doctor has prescribed* because excessive loss of water and salt from your body can cause unpleasant side effects.

This medication should be taken with meals or immediately after eating.

If you forget to take a dose, omit that dose and take only your regular dose at the next scheduled time. *Never take a double dose.*

Your doctor may recommend that you increase the amount of potassium-rich foods (such as bananas and orange juice) in your diet. Be sure to follow these recommendations.

STORAGE

Keep this medication in the container it came in, and keep it out of the reach of children. Do not allow anyone else to take it.

Furosemide

(fur oh′ se mide)

PRODUCT INFORMATION

Brand names: Lasix, SK-Furosemide

USES

Furosemide is a "loop" diuretic that acts on the loops of the tiny filtering tubes in the kidneys. It prevents salt from returning to body tissues and excretes unneeded salt and water in the urine. Furosemide is a strong and effective diuretic that is used to treat high blood pressure and the swelling and water retention caused by a number of medical problems, including heart disease and certain diseases of the kidneys and liver.

Furosemide begins to work as a diuretic about one hour after you take it, and it keeps on working for four to eight hours. It may be useful in treating people who have not responded to other diuretics or whose kidney function is not normal. You may have to take furosemide for a week or two before you know if it is effective in lowering your blood pressure.

UNDESIRED EFFECTS

Frequent urination occurs commonly but usually decreases after a few weeks.

You may experience muscle weakness or cramps, lightheadedness and dizziness. If any of these effects occur, contact your doctor. Furosemide may cause you to excrete too much potassium in your urine; muscle cramps and weakness are signs that your blood level of potassium is too low. If your doctor prescribes a potassium supplement, be sure to take it exactly as instructed. If you have an illness that causes vomiting or diarrhea, the fluid balance in your body may be upset; stop taking furosemide and contact your doctor.

PRECAUTIONS

Because furosemide is a strong medication, your doctor will want to check your response to it carefully. Laboratory tests for liver and kidney function, blood counts and tests to determine the levels of sodium, potassium, sugar and uric acid in your blood will probably be done periodically while you are taking furosemide. Keep in touch with your doctor while you are taking it, and *keep all your appointments for checkups and laboratory tests.*

Weigh yourself at least every day or every other day. If you begin to gain weight rapidly or if your hands and feet begin to get puffy, contact your doctor. If you can pinch the skin on the top of your hand and it remains puckered after you release it, contact your doctor.

Before you take furosemide, tell your doctor what other prescription and nonprescription drugs you are taking, particularly corticosteroids, diabetes medication, diflunisal and indomethacin (arthritis medication), digitalis drugs (e.g., digoxin), lithium, and probenecid and sulfinpyrazone (gout medication). If you do not know the names of the drugs or what they were prescribed for, take the labeled containers to your doctor or pharmacist.

Alcoholic beverages may exaggerate the degree to which furosemide lowers blood pressure, causing lightheadedness or dizziness.

Your doctor may recommend an increase in the amount of potassium-rich foods (such as bananas and orange juice) in your diet. Be sure to follow this recommendation.

Generally, pregnant women, women who might become pregnant during treatment and nursing mothers should not take furosemide.

DOSAGE

Furosemide comes in injection, tablets and liquid to be taken by mouth.

Furosemide is usually taken once or twice a day. Your prescription label gives specific instructions on how much furosemide to take at each dose and how often to take it. Follow these instructions carefully and ask your doctor or pharmacist to explain any part you do not understand. *Do not take more of this drug than your doctor has prescribed* because excessive loss of water and salt from your body can cause unpleasant side effects.

If you are instructed to take furosemide twice a day, take one dose in the morning and one in the middle of the afternoon so you can avoid having to urinate during the night. Use a specially marked measuring spoon to ensure an accurate dose of the liquid.

If you forget to take a dose, take it as soon as you remember and take any remaining doses for the day at evenly spaced intervals. If you are taking furosemide once a day and do not remember a missed dose until the next day, omit the missed dose. *Do not take a double dose to make up for a missed dose.*

STORAGE
Keep this medication in the container it came in, and keep it tightly closed. If the tablets darken in color, discard them and contact your pharmacist to get another supply.

Keep this medication out of the reach of children. Do not allow anyone else to take it.

Metolazone
(me tole' a zone)

PRODUCT INFORMATION
Brand names: Diulo, Zaroxolyn

USES
Metolazone is used to treat high blood pressure and fluid retention that is caused by a number of conditions including heart disease.

Metolazone begins to work as a diuretic, increasing elimination of water and salt, about one hour after it is taken and goes on working for 12 to 24 hours. You may have to take this drug for several weeks before you will know if it is effective in lowering blood pressure. Metolazone is similar to the thiazide diuretics in chemical structure, uses, undesired effects and precautions, but it may be more effective for people with kidney disease. See the general statement titled Thiazide Diuretics.

UNDESIRED EFFECTS
Frequent urination is a common side effect of metolazone, but it should disappear after a few weeks.

You may experience muscle weakness or cramps or lightheadedness on standing or arising from a lying position. Metolazone may cause you to excrete too much potassium in your urine; muscle weakness and cramps are signs that your blood level of potassium is too low. If your doctor prescribes a potassium supplement, be sure to take it as instructed.

Allergic reactions such as skin rash or hives, nausea and vomiting, reduced appetite, stomach cramps, diarrhea, headache or blurred vision may also occur.

You run an increased risk of sunburn while you are taking metolazone. Limit the amount of time you spend in the sun or under a sunlamp. When you go out in the sun, wear sunglasses and be sure your body is covered with clothing or protected by a sunscreen preparation.

Contact your doctor if you experience a sore throat or easy bruising. If you have an illness that causes vomiting or diarrhea, the fluid balance in your body may be upset; stop taking metolazone and contact your doctor.

To relieve dry mouth, drink fluids, chew gum or suck hard candies or lozenges.

Other side effects that may occur include bloating of the abdomen, chest pain, fast heartbeat and chills.

PRECAUTIONS

Laboratory tests for kidney and liver function, tests of the levels of sodium, potassium, sugar and uric acid in your blood and blood counts will probably be done periodically while you are taking this drug. *Keep all appointments with your doctor and at the laboratory.*

Tell your doctor what prescription and nonprescription drugs you are taking, particularly cholestyramine, corticosteroids, digitalis drugs (e.g., digoxin), lithium and medicine for diabetes. If you do not know the names of the drugs or what they were prescribed for, take the labeled containers to your doctor or pharmacist.

Alcoholic beverages may exaggerate the effect of metolazone in lowering your blood pressure and cause lightheadedness or dizziness.

Tell your doctor if you have liver disease or ever had a bad reaction to metolazone or a thiazide diuretic.

DOSAGE

Metolazone comes in tablets and is taken orally. Your prescription label tells you how much to take at each dose and how often to take it. It is usually taken once a day. Follow the instructions carefully and contact your doctor or pharmacist if you have any questions. *Do not take more of this drug than your doctor prescribes* because excessive loss of water and salt from your body can cause unpleasant side effects.

If you are instructed to take this medication once a day, it is best to take it in the morning so that you will not have to urinate during the night.

If you are taking cholestyramine, take it at least one hour after metolazone to prevent problems with absorption (of metolazone).

If you are taking metolazone more than once a day and forget to take a dose, take it as soon as you remember and take the rest of the doses for that day at evenly spaced intervals.

If you are taking this medication once a day and forget to take a dose, take it as soon as you remember. If you do not remember until the next day, omit the missed dose and take only the scheduled dose. *Do not take a double dose to make up for a missed dose.*

Follow your doctor's dietary recommendations. These recommendations may include eating a low-salt or low-sodium diet, taking a potassium supplement or increasing the amount of potassium-rich foods (such as bananas and orange juice) in your diet. The medication will work better and you will feel better.

STORAGE

Keep this medication in the container it came in, and keep it out of the reach of children. Do not allow anyone else to take this medication.

Spironolactone

(speer on oh lak' tone)

PRODUCT INFORMATION

Brand names: Aldactone, Spiractone
Brand names of a combination product containing spironolactone and hydro-chlorothiazide: Aldactazide, Spiractazide, Spironazide

USES

Spironolactone is used alone or in combination with other drugs to treat high blood pressure and water retention caused by conditions such as heart disease, liver disease and lung problems. It acts on the kidneys to eliminate salt and water from the body in the urine.

Spironolactone is known as a potassium-sparing diuretic; it removes much less potassium than other diuretics. Spironolactone is often prescribed in combination with other diuretics and blood pressure medications to minimize potassium loss and reduce blood pressure. The full diuretic effect of spironolactone may not occur for three days and up to four weeks may be required before the full blood pressure lowering effect is evident. Spironolactone also may be used instead of thiazide diuretics to treat high blood pressure in people with gout or diabetes, because these conditions can be made worse by thiazide diuretics.

UNDESIRED EFFECTS

Spironolactone can cause you to retain too much potassium in your body; symptoms of a high blood level of potassium include irregular heartbeat, muscle weakness, fatigue and a "pins and needles" or tingling feeling (usually in the hands and feet). Contact your doctor if you experience any of these effects.

Frequent urination is a common effect of spironolactone, but it will probably decrease after a few weeks.

Spironolactone may cause breast soreness (in females) or an increase in breast size (in males). If these effects are bothersome, contact your doctor. Other side effects of spironolactone include loss of appetite, nausea, vomiting, diarrhea, dry mouth, headache, confusion, drowsiness and lethargy. Contact your doctor if these symptoms persist.

PRECAUTIONS

Weigh yourself every day or every other day, and contact your doctor if you gain weight rapidly or notice puffiness in your hands or feet. If you have an illness that causes vomiting or diarrhea, the fluid balance in your body may be upset; stop taking spironolactone and contact your doctor.

Certain foods should be avoided by people who are taking spironolactone. *Do not use salt substitutes unless your doctor has given you specific instructions for their use. Do not consume grapefruit juice, orange juice, tomato juice, bananas, apricots, coconut, dates, figs, peaches or prunes.* These fruits and juices are high in potassium and could give you more potassium than you need. *Consume these foods only with your doctor's permission.*

Do not take aspirin while you are taking spironolactone. If you need something to relieve minor pain or fever, ask your doctor or pharmacist to recommend an aspirin substitute for you. Tell your doctor what prescription and nonprescription medications you are taking, particularly other diuretics, blood pressure medication and potassium. If you do not know the names of these drugs or what they were prescribed for, take the labeled containers to your doctor or pharmacist.

Alcoholic beverages may exaggerate the degree to which spironolactone lowers blood pressure, causing lightheadedness or dizziness.

Your doctor will want to monitor carefully your response to this medication by testing your kidney function and blood levels of sodium, potassium and chloride. Keep in touch with your doctor while you are taking spironolactone, and *keep all of your appointments for checkups and laboratory tests.*

Tell your doctor if you are pregnant or breast-feeding a baby. Safe use of this drug during pregnancy and while breast-feeding has not been established.

Before you have surgery (including dental surgery) with a general anesthetic, tell the doctor or dentist that you are taking spironolactone.

DOSAGE
Your doctor has determined how often you should take spironolactone tablets and how much you should take at each dose. Follow the instructions on your prescription label carefully and ask your doctor or pharmacist to explain any part you do not understand. *Do not take more of this drug than has been prescribed* by your doctor because excessive loss of water and salt from your body can cause unpleasant side effects.

Spironolactone should be taken with meals or immediately after eating. If you forget to take a dose, take it as soon as you remember and take the rest of the doses for that day at evenly spaced intervals. *Do not take a double dose to make up for a missed dose.*

STORAGE
Keep this medication in the container it came in, and keep it out of the reach of children. Do not allow anyone else to take it.

Triamterene
(trye am′ ter een)

PRODUCT INFORMATION
Brand name: Dyrenium

Brand names of combination products containing triamterene and hydrochloro-thiazide: Dyazide, Maxzide

USES

Triamterene is used to treat water retention caused by such conditions as heart disease, liver disease and lung problems. When used alone, it has little, if any, effect on blood pressure, but it is used in combination with another diuretic (e.g., hydro-chlorothiazide) or other drugs to treat high blood pressure (see the monograph titled Thiazide Diuretics for more information).

Triamterene acts as a diuretic to increase excretion of salt and water by the kidneys. It is known as a potassium-sparing diuretic because it causes a much smaller loss of potassium than most other diuretics. Triamterene begins to work as a diuretic about two to four hours after it is taken and continues to work for about 24 hours. It may take up to three weeks for triamterene to have any effect on blood pressure.

UNDESIRED EFFECTS

Frequent urination occurs commonly, but it usually decreases after a few weeks.

Triamterene can cause you to retain too much potassium in your body. Signs of a high blood level of potassium are muscle weakness, irregular heartbeat, fatigue and a "pins and needles" or a tingling feeling (usually in the hands and feet). Stop taking triamterene and call your doctor immediately if any of these symptoms occur.

If you experience nausea, take triamterene with meals or immediately after eating. Contact your doctor if triamterene causes vomiting or diarrhea, since these effects can upset the fluid balance in your body.

Triamterene can cause skin rash, headache, weakness or dizziness. If you experience any of these effects, contact your doctor.

PRECAUTIONS

Weigh yourself every day or every other day and contact your doctor if you begin to gain weight rapidly.

Triamterene can make certain medical conditions worse. Tell your doctor if you have diabetes or liver or kidney disease.

Certain foods should be avoided by people taking triamterene. *Do not use salt substitutes and do not consume grapefruit juice, orange juice, tomato juice, bananas, apricots, coconut, dates, figs, peaches or prunes.* These are high in potassium and could give you more potassium than you need. *Consume these foods only with your doctor's permission.*

Before taking triamterene, tell your doctor what prescription and nonprescription medications you are taking, particularly other diuretics, lithium, potassium supplements, indomethacin and other nonsteroidal anti-inflammatory agents (arthritis medicine). If you are taking amiloride or spironolactone (other potassium-sparing diuretics), do not take triamterene. If you do not know the names of the drugs or what they were prescribed for, take the labeled containers to your doctor or pharmacist.

Alcoholic beverages may exaggerate the degree to which triamterene lowers blood pressure, causing lightheadedness or dizziness.

Your doctor will want to monitor carefully your response to this medication and will probably ask you to have laboratory tests for kidney and liver function, complete blood counts and tests to determine the levels of sodium, potassium and chloride in your blood. Keep in touch with your doctor while you are taking triamterene, and *keep all of your appointments for checkups and laboratory tests.*

Tell your doctor if you are pregnant or breast-feeding a baby. Safe use of triamterene during pregnancy or while breast-feeding has not been established.

DOSAGE

Triamterene comes as capsules to be taken by mouth. Your doctor will determine how often you should take triamterene and how much you should take at each dose.

Follow the instructions on your prescription label carefully and ask your doctor or pharmacist to explain any part you do not understand. *Do not take more of this drug than your doctor has prescribed* because excessive loss of water and salt or excessive retention of potassium in your body can cause unpleasant side effects.

Note that Dyazide and Maxzide, the combination products containing triamterene and hydrochlorothiazide, are not identical. They contain different amounts of the two component drugs. Therefore, if you are switching from one of these drugs to the other, keep all appointments with your doctor and the laboratory so that your response to the medication can be monitored.

Triamterene should be taken with meals or immediately after eating. If you forget a dose, take the missed dose as soon as you remember and take any remaining doses for that day at evenly spaced intervals. If you do not remember until the next day, omit the missed dose and take only the scheduled dose. *Do not take a double dose to make up for a missed dose.*

STORAGE

Keep this medication in the container it came in, and keep it out of the reach of children. Do not allow anyone else to take it.

ANTIHYPERTENSIVES

Beta Blockers

PRODUCT INFORMATION

Brand name for atenolol (a ten' oh lole): Tenormin
Brand name for metoprolol (me toe' proe lole): Lopressor
Brand name for nadolol (nay doe' lole): Corgard
Brand name for pindolol (pin' doe lole): Visken
Brand name for propranolol (proe pran' oh lole): Inderal
Brand name for timolol (tye' moe lole): Blockadren

Brand name of a combination product containing propranolol and hydrochloro-thiazide: Inderide

USES

Beta blockers are a group of drugs that "block" the action of certain stimulating chemicals in the nervous system. Therefore, the drugs have widespread effects. Beta blockers affect the nerves that control the heart's pumping action and the narrowing (constriction) of the blood vessels.

All of the beta blockers are used to treat high blood pressure because they relax blood vessels, allowing the blood to flow more smoothly through the body and reduce blood pressure. They are often used with a diuretic (water pill) and other blood pressure medication.

Atenolol, metoprolol, pindolol and timolol have been used investigationally and nadolol and propranolol are approved for the treatment of heart pain (angina).

Usually, the treatment for heart pain is medication that increases the supply of blood to the heart, thus providing the heart with more oxygen. However, a person who does not respond to this treatment or who has a decreased blood supply to the heart (sometimes caused by fatty deposits in the vessels) may respond to a beta blocker because its action is entirely different. Rather than increasing the blood supply—and thus the supply of oxygen—to the heart, beta blockers decrease the heart's need for oxygen by decreasing the heart rate. For some people, the medication may reduce the frequency of heart pain attacks; for others, it may allow them to be more active without experiencing heart pain.

Propranolol is sometimes used to treat irregular heartbeat; it slows the transmission (movement) of nerve signals through the electrical system of the heart, which improves the rhythm (beat) of the heart. Propranolol is also used to prevent migraine headaches.

The beta blockers differ in their effect on the lungs. Atenolol and metoprolol may be preferred for people with lung problems such as asthma because they are less likely to cause undesired effects on the lungs (difficulty breathing and wheezing).

Timolol is used to prevent the recurrence of heart attacks (myocardial infarctions); metoprolol and propranolol are used investigationally for this purpose.

UNDESIRED EFFECTS

Beta blockers may have undesired effects on the lungs, particularly in people with lung problems such as hay fever, asthma, bronchitis or emphysema. If you become short of breath, start wheezing or have difficulty breathing while taking this medication, contact your doctor.

A variety of harmful effects on circulation and heart rate can occur depending on your medical condition. Keep in touch with your doctor while taking this medication.

Beta blockers cause some people to become dizzy, lightheaded or drowsy. Do not drive a car or operate dangerous machinery until you know how this drug will affect you.

If this medication upsets your stomach, take it with eight ounces of fluid or with a light snack. If nausea, vomiting or diarrhea persists, contact your doctor. It may be necessary to adjust your dosage.

Some other side effects of beta blockers are cold hands and feet, swelling of the feet and lower legs and unusual tiredness. With long-term therapy, hallucinations (seeing, hearing or feeling things that are not there), mental confusion, nightmares, vivid dreams and sleeping problems can occur. Although these effects are rare, contact your doctor at once if they occur.

Serious blood problems are a rare side effect. Stop taking the medication and contact your doctor if you have unusual bleeding, bruising or weakness.

PRECAUTIONS

Before taking beta blockers, tell your doctor if you have a history of allergy; lung problems such as emphysema, asthma or bronchitis; diabetes; or thyroid, kidney or liver disease.

When taken with other medications, beta blockers may have undesired effects. Before you take this medication, tell your doctor what prescription and nonprescription drugs you are taking, especially medication for your heart condition, high blood pressure, diabetes, asthma, depression or Parkinson's disease; cimetidine; phenothiazines (chlorpromazine, fluphenazine, perphenazine, prochlorperazine, promazine, thioridazine and trifluoperazine); MAO inhibitors (isocarboxazid, pargyline, phenelzine and tranylcypromine); allergy and cold medicines (e.g., phenylpropanolamine); aspirin and nonsteroidal anti-inflammatory agents (particularly phenylbutazone and indomethacin). If you do not know the names of the drugs you are taking or what they were prescribed for, take them in their labeled containers to your doctor or pharmacist.

Your doctor may prescribe a low-salt or low-sodium diet, tell you to stop smoking and restrict your intake of alcohol. It is very important that you follow these instructions to get the greatest benefit from this medication.

Your doctor may ask you to check your pulse (heart rate) every day while you take this medication and will tell you how rapid it should be. Ask your doctor or pharmacist to teach you how to take your pulse. If your pulse is slower than it should be, contact your doctor about taking the drug that day.

Keep all appointments with your doctor so that your response to the medication can be checked. You may have periodic exercise tests, electrocardiograms (EKGs), blood counts and other blood tests.

If you go to a dentist or other doctors, tell them that you are taking a beta blocker. You may want to carry a medical identification card so that, in case of an accident, those treating you will know you are taking a beta blocker.

Before you take this medication, tell your doctor if you are pregnant or nursing a baby. It is not known if it is safe to take a beta blocker during pregnancy or while breast-feeding.

DOSAGE

Beta blockers come as tablets. Your doctor will determine how much you should take at each dose and how often you should take it. Follow the instructions on your prescription label carefully and ask your doctor or pharmacist to explain any part you do not understand.

It is important that you take your medication regularly to be effective in controlling your blood pressure. Do not stop taking this drug without consulting your doctor. When your supply of tablets is getting low, contact your doctor or pharmacist about refilling your prescription.

If you forget to take a dose, take it as soon as you remember and take any remaining doses for that day at evenly spaced intervals. *Do not take a double dose to make up for a missed dose.*

STORAGE

Keep this medication in the container it came in, and keep it out of the reach of children.

Captopril
(kap′ toe pril)

PRODUCT INFORMATION
Brand name: Capoten

USES

Captopril is used to treat moderate to severe high blood pressure and congestive heart failure. It decreases the amount of certain chemicals that constrict the blood vessels so that the vessels remain relaxed and blood flows more smoothly through them. Captopril is usually tried after a combination of a diuretic (water pill), beta blocker and vasodilator has failed to control blood pressure. It is usually used with a diuretic in the treatment of high blood pressure.

Captopril is also taken by people with congestive heart failure who have not responded to digitalis drugs (heart medicine) and diuretics (water pills). A combination of three drugs may work best (see the monographs titled Digitalis Drugs and Thiazide Diuretics for more information).

UNDESIRED EFFECTS

The most common side effect of captopril is a red, itching skin rash which may disappear as your body adjusts to the drug. Contact your doctor if a rash develops; it may be necessary for you to decrease your dosage or take an antihistamine to treat the rash. Do not adjust your dosage or take any medication for the rash without consulting your doctor.

Another common side effect of captopril is a salty or metallic taste or decrease in the ability to taste. This usually goes away within three months while continuing to take the drug.

A less common side effect is a sickness accompanied by rash, fever, difficulty breathing and aching joints. Call your doctor if you experience any of these symptoms.

PRECAUTIONS

Tell your doctor what prescription and nonprescription drugs you are taking, especially amiloride, spironolactone and triamterene (potassium-sparing diuretics); potassium supplements and other medication for high blood pressure. If you do not know the names of the drugs you are taking or what they were prescribed for, take the labeled containers to your doctor or pharmacist.

Because captopril can make certain medical conditions worse, tell your doctor if you have kidney disease or SLE (systemic lupus erythematosis).

Laboratory tests including kidney and liver function tests, blood counts and blood levels of sodium and potassium will probably be done periodically while you are taking this drug. *Keep all appointments with your doctor and the laboratory.*

Contact your doctor if you experience a sore throat, mouth sores, fever or unusual bruising (signs of blood problems); swelling of the feet, ankles or lower legs; fast heartbeat or chest pain.

Captopril may cause dizziness, lightheadedness or fainting, particularly when you get out of bed or rise from a chair. Get up slowly to give your body time to adjust to the change in position.

If you have an illness that causes vomiting or diarrhea, the fluid balance in your body may be upset resulting in dizziness or fainting. Avoid strenuous exercise, exposure to hot weather and activities that result in excessive sweating because lightheadedness or fainting could result.

You run an increased risk of sunburn while taking captopril. Limit the amount of time you spend in the sun and wear sunglasses and protective clothing or a sunscreen preparation.

Your doctor may prescribe a low-sodium or low-salt diet. Do not use salt substitutes unless your doctor has given you specific instructions for their use. Salt substitutes contain potassium and could give you more potassium than you need. Follow your doctor's instructions on diet.

Inform your dentist or doctor that you are taking captopril if you plan on having surgery or any treatment with general anesthesia because this could result in a sudden, sharp drop in blood pressure and dizziness, lightheadedness or fainting.

Tell your doctor if you are pregnant or breast-feeding a baby. Captopril is passed from a mother to an unborn baby and through the milk to a breast-fed baby. It is not known if it is safe to take captopril during pregnancy or while breast-feeding.

DOSAGE

Captopril comes in tablets to be taken by mouth. Your doctor will determine how much you should take at each dose or how often you should take it. Follow the instructions on your prescription label carefully and ask your doctor or pharmacist to explain any part you do not understand. Captopril is usually taken three times a day. It should be taken on an empty stomach, one hour before or two hours after meals.

If you forget to take a dose, take it as soon as you remember and take the rest of the doses for that day at evenly spaced intervals. *Do not take a double dose to make up for a missed dose.*

Do not stop taking captopril without consulting your doctor. It will take several weeks for the full effect of the medication to be seen.

STORAGE
Captopril tablets may have a slight sulfur odor (like hard-boiled eggs). Keep captopril in the container it came in and keep it tightly closed and protected from moisture. Keep it out of the reach of children. Do not allow anyone else to take your medication.

Clonidine
(kloe' ni deen)

PRODUCT INFORMATION
Brand name: Catapres
Brand name of a combination product containing clonidine and chlorthalidone:
Combipres

USES
The nerves that control the blood vessels and are responsible for contracting and expanding the blood vessels are governed by a collection of nerve cells in the brain called the vasomotor center. Clonidine acts on the vasomotor center and helps keep the blood pressure normal by preventing the nerves from allowing the blood vessels to contract or narrow too much. The vessels remain more relaxed and open, and blood flows more smoothly through the body. This drug works very quickly, causing a decrease in blood pressure usually within an hour.

Although clonidine may be used alone to reduce blood pressure, it appears to be more effective when prescribed with a diuretic (water pill) such as chlorthalidone (see the monographs titled Thiazide Diuretics and Chlorthalidone for more information). Clonidine is also used with other medications that lower blood pressure, which often makes it possible to reduce the amount of each drug given.

Clonidine is sometimes prescribed for people who have experienced severe dizziness with other medications taken to lower blood pressure. It has also been used investigationally to prevent migraine headaches.

UNDESIRED EFFECTS
Clonidine makes many people drowsy or less alert than usual. Do not drive a car or operate dangerous machinery until you know how this drug will affect you.

Some of the common side effects of clonidine are dry nose, mouth and throat, headache and constipation. These effects tend to disappear as treatment continues. However, if they continue or are bothersome, tell your doctor at your next visit.

Contact your doctor if you experience swelling of the feet and lower legs, weight gain, depression, insomnia or nightmares. Although these effects do not occur very often, they may require medical attention.

PRECAUTIONS

Before you take clonidine, tell your doctor if you have heart or blood vessel disease or kidney disease. Your doctor needs this information to select the best treatment for you.

Do not drink alcoholic beverages, particularly at the start of treatment. They exaggerate the side effects of clonidine, especially drowsiness.

If you take medication for depression while taking clonidine, the effect of clonidine on blood pressure may be decreased. Other drugs may increase clonidine's effect on blood pressure, causing it to go too low. Some of these drugs are antihistamines for hay fever or other allergies, cold remedies, sleeping pills, tranquilizers, drugs for seizures and other blood pressure medications. Tell your doctor what prescription and nonprescription drugs you are taking including digitalis (digoxin), beta blockers and guanethidine. If you do not know the names of the medications you are taking or what they were prescribed for, take the labeled containers to your doctor or pharmacist.

If your doctor recommends a low-salt or low-sodium diet, it is important for you to follow this recommendation. Restricting the intake of salt helps clonidine to work as it should. Be careful about exposure to cold because it can cause paleness and pain in your fingers and toes.

Women who are pregnant or think they may be should tell their doctors before beginning to take clonidine. Nursing mothers should ask their doctor's advice about continuing to nurse if they are to take clonidine.

DOSAGE

Clonidine comes as tablets. Your doctor will determine how much you should take at each dose and how often you should take it. Follow the instructions on your prescription label carefully and ask your doctor or pharmacist to explain any part you do not understand. Clonidine is usually taken two or three times a day. Take the last dose of the day at bedtime to control blood pressure during the night.

If you forget to take a dose, take it as soon as you remember and take any remaining doses for that day at evenly spaced intervals. If you remember a missed dose at the time you are to take another, take only one dose. *Do not take a double dose to make up for a missed dose.*

It is important that you take this drug regularly. When your supply of tablets is getting low, contact your doctor or pharmacist about refilling the prescription. Make sure you have enough medication on hand. Check your supply before vacations, holidays and other occasions when you may be unable to obtain a refill. *Do not stop taking clonidine without consulting your doctor.* If you stop taking clonidine suddenly, your blood pressure may "rebound" or rise to a dangerously high level.

STORAGE
Keep the medication in the container it came in, and keep it tightly closed and protected from moisture. Keep clonidine out of the reach of children. Do not allow anyone else to take it.

Guanethidine
(gwahn eth′ i deen)

PRODUCT INFORMATION
Brand name: Ismelin
Brand name of a combination product containing hydrochlorothiazide and guanethidine: Esimil

USES
Guanethidine is a powerful and effective drug that lowers blood pressure. It reduces the supply of certain chemicals that stimulate the nerves of the blood vessels and cause those vessels to contract or narrow. When these chemicals do not reach the nerves, the blood vessels relax, blood flows more easily through the open vessels and the blood pressure becomes more normal.

Guanethidine is usually prescribed with a diuretic (water pill) such as hydrochlorothiazide (see the monographs titled Thiazide Diuretics and Hydrochlorothiazide for more information). It may also be used with other medications that lower blood pressure.

UNDESIRED EFFECTS
Guanethidine frequently causes lightheadedness, dizziness or fainting, particularly when you get out of bed or rise from a chair. It may help if you get up slowly to give your body time to adjust to the change in position. However, if this problem continues or gets worse, contact your doctor.

Lightheadedness, dizziness and fainting are more likely to occur during hot weather or when you drink alcohol, stand in one position too long or exercise suddenly or excessively. While taking guanethidine, use alcohol sparingly and avoid strenuous exercise and exposure to a hot environment.

If you become dizzy or weak while standing, sit down. Dizziness is usually worse when you first start to take this medication.

Frequent bowel movements and diarrhea are common side effects of this medication. Contact your doctor if these problems persist. Occasionally, men may have difficulty ejaculating while taking guanethidine.

Guanethidine occasionally will cause blood problems that require immediate medical attention. Symptoms of these blood problems are chills, fever, sore throat, difficulty swallowing and sores in the mouth. If you experience any of these symptoms, contact your doctor. Do not stop taking the medication until your doctor advises you to do so.

If you experience swelling of the feet, ankles or lower legs with weight gain, chest pains or difficulty in breathing, contact your doctor. Although these effects do not occur very often, they may require medical attention. They may indicate that the drug is having a bad effect on your heart; your doctor probably will want to change your medication.

PRECAUTIONS

Before taking guanethidine, inform your doctor if you have a history of asthma, heart disease, stroke, diabetes, ulcers or chronic indigestion. Guanethidine may worsen these conditions.

Certain prescription drugs, particularly those given for depression, certain mental illnesses and weight reduction, can decrease the effectiveness of guanethidine. Oral contraceptives (birth-control pills) may also interfere with the lowering of blood pressure. Before taking guanethidine, tell your doctor what prescription and nonprescription drugs you are taking, including digitalis drugs (heart medication), levodopa (medicine for tremors), decongestants, haloperidol, thiothixene, MAO inhibitors (isocarboxazid, pargyline, phenelzine and tranylcypromine), phenylephrine eyedrops, reserpine, minoxidil and other blood pressure medications. Consult your doctor before taking any other medication especially medicine for colds. If you do not know the names of the medications you are taking or what they were prescribed for, take the labeled containers to your doctor or pharmacist.

If your doctor prescribes a low-salt or low-sodium diet or tells you to stop smoking, *follow these instructions.*

If you are a diabetic, guanethidine may cause your blood sugar to drop.

Before having any surgery (including dental surgery) or procedures requiring anesthesia, tell the doctor or dentist that you are taking guanethidine.

Keep all appointments with your doctor and the laboratory for tests (such as a blood count) to determine your response to this medication.

Safe use of guanethidine during pregnancy and while breast-feeding has not been established. Therefore, if you are pregnant or breast-feeding a baby, tell your doctor.

DOSAGE

Guanethidine comes as tablets. Your doctor will determine how much you should take at each dose and how often you should take it. Follow the instructions on your prescription label and ask your doctor or pharmacist to explain any part you do not understand. Guanethidine is usually taken once a day.

It is important to take this medication regularly on the schedule your doctor prescribes. Take it at the same time every day. It will be easier to remember if you take the medication at the same time you do something else every day, such as brushing your teeth in the morning or going to bed at night. Guanethidine usually must be taken for two to seven days before it is fully effective.

If you forget to take a dose, take it as soon as you remember. However, if you remember a missed dose at the time you are scheduled to take another dose, omit the missed dose and take the scheduled dose. *Do not take a double dose to make up for a missed dose.*

Do not stop taking this medication without consulting your doctor. Make sure you have enough guanethidine on hand so you can take it exactly as prescribed. Check your supply before holidays and vacations, when it may be difficult to refill your prescription.

STORAGE
Keep this medication in the container it came in, and store it out of the reach of children. Do not allow anyone else to take it.

Hydralazine
(hye dral' a zeen)

PRODUCT INFORMATION
Brand name: Apresoline
Brand names of combination products containing hydrochlorothiazide: Apresazide, Apresodex, Apresoline-Esidrix, Hydralazine Plus, Hydralazine-Thiazide
Brand name of a combination product containing reserpine: Serpasil-Apresoline
Brand names of a combination product containing hydrochlorothiazide, reserpine and hydralazine: Ser-Ap-Es and others

USES
Hydralazine is used to treat high blood pressure. It relaxes the muscles in the walls of the blood vessels so that they expand and the blood flows more smoothly through them. To achieve best blood pressure control, hydralazine usually is prescribed with another drug that lowers blood pressure (usually a beta blocker or reserpine) and a diuretic (water pill) such as hydrochlorothiazide (see the monographs titled Beta Blockers, Reserpine, Thiazide Diuretics and Hydrochlorothiazide for more information).

UNDESIRED EFFECTS
Headache and rapid heartbeat are the most common side effects during the first few weeks of therapy with hydralazine. If these side effects occur, contact your doctor.

Heart pain (angina), dizziness, loss of appetite, nausea, vomiting, diarrhea and swelling of the feet and lower legs may occur occasionally. Contact your doctor if these effects persist or are bothersome.

In some patients who take large doses of hydralazine for long periods of time, the drug can cause a condition that resembles rheumatoid arthritis. The symptoms are fever, chest pain, joint pain, general feeling of discomfort or weakness, muscle aches, skin rash or itching, swelling of the feet and lower legs and swelling of the lymph glands. This condition requires medical treatment. Contact your doctor if you experience these symptoms.

Numbness or tingling of the fingers or toes occurs rarely but may be signs of pyridoxine deficiency. Contact your doctor if you experience these symptoms.

Hydralazine rarely causes blood problems. Symptoms are chills, fever, sore throat, difficulty in swallowing and sores in the mouth. Stop taking hydralazine and contact your doctor immediately if you experience these symptoms.

PRECAUTIONS

Before you take hydralazine, tell your doctor if you have heart disease (especially coronary artery disease), because hydralazine may cause severe heart pain. If you have kidney disease or a history of stroke or allergies to aspirin or tartrazine (yellow dye in some foods and medications including certain strengths of hydralazine tablets), tell your doctor.

Certain other drugs can add to the blood pressure lowering effect of hydralazine resulting in dizziness, lightheadedness or fainting especially when getting out of bed or rising from a sitting position to a standing position. Tell your doctor what prescription and nonprescription drugs you are taking particularly MAO inhibitors (isocarboxazid, pargyline, phenelzine and tranylcypromine) and other blood pressure medication. If you do not know the names of the drugs you are taking or what they were prescribed for, take the labeled containers to your doctor or pharmacist.

It is important that you follow your doctor's instructions concerning a low-salt or low-sodium diet. High salt intake can keep hydralazine from working the way it should.

Keep all your appointments with your doctor for the tests (such as blood counts, liver function tests and electrocardiograms) needed to check your response to hydralazine.

It is not known whether this drug is safe for a pregnant woman and her unborn child. Therefore, if you are pregnant, tell your doctor. If you are nursing a baby, ask your doctor about continuing to nurse before taking hydralazine.

DOSAGE

Hydralazine comes as tablets. Your doctor will determine how much you should take at each dose and how often you should take it. Follow the instructions on your prescription label carefully and ask your doctor or pharmacist to explain any part you do not understand. Hydralazine is taken two to four times a day. You may start with a small dose and increase it gradually. *It is important that you follow your dosage schedule.* Hydralazine should be taken with meals or a snack. It may take several weeks before the medication is fully effective.

If you miss a dose, take the missed dose when you remember it. However, if you do not remember a missed dose until it is time for a scheduled dose, omit the missed dose and take only the scheduled dose. *Do not take a double dose to make up for a missed dose.*

Do not stop taking this medication without consulting your doctor. Make sure you have enough medication on hand to allow you to take it exactly as prescribed, particularly when you will be away from home and may not be able to refill your prescription.

STORAGE
Keep hydralazine in the container it came in, and keep it out of the reach of children. Do not allow anyone else to take it.

Methyldopa
(meth ill doe' pa)

PRODUCT INFORMATION
Brand name: Aldomet
Brand name of a combination product containing chlorothiazide: Aldoclor
Brand name of a combination product containing hydrochlorothiazide: Aldoril

USES
Methyldopa is used to treat moderate to severe high blood pressure. It acts on a center in the brain to decrease the activity of the nerves governing the blood vessels allowing them to relax and open. This permits the blood to flow more evenly through the body and lowers the blood pressure.

Methyldopa is generally given with a diuretic (water pill) such as chlorothiazide or hydrochlorothiazide (see the monographs titled Thiazide Diuretics, Chlorothiazide and Hydrochlorothiazide). In more severe cases of high blood pressure, methyldopa may be prescribed with other drugs that lower blood pressure to achieve the desired control.

UNDESIRED EFFECTS
Drowsiness is the most common side effect of methyldopa and usually occurs 48 to 72 hours after you begin to take the drug or the dosage is increased. Drowsiness should disappear as your body adjusts to methyldopa. Do not drive a car, operate dangerous machinery or perform activities that require alertness until you know how this drug will affect you.

Methyldopa frequently causes headache, stuffy nose and dry mouth. You can relieve dry mouth by sucking hard candy, chewing gum or drinking fluids.

Dizziness or lightheadedness may occur when you get out of bed or rise from a chair. Get up slowly to give your body time to adjust to the change in position. Check with your doctor if this problem continues or gets worse.

Less common side effects are diarrhea, nausea or vomiting, numbness or tingling of the hands or feet, skin rash, swelling of the breasts or unusually slow heartbeat. These effects tend to disappear as your body becomes accustomed to the drug. However, if they continue or are bothersome, tell your doctor.

If you develop a fever for no apparent reason, contact your doctor. This is particularly important during the first few weeks when you are taking methyldopa.

If your feet and lower legs swell, contact your doctor. This may be an indication that methyldopa is having a bad effect on your heart.

Other effects, which are rare but require medical attention, are flu-like illness, mood and mental changes, severe or continuing diarrhea and stomach cramps, unusual bleeding or bruising and yellowing of the skin and eyes.

Long-term therapy with methyldopa may cause weight gain and blood problems such as anemia.

PRECAUTIONS

If you ever had liver disease or jaundice (yellowing of the skin and eyes), tell your doctor before taking methyldopa. This drug has caused jaundice and liver disorders, so your doctor will probably test your liver function after several months. *Keep all appointments with your doctor* and the laboratory for tests (such as blood counts and liver function tests) needed to check your response to methyldopa.

Certain drugs, such as those for depression or weight reduction (amphetamines) can decrease the effect of methyldopa on blood pressure. Levodopa, diuretics (water pills) and other blood pressure medication can increase the effect of methyldopa. Before taking methyldopa, tell your doctor what prescription and nonprescription drugs you are taking including amphetamines, antidepressants, chlorpromazine, diuretics, haloperidol, levodopa, lithium, MAO inhibitors (isocarboxazid, pargyline, phenelzine and tranylcypromine), and medication for high blood pressure. If you do not know the names of the drugs you are taking or what they were prescribed for, take the labeled containers to your doctor or pharmacist.

Follow your doctor's instructions on alcohol, salt and sodium consumption and smoking so that this medication will work as it should.

If you are pregnant or think you may be, tell your doctor before you take methyldopa. Methyldopa has been used safely by some pregnant women with high blood pressure without harm to the unborn baby. If you are nursing a baby, ask your doctor about continuing to nurse. Methyldopa is passed from a mother to her breast-fed baby through the milk.

Before you have surgery (including dental surgery) or procedures requiring anesthesia, tell the doctor or dentist in charge that you are taking methyldopa.

DOSAGE

Methyldopa comes as film-coated tablets and suspension (liquid) to be taken by mouth. Your doctor will determine how much you should take at each dose and how often you should take it. *Take methyldopa exactly as prescribed.* Follow the instructions on your prescription label carefully and ask your doctor or pharmacist to explain any part you do not understand. Methyldopa is usually taken two to four times a day. Measure the suspension with a specially marked spoon or dropper from your pharmacist to ensure an accurate dose.

Methyldopa usually begins to work six to 12 hours after it is taken, but you may have to take it for four days before it is fully effective.

If you forget a dose, take it as soon as you remember. Take the remaining doses for that day at evenly spaced intervals. If you remember a missed dose when it is almost time for a scheduled dose, omit the missed dose and take only the scheduled dose. *Do not take a double dose to make up for a missed dose.*

Do not stop taking this medication without consulting your doctor. Make sure you have enough medication on hand to allow you to take it exactly as prescribed. Check your supply before going away from home if it may be difficult to refill your prescription.

STORAGE
Keep this medication in the container it came in, and keep it out of the reach of children. Do not allow anyone else to take it.

Minoxidil
(mi nox′ i dill)

PRODUCT INFORMATION
Brand name: Loniten

USES
Minoxidil is used to treat severe high blood pressure that has not responded to treatment with other blood pressure medication. It acts directly on the blood vessel walls to relax them so that blood flows more smoothly through them. Minoxidil is usually used with a beta blocker and a diuretic (usually furosemide or ethacrynic acid) which act to reduce blood pressure and to offset some of the side effects (sodium and water retention, swelling of the lower legs and feet, heart pain and rapid heartbeat) of minoxidil. See the monographs titled Beta Blockers, Furosemide and Thiazide Diuretics for more information.

UNDESIRED EFFECTS
Rapid heartbeat, angina (heart pain), sodium (salt) and water retention and swelling of the feet, ankles and lower legs may occur. Contact your doctor if you experience any of these symptoms. If you are not already taking a diuretic and beta blocker, it may be necessary for your doctor to prescribe additional medication or adjust the dosages of these medications. Diuretics (water pills) are taken to reduce the sodium and water retention, and beta blockers are taken to slow the rapid heartbeat and decrease the angina (heart pain) caused by minoxidil.

Lengthening, thickening and darkening of fine body hair occur commonly three to six weeks after starting to take minoxidil. This is seen first on the face and appears later on the back, arms, legs, scalp and chest. It may be accompanied by itchiness also. This effect may be controlled with the use of hair removers or by shaving and will go away when the drug is discontinued (it may take up to six months for hair to grow out and for normal appearance to return).

Other more rare side effects include breast tenderness and enlargement, headache, nausea and skin rash.

PRECAUTIONS
Tell your doctor if you have heart disease, congestive heart failure or kidney

disease or if you have had a recent heart attack. Keep in close contact with your doctor and *keep all scheduled appointments*. Weigh yourself every day and follow your doctor's instructions for diet and the use of salt.

Your doctor may instruct you to measure your heart rate (pulse) daily; your doctor or pharmacist can show you how to do this. If your heart rate increases by more than 20 beats per minute while at rest, if breathing becomes difficult (especially while lying down) or if dizziness, lightheadedness, fainting, heart pain, rapid weight gain or swelling or puffiness of the face, hands, ankles or stomach area occurs, contact your doctor.

Tell your doctor if you are pregnant or breast-feeding a baby. It is not known whether it is safe to take minoxidil during pregnancy or while nursing a baby.

Tell your doctor what prescription and nonprescription drugs you are taking, especially guanethidine (even if you stopped taking it in the last three weeks), diuretics and other medications for high blood pressure. If you do not know the names of the drugs or what they were prescribed for, take the labeled containers to your doctor or pharmacist.

DOSAGE
Minoxidil comes as tablets to be taken by mouth. Your doctor will determine how much you should take at each dose and how often you should take it. Follow the instructions on your prescription label carefully and ask your doctor or pharmacist to explain any part you do not understand. Minoxidil is usually taken once or twice a day. *It is important that you take this medication regularly to be effective.* Try to take this medication at the same time you do something else every day, such as brushing your teeth in the morning, to help you to remember to take it.

If you forget to take a dose, take it as soon as you remember and take any remaining doses for that day at evenly spaced intervals. If it is almost time for the next scheduled dose, omit the missed dose and take only the scheduled dose. *Do not take a double dose to make up for a missed dose.*

STORAGE
Keep this medication in the container it came in and keep it out of the reach of children. Do not let anyone else take it.

Prazosin
(pra zoe' sin)

PRODUCT INFORMATION
Brand name: Minipress
Brand name of a combination product containing polythiazide (a thiazide diuretic): Minizide

USES
Prazosin is used to treat high blood pressure. It relaxes the muscles in the walls

of blood vessels so the blood flows more easily and blood pressure is decreased. Prazosin is often used with other blood pressure medications especially diuretics (see the monograph titled Thiazide Diuretics for more information).

Prazosin has also been used investigationally with digitalis drugs (heart medicine) and diuretics (water pills) to treat severe congestive heart failure.

UNDESIRED EFFECTS

Prazosin can cause dizziness, lightheadedness or fainting (sometimes preceded by fast heartbeat), particularly when you get up suddenly from a sitting or lying position. If this occurs, sit or lie down until the dizziness passes and arise slowly to give your body time to adjust to the change in position. Take prazosin with food to prevent this problem. Dizziness caused by prazosin is most common when you start to take the drug or increase your dosage and usually disappears as your body adjusts to the drug. Do not drive a car or operate dangerous machinery until you determine how this drug affects you. Contact your doctor if you continue to experience problems with dizziness or fainting; it may be necessary to decrease your dosage.

Prazosin may also cause drowsiness, weakness, lack of energy, palpitation, headache and nausea. These effects usually disappear as your body adjusts to prazosin. If these effects are persistent or severe, contact your doctor; it may be necessary to reduce your dosage.

PRECAUTIONS

Before you take prazosin, tell your doctor if you have heart or kidney disease. Tell your doctor what prescription and nonprescription medications you are taking, particularly beta blockers (atenolol, metoprolol, nadolol, pindolol, propranolol and timolol), diuretics (water pills) or other blood pressure medication. Prazosin controls high blood pressure but does not cure it. Therefore, it is important that you take prazosin regularly as prescribed by your doctor. Follow your doctor's instructions on diet and avoid the use of salt (sodium). If you experience swelling of the feet and lower legs or rapid weight gain (sodium and water retention), contact your doctor.

Tell your doctor if you are pregnant or breast-feeding a baby. It is not known if it is safe to take prazosin during pregnancy or while breast-feeding.

DOSAGE

Prazosin comes as capsules to be taken by mouth. Your doctor will determine how much you should take at each dose and how often you should take it. Follow the instructions on your prescription label and ask your doctor or pharmacist to explain any part you do not understand. Prazosin is usually taken two or three times a day.

If you forget to take a dose, take it as soon as you remember and take any remaining doses for that day at evenly spaced intervals. *Do not take a double dose to make up for a missed dose.*

STORAGE

Keep prazosin in the container it came in and store it out of the reach of children. Do not allow anyone else to take your medication.

Reserpine
(re ser' peen)

PRODUCT INFORMATION

Brand names: Sandril, Serpalan, Serpasil, Serpate and others

Brand names of combination products containing the diuretic chlorthalidone: Demi-Regroton, Regroton

Brand names of combination products containing the thiazide diuretic hydro-chlorothiazide: Hydropres, Serpasil-Esidrix and others

Brand names of combination products containing the thiazide diuretic hydro-flumethiazide: Salutensin and others

USES

Reserpine is used to treat high blood pressure. It decreases the amount of certain chemicals in the nerves that control the blood vessels. It helps keep blood pressure normal by relaxing the blood vessels to permit the blood to flow more easily through the body.

Reserpine is generally more effective when used with a diuretic (water pill) and may also be prescribed with other drugs that lower blood pressure (e.g., hydralazine) to achieve better blood pressure control (see the monographs titled Thiazide Diuretics and Hydralazine for more information).

Reserpine is also used to treat mental illness, particularly when the person is agitated.

UNDESIRED EFFECTS

Dry mouth, stuffy nose, tiredness, lethargy and red eyes are some of the more common undesired effects of reserpine. To relieve dry mouth, suck on hard candies, chew gum or drink fluids.

Reserpine causes some people to become drowsy. Do not drive a car or operate dangerous machinery until you know how this medication will affect you. Avoid the use of alcohol and sleeping pills because they can increase the drowsiness.

Depression is the most serious side effect of reserpine. Stop taking it if you begin to feel "blue" or despondent, lose your appetite or wake much earlier than usual in the morning. Contact your doctor right away and describe how you feel.

If reserpine upsets your stomach or gives you diarrhea or stomach cramps, take it with meals or a snack. Contact your doctor if these effects continue or are bothersome.

After you take reserpine, you may experience dizziness when you stand. If you become dizzy, move slowly from a sitting to a standing position. Contact your doctor if the dizziness is severe or persists.

Reserpine can cause nightmares, mood changes, weight gain and decreased sexual drive. Contact your doctor if any of these effects occur.

Although allergic reactions to reserpine are rare, it may cause asthma attacks in people who suffer from asthma.

PRECAUTIONS

Reserpine (in large doses) has caused cancer in laboratory test animals. However, it is not known whether it has this effect on humans. Tell your doctor if you or any members of your family have a history of cancer especially breast cancer. Discuss this with your doctor.

Before taking this medication, tell your doctor if you have a history of kidney disease, peptic ulcer, colitis, mental depression, epilepsy or gallstones. Reserpine can make these conditions worse or cause problems to recur. Tell your doctor if you are having shock treatments (electroconvulsive therapy) for mental illness.

Tell your doctor what prescription and nonprescription drugs you are taking, especially digitalis drugs (e.g., digoxin), beta blockers (atenolol, metoprolol, nadolol, pindolol, propranolol and timolol), diuretics (water pills), quinidine, levodopa, procainamide, barbiturates, sedatives, tranquilizers, methotrimeprazine, MAO inhibitors (isocarboxazid, pargyline, phenelzine and tranylcypromine), sleeping pills, decongestants, medicine for depression and other blood pressure medication. If you do not know the names of the drugs you are taking or what they were prescribed for, take the labeled containers to your doctor or pharmacist.

Follow carefully your doctor's instructions for a low-salt or low-sodium diet, the use of alcohol and smoking.

Keep all appointments with your doctor so your response to reserpine can be checked. Your doctor may ask you to have your eyes examined and to have blood tests periodically.

Tell your doctor if you are pregnant or breast-feeding a baby. Reserpine should not be taken during pregnancy or while nursing a baby.

DOSAGE

Reserpine comes as tablets to be taken by mouth. Your doctor will determine how much you should take at each dose and how often you should take it. Follow the instructions on your prescription label carefully and ask your doctor or pharmacist to explain any part you do not understand.

Reserpine is usually taken once or twice a day. Take it at the same time you do something else each day, such as brushing your teeth in the morning, eating dinner or going to bed at night.

If you forget a dose, *do not take the missed dose when you remember it.* Omit the missed dose and take only the next scheduled dose. *Do not take a double dose to make up for a missed dose. It is important that you take reserpine regularly as prescribed by your doctor. Do not stop taking this medication without consulting your doctor.*

Make sure you have enough medication on hand so you can take it exactly as directed. Be sure to check your supply before vacations and holidays, when it may be difficult to refill your prescription.

STORAGE
Keep this medication in the container it came in, and keep it out of the reach of children. Do not allow anyone else to take it.

Irregular Heartbeat or Arrhythmia

A variation from the normal rhythm of the heartbeat is called an arrhythmia (a rith' me a). An irregular heartbeat can be caused by disease (e.g., infection and high blood pressure), drugs (e.g., nicotine and caffeine) or by damage to the heart muscle from a heart attack. When the heart loses its normal, rhythmic beat, the efficiency of its pumping action decreases.

There are three principal types of cardiac arrhythmias: slow beat (less than 55 beats per minute), fast beat (more than 100 beats per minute) and an early beat (often described as a "skipped" beat).

Antiarrhythmic drugs are given orally primarily to prevent or treat fast beats and early beats or by injection in a hospital to treat more severe irregular heartbeat problems. They regulate the rhythm of the heartbeat. Artificial pacemakers are also used to correct the very slow heartbeats.

ANTIARRHYTHMICS

Disopyramide
(dye soe peer' a mide)

PRODUCT INFORMATION
Brand name: Norpace

USES
Disopyramide is used to treat arrhythmias (irregular heartbeat). It relaxes an overactive heart by acting on heart muscle and nerves, thus allowing the heart to beat at a normal rate. This improves the efficiency of the heart's pumping action. Disopyramide suppresses and prevents the recurrence of early heartbeats.

UNDESIRED EFFECTS
Disopyramide commonly causes dry mouth. This effect tends to disappear as your body adjusts to the drug. To relieve dry mouth, drink fluids, chew gum or suck hard candy or lozenges. Other side effects of disopyramide include dry nose and eyes, blurred vision, constipation, difficulty breathing, weight gain, swelling of the feet and lower legs and frequent and difficult urination. Disopyramide affects the heartbeat and can also cause a drop in blood pressure and dizziness, lightheadedness or

fainting, especially if you sit or stand up too quickly. Contact your doctor if these effects are severe or persist. It may be necessary to adjust your dosage.

PRECAUTIONS

Before taking disopyramide, tell your doctor if you have myasthenia gravis; heart, kidney, liver or prostate disease; glaucoma (or a family history of glaucoma) or difficulty urinating.

Tell your doctor what prescription and nonprescription drugs you are taking particularly phenobarbital, phenytoin, procainamide, quinidine, rifampin, verapamil and warfarin. If you do not know the names of the drugs or what they were prescribed for, take the labeled containers to your doctor or pharmacist.

Avoid alcoholic beverages while taking disopyramide.

Keep in close touch with your doctor while taking this medication. *Keep all appointments with your doctor* so your response to this drug can be determined. You will probably have an EKG (electrocardiogram) done periodically.

Tell your doctor if you are pregnant or breast-feeding a baby. It is not known if it is safe to take disopyramide during pregnancy or while breast-feeding. Follow your doctor's advice on diet and smoking. Cigarettes and caffeine-containing beverages may increase the irritability of the heart and interfere with the action of this drug.

DOSAGE

Disopyramide comes as regular and extended-release capsules to be taken by mouth. The regular capsules are usually taken every six hours, and the extended-release capsules are usually taken every 12 hours. Your doctor will determine which form you should take, how often you should take it and how much you should take at each dose. Follow the instructions on your prescription label carefully and ask your doctor or pharmacist to explain any part you do not understand. *It is extremely important that you take disopyramide on the exact schedule prescribed even if you must awaken at night to take it.* Try not to skip doses because missing doses may allow irregular heartbeats to develop.

If you forget a dose, take it as soon as you remember. However, if it is less than four hours before your next scheduled dose, omit the missed dose and take only the scheduled dose. *Do not take a double dose to make up for a missed dose.* Do not stop taking this medication without consulting your doctor.

Be sure you have enough of this medication on hand to permit you to take all of the prescribed doses. Check your supply before vacations and holidays.

STORAGE

Keep this medication in the container it came in and keep it out of the reach of children. Do not allow anyone else to take your medication.

Procainamide
(proe kane a' mide)

PRODUCT INFORMATION
Brand names: Procan, Promine, Pronestyl

USES
Procainamide is used to treat arrhythmias. It relaxes an overactive heart by acting on the heart muscle and nerves, allowing the heart to beat at a normal rate and rhythm. This improves the efficiency of the heart's pumping action.

Procainamide is used to maintain normal heart rate and rhythm after they have been established by other means (with an injectable antiarrhythmic drug or electric shock) and to prevent recurrence of irregular or fast beats. Procainamide is also used to treat early beats.

UNDESIRED EFFECTS
Procainamide can cause nausea, vomiting, diarrhea, bitter taste and loss of appetite. Usually these effects are mild, but if they are severe, contact your doctor.

If you experience chills, unexplained fever, joint pain, sore throat, mouth or gums, fatigue, unusual bleeding or bruising, difficulty breathing, itching, skin rash or coughing up of thick yellow or green sputum while you are taking procainamide, contact your doctor. Report these symptoms to your doctor promptly, since they may indicate a potentially serious condition.

PRECAUTIONS
If you ever had an allergic reaction to a local anesthetic such as procaine (Novocain), which is commonly used in dental procedures, or to sulfite-containing foods, drugs or beverages, tell your doctor before you take procainamide.

Tell your doctor what prescription and nonprescription drugs you are taking particularly blood pressure medication, disopyramide, neostigmine, phenytoin, propranolol, pyridostigmine and quinidine. If you do not know the names of the drugs you are taking or what they were prescribed for, take the labeled containers to your doctor or pharmacist.

Tell your doctor if you have myasthenia gravis or heart (congestive heart failure), kidney or liver disease. Keep in close touch with your doctor and pharmacist while taking procainamide. You may have an electrocardiogram (EKG) or blood tests done periodically.

Cigarettes and caffeine-containing beverages may increase irritability of the heart and interfere with the action of procainamide. Follow your doctor's advice about smoking and dietary restrictions.

Tell your doctor if you are pregnant or breast-feeding a baby. It is not known whether it is safe to take procainamide during pregnancy or while breast-feeding.

Before having surgery with an anesthetic, tell the doctor or dentist in charge that you are taking procainamide.

DOSAGE

Procainamide comes as capsules, regular tablets and extended-release tablets to be taken by mouth. Your doctor will determine how often you should take it and how much you should take at each dose. Carefully follow the instructions on your prescription label and ask your doctor or pharmacist to explain any part you do not understand.

Procainamide is usually taken four to six times a day (extended-release tablets are usually taken four times a day). Do not chew or crush extended-release tablets; they should be swallowed whole. *It is extremely important that you take this medication on the exact schedule prescribed by your doctor, even if you must awaken during the night to take it.* Procainamide must be taken regularly around the clock to keep the heart beating at a normal rate.

If you forget to take a dose, take it as soon as you remember and go back to your regular schedule. However, if it is less than two hours (four hours for extended-release tablets) before your next scheduled dose, omit the missed dose and follow your regular schedule. *Do not take a double dose to make up for a missed dose.*

Be sure you have enough of this medication on hand at all times to take all of your prescribed doses. Check your supply before holidays, vacations or other times when it may be difficult to obtain more.

STORAGE

Keep procainamide in the container it came in, and keep it out of the reach of children. Do not let anyone else take it.

Propranolol

Propranolol is a member of the group of drugs known as "beta blockers." It is used to treat irregular heartbeat as well as high blood pressure, heart pain (angina) and certain other medical conditions. See the section titled Beta Blockers (page 27) for more information.

Quinidine
(kwin' i dine)

PRODUCT INFORMATION

Brand names: Cardioquin, Duraquin, Quinaglute, Quinidex, Quinora, SK-Quinidine and others

USES

Quinidine is used to treat arrhythmias. It relaxes an overactive heart by working on the heart muscles and nerves, slowing down the heart and allowing it to beat at a normal rate and rhythm. This improves the efficiency of the heart's pumping action.

Quinidine is used to maintain normal heart rate and rhythm after it has been established by other means (with an injectable antiarrhythmic drug or electric shock) and to prevent recurrence of irregular or fast beats.

Quinidine is extracted from the bark of the cinchona tree in South America. This tree also yields quinine, a drug used to treat malaria. Quinidine is available in three chemical preparations (quinidine gluconate, quinidine polygalacturonate and quinidine sulfate) and has a bitter taste.

UNDESIRED EFFECTS

Quinidine can cause skin rash, unusual bleeding or bruising, fever, ringing in the ears or changes in hearing, changes in vision, feeling of excitement or apprehension, delirium, dizziness and severe headache. If you experience any of these symptoms, contact your doctor.

Quinidine affects the heartbeat and can also cause a drop in blood pressure and dizziness, lightheadedness or fainting, especially if you sit or stand up too quickly.

Quinidine may cause loss of appetite, stomach pain and cramps, nausea, bitter taste or diarrhea. Take the medication with food or antacids if these problems occur, and contact your doctor if they persist or are severe. Do not take baking soda for stomach upset.

PRECAUTIONS

Tell your doctor if you ever had an allergic reaction to quinidine or quinine (a substance used to treat malaria and found in tonic water and some nonprescription cold remedies).

Tell your doctor if you have asthma or other lung problems, muscle weakness, infection, thyroid disease, myasthenia gravis or kidney or liver disease before taking quinidine.

Tell your doctor what prescription and nonprescription drugs you are taking (or have taken in the past month) particularly anticoagulants (blood thinners), blood pressure medication, digitalis (heart medication), neostigmine, phenobarbital, phenytoin, procainamide, propranolol, reserpine and pyridostigmine. If you do not know the names of the drugs you are taking or what they were prescribed for, take the labeled containers to your doctor or pharmacist. Keep in close touch with your doctor while taking quinidine. You may have an electrocardiogram (EKG) and blood tests periodically.

Before having surgery with an anesthetic, tell the doctor or dentist in charge that you are taking quinidine.

Cigarettes and caffeine-containing beverages may increase the irritability of the heart and interfere with the action of quinidine. Follow your doctor's advice about smoking and dietary restrictions.

Tell your doctor if you are pregnant or breast-feeding a baby. Quinidine is chemically related (similar) to quinine which has caused blindness and may cause deafness in unborn babies. Quinidine passes from a mother to her breast-fed baby through the milk. It is not known if it is safe to take this drug while breast-feeding a baby.

DOSAGE

Quinidine comes as capsules, regular tablets and extended-release tablets to be taken by mouth. Your doctor will determine how often you should take it and how much you should take at each dose. Follow the instructions on your prescription label carefully and ask your doctor or pharmacist to explain any part you do not understand.

Quinidine usually is taken three or four times a day (extended-release tablets are usually taken two or three times a day). *It is extremely important that you take this medication on the exact schedule prescribed by your doctor, even if you must awaken during the night to take it.* Quinidine must be taken regularly to keep the heart beating at a normal rate.

Do not chew or crush extended-release tablets; they should be swallowed whole.

Take quinidine with food or antacids to lessen stomach upset.

If you forget to take a dose, take it as soon as you remember. If you are more than two hours late, omit the missed dose. Take the next dose at the regularly scheduled time. *Do not take a double dose to make up for a missed dose.*

Be sure you have enough of this medication on hand at all times to take all of your prescribed doses. Be sure to check your supply before holidays or at any other time that it may be difficult to obtain more.

STORAGE

Keep this medication in the light-resistant container it came in. When quinidine is exposed to light, it darkens. Keep quinidine out of the reach of children. Do not let anyone else take it.

Angina Pectoris (Heart Pain)

Angina pectoris (an ji' nah peck' tore us) is heart pain that occurs when the heart's need for oxygen is greater than its supply. It may be brought on by exercise or emotional stress (both of which increase the heart's need for oxygen), or any disease that causes a decrease in blood flow to the heart. A common cause of reduced blood flow to the heart is fatty deposits that narrow the blood vessels of the heart (athero-sclerosis).

Heart pain is experienced as a crushing or squeezing sensation in the area of the breastbone. Occasionally the pain is felt in the neck, shoulder or upper abdomen, where it is often confused with indigestion. The pain frequently spreads down the left arm.

Treatment for angina attacks includes rest and drug therapy. Drugs known as vasodilators open blood vessels to permit more oxygen to reach the heart. Calcium channel blockers, drugs that reduce the heart's oxygen needs in addition to opening blood vessels, are also used.

Your doctor will probably ask you to stop smoking, lose weight, get plenty of rest and avoid situations that cause heart pain (exertion, overeating, exposure to cold weather and emotional upset).

CALCIUM CHANNEL BLOCKERS
Diltiazem
(dil tye' a zem)

PRODUCT INFORMATION
Brand name: Cardizem

USES
Diltiazem is used to treat angina (heart pain). It is a member of the class of drugs known as calcium channel blockers. It "blocks" the movement of calcium into muscle cells of the heart and blood vessels. This opens the blood vessels allowing blood to flow more smoothly so that the heart receives more oxygen. Diltiazem also lowers blood pressure slightly and relaxes the heart so that it does not have to pump as hard and requires less oxygen.

UNDESIRED EFFECTS
Common side effects of diltiazem include fatigue, nausea, loss of appetite and

headache. If these effects are persistent or severe, contact your doctor. If you experience swelling of the feet, ankles or lower legs, skin rash or irregular (slow) heartbeat or if the duration, frequency or severity of heart pain attacks increases, contact your doctor immediately.

PRECAUTIONS

Tell your doctor if you have heart (congestive heart failure), liver or kidney disease.

Diltiazem may cause dizziness, lightheadedness or fainting. Sit or stand up slowly to allow your body to adjust to the change in position. Also, alcohol may add to the blood pressure-lowering effect of diltiazem resulting in dizziness, lightheadedness or fainting.

Tell your doctor what prescription and nonprescription medications you are taking, especially beta blockers (atenolol, metoprolol, nadolol, pindolol, propranolol and timolol) and digitalis drugs (e.g., digoxin).

Use caution during exercise or physical exertion. *Keep all appointments with your doctor*. This medication must be taken regularly to be effective. Do not suddenly stop taking it.

Tell your doctor if you are pregnant or breast-feeding a baby. It is not known if it is safe to take diltiazem during pregnancy or while breast-feeding.

DOSAGE

Diltiazem comes as tablets. Your doctor has determined how much you should take at each dose and how often you should take this medication. Follow the instructions on your prescription label carefully and ask your doctor or pharmacist to explain any part you do not understand.

Diltiazem is usually taken four times a day, before meals and at bedtime.

If you forget to take a dose, take it as soon as you remember. However, if it is less than three hours before your next dose, omit the missed dose and take only the scheduled dose. *Do not take a double dose to make up for a missed dose.*

STORAGE

Keep diltiazem in the container it came in and keep it out of the reach of children. Do not allow anyone else to take this medication.

Nifedipine
(nye fed′ i peen)

PRODUCT INFORMATION
Brand name: Procardia

USES

Nifedipine is used to treat angina (heart pain). Nifedipine is a member of the class of drugs known as calcium channel blockers. It "blocks" the movement of calcium into muscle cells of the heart and blood vessels. This opens the blood vessels allowing blood to flow more smoothly so that the heart receives more oxygen. Nifedipine also lowers blood pressure slightly and relaxes the heart so that it does not have to pump as hard and requires less oxygen.

UNDESIRED EFFECTS

Common side effects of nifedipine include nervousness, muscle cramps, flushing (feeling of warmth), weakness, headache, nausea, heartburn, coughing, nasal congestion and sore throat. If these are severe or persist, contact your doctor. If you experience an increase in the frequency, duration or severity of heart pain or swelling of the lower legs, feet or ankles, difficulty breathing, wheezing or fast or pounding heartbeat, contact your doctor immediately.

PRECAUTIONS

Tell your doctor if you have heart (congestive heart failure), liver or kidney disease.

Nifedipine may cause dizziness, lightheadedness or fainting. Sit or stand up slowly to allow your body to adjust to the change in position. Also, alcohol may add to the blood pressure-lowering effect of nifedipine resulting in dizziness, lightheadedness or fainting.

Tell your doctor about all prescription and nonprescription medications that you are taking, especially beta blockers (atenolol, metoprolol, nadolol, pindolol, propranolol and timolol), digitalis drugs (e.g., digoxin) and medicine for high blood pressure. Before having surgery, tell the doctor in charge that you are taking nifedipine.

Use caution during exercise or physical exertion. *Keep all appointments with your doctor*. Nifedipine must be taken regularly to be effective. Do not suddenly stop taking this medication.

Tell your doctor if you are pregnant or breast-feeding a baby. It is not known if it is safe to take nifedipine during pregnancy or while breast-feeding.

DOSAGE

Nifedipine comes as capsules. Your doctor will determine how much you should take at each dose and how often you should take it. Follow the instructions on your prescription label and ask your doctor or pharmacist to explain any part you do not understand. Nifedipine is usually taken three or four times a day.

If you forget to take a dose, take it as soon as you remember. However, if it is less than three hours before your next dose, omit the missed dose and take only the scheduled dose. *Do not take a double dose to make up for a missed dose.*

STORAGE

Keep nifedipine in the container it came in and keep it out of the reach of children. Do not allow anyone else to take this medication.

Verapamil
(ver ap' a mill)

PRODUCT INFORMATION
Brand names: Calan, Isoptin

USES
Verapamil is used to treat angina (heart pain). It is also given by injection to treat arrhythmias (irregular heartbeat).

Verapamil is a member of the class of drugs known as calcium channel blockers. It "blocks" the movement of calcium into muscle cells of the heart and blood vessels. This opens the blood vessels allowing blood to flow more smoothly so that the heart receives more oxygen. Verapamil also lowers blood pressure slightly and relaxes the heart so that it does not have to pump as hard and requires less oxygen.

UNDESIRED EFFECTS
Common side effects of verapamil include constipation, fatigue, dizziness, headache and nausea. If these are severe or persist, contact your doctor. If you experience swelling of the lower legs, feet or ankles, difficulty breathing or irregular heartbeat (fast or slow), contact your doctor immediately.

PRECAUTIONS
Tell your doctor if you have heart (congestive heart failure), liver or kidney disease.

Verapamil may cause dizziness, lightheadedness or fainting. Sit or stand up slowly to allow your body to adjust to the change in position. Also, alcohol may add to the blood pressure-lowering effect of verapamil resulting in dizziness, lightheadedness or fainting.

Tell your doctor what prescription and nonprescription medications you are taking, especially anticoagulants (blood thinners), beta blockers (atenolol, metoprolol, nadolol, pindolol, propranolol and timolol), digitalis drugs (e.g., digoxin), disopyramide, medication for arthritis, diabetes, glaucoma or high blood pressure, phenytoin (seizure medication), quinidine and "sulfa" drugs (antibiotics).

Use caution during exercise or physical exertion. *Keep all appointments with your doctor and the laboratory.* You may have electrocardiograms (EKG) and liver function tests done periodically. Tell your doctor if you are pregnant or breast-feeding a baby. It is not known if it is safe to take verapamil during pregnancy. Do not breast-feed while taking verapamil.

DOSAGE
Verapamil comes as tablets and injection. Your doctor will determine how much you should take at each dose and how often you should take it. Follow the instructions on your prescription label and ask your doctor or pharmacist to explain any part you do not understand. Verapamil is usually taken three or four times a day.

Verapamil must be taken regularly to be effective. Do not suddenly stop taking this medication.

If you forget to take a dose, take it as soon as you remember. However, if it is less than three hours before your next scheduled dose, omit the missed dose and take only the scheduled dose. *Do not take a double dose to make up for a missed dose.*

Your doctor may ask you to check your pulse (heart rate) daily while taking this medication and will tell you how fast it should be. Ask your doctor or pharmacist to teach you how to do this. If your pulse is slower than it should be, contact your doctor about taking the drug that day.

STORAGE
Keep verapamil in the container it came in, and keep it out of the reach of children. Do not allow anyone else to take your medication.

VASODILATORS
Dipyridamole
(dye peer id' a mole)

PRODUCT INFORMATION
Brand names: Persantine, Pyridamole, SK-Dipyridamole

USES
Dipyridamole is a member of the group of drugs known as vasodilators that open blood vessels to permit more blood to flow to the heart and thus increase the heart's oxygen supply. Dipyridamole is prescribed for long-term treatment of heart pain (angina) caused by insufficient oxygen. It may reduce the frequency or eliminate angina attacks. *It will not relieve pain if taken during an attack.* It is also used in combination with other drugs, particularly aspirin, to prevent clots from forming in blood vessels.

UNDESIRED EFFECTS
Dipyridamole can cause headache, dizziness, weakness, fainting, skin rash and flushing. Contact your doctor if these effects are bothersome or persist. Nausea, vomiting, diarrhea and stomach irritation may occur. If this medication upsets your stomach, try taking it with a light snack.

PRECAUTIONS
Tell your doctor if you have ever had an allergic reaction to aspirin or tartrazine (a yellow dye present in some foods and medications including dipyridamole).

Before you take this medication, tell your doctor what other prescription and nonprescription drugs you are taking, especially heart medication and anticoagulants (blood thinners). If you do not know the names of the drugs you are taking or what they were prescribed for, take the labeled containers to your doctor or pharmacist.

You should not take this drug if you have low blood pressure or have had a recent heart attack. If you experience an increase in the frequency or severity of heart pain, stop taking the drug and contact your doctor immediately.

Follow your doctor's advice about smoking and about use of alcoholic beverages while taking dipyridamole.

Tell your doctor if you are pregnant. It is not known whether this drug is safe for a pregnant woman or her unborn child.

DOSAGE

Dipyridamole comes as tablets. It is usually taken three times a day. Your prescription label tells you how often to take dipyridamole and how much to take at each dose. Follow the instructions carefully and ask your doctor or pharmacist to explain any part you do not understand.

Dipyridamole should be taken on an empty stomach, at least one hour before meals. Take it with a full eight-ounce glass of fluid such as water, coffee, tea, milk or fruit juice. You may take dipyridamole with a light snack if it upsets your stomach.

If you forget to take a dose, do not take it when you remember. Omit the missed dose and take only your regular dose at the next scheduled time. This medication must be taken regularly for up to three months to be effective. Therefore, take it according to the schedule prescribed by your doctor and keep in touch with your doctor while taking it. Do not take more than the amount specified on your prescription label.

STORAGE

Keep this medication in the container it came in, and keep it out of the reach of children. Do not allow anyone else to take it.

Erythrityl Tetranitrate
(e ri' thri till tet rah nye' trate)

PRODUCT INFORMATION
Brand name: Cardilate

USES

Erythrityl tetranitrate is a member of the nitrate group of vasodilators. It relaxes and opens blood vessels increasing blood flow and the oxygen supply to the heart. It is prescribed for long-term prevention of angina (heart pain) attacks and may reduce the frequency and the severity of pain. It is also used to prevent angina attacks in situations likely to provoke attacks. *It is not used to relieve heart pain once an attack has started.*

UNDESIRED EFFECTS

Erythrityl tetranitrate can cause headache, rapid heartbeat, flushing, redness of the skin, dizziness, weakness and fainting. These side effects are usually temporary and disappear as your body adjusts to the drug. If these effects persist or keep you from resuming normal activities, contact your doctor. If dizziness or rapid heartbeat occurs when you take this drug, sit down for a few minutes.

If you develop a severe skin rash and peeling, you may be allergic to this drug. Stop taking it and contact your doctor if you experience these symptoms.

Tablets placed under the tongue (sublingual) or between the cheek and gums to dissolve usually produce a tingling or burning sensation indicating that they are being absorbed by the lining of the mouth.

PRECAUTIONS

Tell your doctor what prescription and nonprescription drugs you are taking, especially other drugs to treat your heart condition or blood pressure, beta blockers (atenolol, metoprolol, nadolol, pindolol, propranolol and timolol), phenothiazines (chlorpromazine, fluphenazine, perphenazine, prochlorperazine, promazine, thioridazine and trifluoperazine) and drugs to treat colds, allergies or cough. If you do not know the names of the drugs or what they were prescribed for, take the labeled containers to your doctor or pharmacist.

Follow your doctor's advice about smoking and drinking alcoholic beverages. Alcohol may increase the dizziness caused by this drug. Avoid exposure to cold environments; this may reduce the effectiveness of this drug.

Tell your doctor if you ever had an allergic reaction to amyl nitrite, isosorbide dinitrate, nitroglycerin or pentaerythritol tetranitrate. Also, tell your doctor if you have severe anemia, intestinal disease or glaucoma.

You may develop ''tolerance'' to this drug after you have been taking it for awhile. This means that the dose your doctor has prescribed for you loses its effectiveness. Discuss this with your doctor.

Keep in close touch with your doctor while taking this medication. You may have periodic examinations and various blood tests. *Keep all appointments with your doctor and the laboratory.*

DOSAGE

Erythrityl tetranitrate comes as tablets to be chewed, swallowed or placed under the tongue (sublingual) or between the cheek and gums.

Your doctor will select the best form for you and will determine how often you should take it and how much you should take at each dose. Follow the instructions on your prescription label carefully and ask your doctor or pharmacist to explain any part you do not understand. Be sure you understand whether your tablets should be swallowed whole, chewed or dissolved in the mouth.

If chewable tablets have been prescribed for you, chew them thoroughly before you swallow them. If your doctor has prescribed tablets that dissolve in the mouth, place them under the tongue or between the cheek and gum and leave them there until completely dissolved. Try not to swallow saliva too often until the tablet has completely dissolved.

Take the chewable tablets or tablets to be dissolved in the mouth 30 to 45 minutes prior to exercise or other activities that may provoke an angina attack.

Tablets that are chewed or dissolved in the mouth start to take effect within five minutes and go on working for up to two hours. Tablets that are swallowed begin to work after 30 minutes; their effect lasts for up to 90 minutes.

Contact your doctor if you continue to experience angina attacks in spite of taking this medication to prevent them. If you forget to take a dose, take it as soon as you remember. However, if you remember a missed dose when it is almost time to take the next scheduled dose, omit the missed dose and take only the scheduled dose. *Do not take a double dose to make up for a missed dose.*

STORAGE
Keep erythrityl tetranitrate in a tightly closed container away from excessive heat. Keep this medication out of the reach of children, and do not allow anyone else to take it.

Isosorbide Dinitrate
(eye soe sor′ bide dye nye′ trate)

PRODUCT INFORMATION
Brand names: Dilatrate, Iso-Bid, Isonate, Isordil, Isotrate, Onset, Sorate, Sorbitrate and others

USES
Isosorbide dinitrate is a member of the nitrate group of vasodilators. It relieves angina (heart pain) by relaxing and opening blood vessels, thus increasing the blood flow and the oxygen supply to the heart.

Isosorbide dinitrate is available in various forms: chewable tablets and tablets to be dissolved in the mouth (sublingual) for quick relief of angina attacks when they occur and regular tablets, extended-release tablets and capsules to be swallowed on a regular schedule for prevention of heart pain. Chewable tablets and tablets to be dissolved in the mouth begin to give relief within three minutes and go on working for up to two hours. The tablets or capsules to be swallowed begin to work in 30 to 60 minutes; their effectiveness lasts up to eight hours.

UNDESIRED EFFECTS
Isosorbide dinitrate can cause headache, rapid heartbeat, flushing, redness of the skin, dizziness, weakness and fainting. These side effects usually are temporary and disappear as your body adjusts to the drug. If these side effects persist or keep you from resuming normal activities, contact your doctor. If dizziness or rapid heartbeat occurs when you take this drug, sit down for a few minutes.

Allergic reactions may occur, with severe skin rash and peeling of the skin. Stop taking the medication and contact your doctor if you experience these symptoms.

Tablets placed under the tongue (sublingual) or between the cheek and gums to dissolve usually produce a tingling or burning sensation indicating that they are being absorbed by the lining of the mouth.

PRECAUTIONS

Tell your doctor what prescription and nonprescription drugs you are taking, especially other drugs for your heart condition or blood pressure, beta blockers (atenolol, metoprolol, nadolol, pindolol, propranolol and timolol), phenothiazines (chlorpromazine, fluphenazine, perphenazine, prochlorperazine, promazine, thioridazine and trifluoperazine) and medication to treat coughs, colds or allergy.

Follow your doctor's advice about smoking and drinking alcoholic beverages while taking this drug. Alcohol can add to the dizziness caused by this drug. Avoid exposure to cold environments; this may reduce the effectiveness of this drug.

Tell your doctor if you have severe anemia, intestinal disease or glaucoma.

You may develop "tolerance" to isosorbide dinitrate after you have been taking it for awhile. This means that you may no longer get relief from the dose your doctor has prescribed for you. Discuss this with your doctor.

Keep in close touch with your doctor while taking this medication. You may have periodic examinations and various blood tests. *Keep all appointments with your doctor and the laboratory.*

Tell your doctor if you ever had an allergic reaction to amyl nitrite, erythrityl tetranitrate, nitroglycerin or pentaerythritol tetranitrate.

DOSAGE

Tablets for quick relief of pain: Isosorbide dinitrate comes in two types of tablets to be taken for quick relief when a pain attack occurs—chewable tablets and tablets to be dissolved under the tongue or between the cheek and gums. Your doctor will select the best form for you and tell you how many tablets to take for each attack and how often to take them if pain is not relieved. It is usually taken every five or 10 minutes until pain is relieved.

If your doctor has prescribed tablets that dissolve in the mouth, place them under the tongue or between the cheek and gum and leave them there until completely dissolved. Try not to swallow saliva too often until the tablet has completely dissolved.

If chewable tablets have been prescribed for you, chew them thoroughly before you swallow them.

When an attack occurs, stop whatever you are doing, sit down and take a tablet as instructed. If the pain is not relieved after waiting five or 10 minutes (see the instructions on your prescription label), take another dose. Contact your doctor immediately or go to a hospital if the pain has not been relieved after you have taken three tablets. Do not take more tablets or take them more often than as directed on your prescription label.

Carry isosorbide dinitrate tablets with you at all times. You may learn through experience what activities cause heart pain (angina). Take a tablet before any activity or stressful situation that may provoke pain. Discuss this with your doctor and follow your doctor's advice for avoiding pain.

Tablets for prevention of angina attacks: Regular tablets and extended-release tablets and capsules are used to prevent attacks of heart pain. They do not relieve the pain of an angina attack once it occurs.

Isosorbide dinitrate tablets usually are taken four times a day. Your prescription label tells you how often to take them and how much to take at each dose. Follow the instructions carefully and ask your doctor or pharmacist to explain any part you do not understand.

Contact your doctor if you continue to experience angina attacks in spite of taking medication to prevent them. If you forget to take a dose, take it as soon as you remember. However, if you remember a missed dose when it is almost time to take the next scheduled dose, omit the missed dose and take only the scheduled dose. *Do not take a double dose to make up for a missed dose.*

STORAGE
Keep isosorbide dinitrate tablets in the container they came in, and keep it tightly closed and away from excessive heat. Keep this medication out of the reach of children and do not allow anyone else to take it.

Nitroglycerin
(ny troe gli′ ser in)

PRODUCT INFORMATION
Brand names: Ang-O-Span, Cardabid, Nitro-Bid, Nitrodisk, Nitro-Dur, Nitroglyn, Nitrol, Nitrong, Nitrospan, Nitrostat, Susadrin, Transderm-Nitro, Trates and others

USES
Nitroglycerin is a vasodilator drug used to relieve and prevent angina (heart pain). It reduces the frequency, duration and severity of angina attacks. Nitroglycerin is available in several forms: tablets to be dissolved in the mouth at the time of an angina attack for quick relief; slow-release tablets and capsules swallowed on a regular schedule for prevention of angina attacks; ointment applied to the skin; and skin patches containing a premeasured amount of ointment to be absorbed through the skin over a 24-hour period to prevent heart pain and injection.

Nitroglycerin relieves heart pain by relaxing and opening the blood vessels allowing more blood and oxygen to reach the heart. Tablets dissolved in the mouth begin to give relief within two minutes and go on working for up to 30 minutes. The ointment begins to take effect after about 30 minutes.

UNDESIRED EFFECTS
Nitroglycerin can cause headache, flushing, rapid heartbeat, redness of the skin, dizziness, weakness and fainting. These side effects usually are temporary and disappear as your body adjusts to the drug. If these effects persist or keep you from resuming normal activities, contact your doctor. If dizziness or rapid heartbeat occurs when you take this drug, sit down for a few minutes.

Severe skin rash and peeling may be indications of an allergic reaction. Stop taking nitroglycerin and contact your doctor if these symptoms occur.

Nitroglycerin tablets placed under the tongue or between the cheek and gums usually produce a tingling or burning sensation indicating that they are being absorbed as they should.

PRECAUTIONS

Before you start taking nitroglycerin, tell your doctor what prescription and nonprescription drugs you are taking, especially other drugs for your heart condition or blood pressure, beta blockers (atenolol, metoprolol, nadolol, pindolol, propranolol and timolol), phenothiazines (chlorpromazine, fluphenazine, perphenazine, prochlorperazine, promazine, thioridazine and trifluoperazine), medicine for depression and medications for colds, cough or allergy.

Tell your doctor if you have severe anemia, thyroid disease, glaucoma or intestinal disease. Also, tell your doctor if you ever had an allergic reaction to amyl nitrite, erythrityl tetranitrate, isosorbide dinitrate or pentaerythritol tetranitrate.

Follow your doctor's advice about smoking and drinking alcoholic beverages. Alcohol can add to the dizziness caused by this drug. Avoid exposure to cold environments, since the effectiveness of nitroglycerin is reduced in cold environments.

You may develop "tolerance" to nitroglycerin after you have been taking it for awhile. This means that you may no longer get relief from the dose your doctor has prescribed for you. Discuss this with your doctor.

Keep in close touch with your doctor while taking this medication. You may have periodic examinations and various blood tests. *Keep all appointments with your doctor and the laboratory.*

DOSAGE

The tablets to be dissolved in the mouth are absorbed by the lining of the mouth to give fast pain relief.

When an attack occurs, stop whatever you are doing, sit down and place a tablet under your tongue or between your cheek and gum. Leave it there until it dissolves completely. Try not to swallow saliva too often until the tablet has completely dissolved. Do not swallow the tablet. Your doctor will tell you how many tablets to take for each attack and how often to take them. If the pain is not relieved within five minutes, take another dose. Contact your doctor immediately or go to a hospital if the pain is not relieved after you have taken three doses and 15 minutes have passed.

Carry nitroglycerin tablets with you at all times. Be sure your supply is fresh. Throw away tablets that do not cause a tingling or burning sensation in your mouth or are more than six months old; these tablets are not fresh. Contact your doctor or pharmacist to obtain a fresh supply. You may learn through experience what activities cause heart pain. Take a nitroglycerin tablet before any activity or stressful situation you know may provoke heart pain. Talk this over with your doctor and follow your doctor's advice for avoiding pain.

The slow-release tablets and capsules are swallowed whole. They are usually taken two or three times a day. Your prescription label tells you how often to take them and how much to take at each dose. Follow the instructions carefully and ask your doctor or pharmacist to explain any part you do not understand.

Contact your doctor if you continue to experience angina attacks in spite of taking nitroglycerin to prevent them. If you forget to take a dose, take the missed dose as soon as you remember. However, if you do not remember until it is less than six hours before your next scheduled dose, omit the missed dose and take only the scheduled dose. *Do not take a double dose to make up for a missed dose.*

Nitroglycerin *ointment* is used to prevent angina, especially at night. It is not used to relieve heart pain during an attack because it takes 30 minutes for the ointment to take effect.

The tube of ointment comes with papers with a ruled line for measuring the dose (in inches). Carefully follow the instructions on your prescription label for application of the ointment. It is usually applied every three or four hours and at bedtime. Squeeze the ointment onto the paper, carefully measuring the amount specified on your prescription label. Use the paper to spread the ointment in a thin layer on a relatively hair-free area of skin (an area at least two inches by three inches), such as the chest. Do not rub the ointment in. Cover the area with plastic wrap and tape it in place. Do not use more ointment or use it more often than as instructed. Contact your doctor if you experience headaches or heart pain while using the ointment. Do not suddenly stop using the ointment.

Nitroglycerin *skin patches* (Nitrodisk, Nitro-Dur and Transderm-Nitro) contain a 24-hour supply of ointment in a specially designed material that releases the drug for absorption through the skin. The patches are used to prevent heart pain. They are not used to relieve pain during an attack.

Follow the instructions included in the package for use of the skin patches. Apply a fresh patch once a day (preferably at the same time every day) to an area of skin that is clean, dry, intact and relatively free of dense hair, such as the upper arm. Apply patches to a different site each day to prevent skin irritation. Some manufacturers claim that the patches are resistant to moisture and may even be worn in the shower without falling off. If a patch falls off, put a new one on.

STORAGE

Keep nitroglycerin in the container it came in and keep it in a cool, dark place. Protect the tablets and capsules from air, moisture, heat and light. Nitroglycerin tablets must be kept in glass containers with tightly fitting metal caps. Keep the bottle tightly closed and do not put cotton or any other medications in the bottle. Do not carry nitroglycerin tablets loose in your pocket or purse. Keep nitroglycerin out of the reach of children.

Pentaerythritol Tetranitrate

(pen tah eh rith′ ri tall tet rah nye′ trate)

PRODUCT INFORMATION
Brand names: Duotrate, Peritrate

USES

Pentaerythritol tetranitrate is a member of the nitrate group of vasodilators. It relaxes and opens blood vessels increasing blood flow and the oxygen supply to the heart. It is prescribed for long-term prevention of angina attacks and may reduce the frequency and severity of pain. However, it is not used for quick relief of heart pain when an attack occurs.

Pentaerythritol tetranitrate begins to work 20 to 60 minutes after it is taken and goes on working for four to five hours.

UNDESIRED EFFECTS

Pentaerythritol tetranitrate can cause headache, rapid heartbeat, flushing, redness of the skin, dizziness, weakness and fainting. These side effects are usually temporary and disappear as your body adjusts to the drug. If these effects persist or keep you from performing your normal activities, contact your doctor. If dizziness or rapid heartbeat occurs when you take this drug, sit down for a few minutes.

If you develop a severe skin rash and peeling, you may be allergic to this drug. Stop taking it and contact your doctor if you experience these symptoms.

PRECAUTIONS

Inform your doctor what prescription and nonprescription drugs you are taking, especially other drugs to treat your heart condition or blood pressure, beta blockers (atenolol, metoprolol, nadolol, pindolol, propranolol and timolol), phenothiazines (chlorpromazine, fluphenazine, perphenazine, prochlorperazine, promazine, thioridazine and trifluoperazine) and drugs to treat colds, allergies or cough. If you do not know the names of the drugs or what they were prescribed for, take the labeled containers to your doctor or pharmacist.

Follow your doctor's advice about smoking and drinking alcoholic beverages. Alcohol may increase the dizziness caused by this drug. Avoid exposure to cold environments; this may reduce the effectiveness of this drug.

Tell your doctor if you have severe anemia, intestinal disease or glaucoma.

Tell your doctor if you ever had an allergic reaction to amyl nitrite, erythrityl tetranitrate, isosorbide dinitrate or nitroglycerin.

You may develop "tolerance" to this drug after you have been taking it for awhile. This means that the dose your doctor has prescribed for you loses its effectiveness. Discuss this with your doctor.

Keep in close touch with your doctor while taking this medication. You may have periodic examinations and various blood tests. *Keep all appointments with your doctor and the laboratory.*

DOSAGE

Pentaerythritol tetranitrate comes in regular tablets and extended-release capsules and tablets. The tablets are usually taken four times a day—at least 30 minutes before or an hour after meals and at bedtime. The extended-release tablets or capsules are usually taken twice a day.

Your doctor will select the best form for you and will determine how often you should take it and how much you should take at each dose. Follow the instructions on your prescription label carefully and ask your doctor or pharmacist to explain any part you do not understand.

Contact your doctor if you continue to experience angina attacks in spite of taking this medication to prevent them. If you forget to take a dose, take the missed dose as soon as you remember. Take the remaining doses for that day at regularly spaced intervals. However, if you do not remember a missed dose until you are scheduled to take the next one, take only one dose. *Do not take a double dose to make up for a missed dose.*

STORAGE
Keep pentaerythritol tetranitrate in a tightly closed container away from excessive heat. Keep this medication out of the reach of children, and do not allow anyone else to take it.

BETA BLOCKERS

The beta blockers have been used to treat angina (heart pain). See the section titled Beta Blockers (page 27) for more information.

Blood Clots

Blood clots can form in the veins of the legs, heart, lungs or brain as a result of inflammation of the veins, a heart attack or poor circulation when the heart is not pumping blood efficiently. Blood clots can be life-threatening. Even those that form in the legs carry the risk that part of the clot may break off and be carried by the bloodstream to a vital organ such as the lungs. Blood clots can also cause a heart attack or stroke.

Because they are so serious, blood clots are treated with anticoagulants (blood thinners), drugs that slow up the clotting process. The goal of treatment is to prevent formation of new clots and to prevent existing clots from getting larger without causing bleeding. This delicate balance can only be achieved with frequent blood tests that check the time required for the blood to clot (prothrombin time).

Even when anticoagulants are taken as prescribed serious bleeding can occur. Call your doctor immediately if any of the following signs of bleeding occur while you are taking anticoagulants:

- unusual nosebleed or bloody gums after brushing your teeth
- prolonged bleeding from cuts, a heavy menstrual period or blood oozing from a clot
- vomiting or spitting up blood that looks either red or brown and resembles coffee grounds
- sudden appearance of bruises or black and blue marks on the skin
- black or bloody bowel movements or red or dark brown urine
- new or unexpected pain such as headaches, stomach pain or backaches

Warfarin/Oral Anticoagulants

PRODUCT INFORMATION
Brand name for anisindione (an iss in dye' one): Miradon
Brand name for dicumarol (dye koo' ma role): Dicumarol
Brand name for phenprocoumon (fen proe koo' mon): Liquamar
Brand names for warfarin (war' far in): Athrombin-K, Coufarin, Coumadin, Panwarfin

USES
The most commonly prescribed oral anticoagulant drug (blood thinner) is warfarin. The uses, undesired effects, precautions, dosage, instructions and storage of anisindione, dicumarol and phenprocoumon are generally the same as for warfarin.

Oral anticoagulants prevent blood clots from forming or from getting larger by interfering with the action of vitamin K in the formation of blood clotting factors. They do not dissolve blood clots. They are used to treat conditions in which a blood clot may occur (lengthy periods of immobilization, diseased heart valves and irregular heartbeat) or has occurred, particularly pulmonary embolism (a blood clot in the lung) and thrombophlebitis (a clot in a blood vessel, usually in the leg).

For people with artificial heart valves, warfarin is sometimes used with the drug dipyridamole (or aspirin) to minimize the chance of clot formation (see the monograph titled Dipyridamole for more information). When the injectable drug heparin has been used in the hospital to prevent blood clots, warfarin is frequently the oral drug taken to maintain this effect. *It is very important to take warfarin exactly on schedule in the precise amount your doctor has prescribed.*

UNDESIRED EFFECTS

Bleeding is the most common undesired effect of anticoagulants. Contact your doctor at the first sign of bleeding such as bruising or black and blue marks, blood in the urine (red or dark brown urine) or nosebleed. Also, let your doctor know if you develop unusual pains in your lower back or abdomen or a prolonged headache. *In the event of accidental overdose, contact your doctor, poison control center or nearest hospital emergency room immediately.*

Bothersome side effects include rash, hives, loss of hair, fever, nausea, vomiting and diarrhea. Any illness that causes vomiting, diarrhea or fever can change the effect of this medication, so if any of these problems last for more than a few days, contact your doctor.

PRECAUTIONS

Tell your doctor if you are allergic to aspirin or tartrazine (a yellow dye present in some processed foods and medications including certain brands of warfarin). Do not switch to a different brand name warfarin product because it may differ in absorption.

Periodic laboratory tests, especially prothrombin time (a test that measures the time it takes for your blood to clot), must be done to check your response to this drug so that your dose can be adjusted if necessary. *Keep all appointments with your doctor and the laboratory.*

Prothrombin time (PT) tests are repeated more frequently—perhaps daily—when therapy is first started. Once the proper drug dosage is established and you take your medication properly, the tests can be done less frequently. Failure to keep appointments for these tests could result in the improper control of your anticoagulant therapy.

A large number of drugs increase or decrease the anticoagulant effects of your medication. Tell your doctor what prescription and nonprescription drugs you are taking. If you do not know the names of the drugs or what they were prescribed for, take the labeled containers to your doctor or pharmacist. Among the drugs that may alter the effect of warfarin and the other anticoagulants are antibiotics, aspirin, barbiturates, birth-control pills, chloral hydrate, cholestyramine, clofibrate, disopyramide, disulfiram, drugs for arthritis and muscle pains, glutethimide, oral diabetes drugs, oxyphenbutazone, phenylbutazone, phenytoin and thyroid hormones.

Do not stop taking any of the medications you are currently taking unless directed to do so by your doctor. Do not take any other drugs unless you have your doctor's permission.

It is important that all of the doctors and dentists taking care of you know that you are taking an anticoagulant so they can avoid prescribing medications that interfere with its effect.

Tell your doctor about any other medical conditions you have, especially those involving bleeding (ulcers or lengthy or heavy menstrual periods), diabetes, kidney or liver disease or high blood pressure.

Vitamin K can decrease the therapeutic effect of warfarin and other oral anticoagulants. Therefore, ask your doctor about eating foods that contain vitamin K, including fish, asparagus, bacon, liver, broccoli, cabbage, cauliflower, kale, lettuce, spinach, turnip greens, watercress and onions. Once your doctor has determined the proper dosage for you, do not change your diet.

Women who become pregnant while taking an anticoagulant should promptly notify their doctors. Warfarin and other anticoagulants should not be taken during pregnancy because they pass to the unborn baby and may cause fatal bleeding. Tell your doctor (and pediatrician) if you are breast-feeding a baby. Anticoagulants pass from a mother to her breast-fed baby through the milk. The baby should be watched for signs of bleeding.

Avoid any activities that have a high risk of injury. You may want to carry a card or wear a bracelet indicating that you are taking an anticoagulant, so those treating you will know this in the event of an accident.

Avoid excessive consumption of alcoholic beverages. Ask your doctor how much, if any, alcohol you may consume.

DOSAGE

Oral anticoagulant tablets are usually taken once every 24 hours. Your doctor has determined how much you should take at each dose. *Carefully follow the instructions on your prescription label,* and ask your doctor or pharmacist to explain any part you do not understand. Your doctor may change your dosage frequently depending on side effects (bleeding) and your prothrombin time (PT). If your dose is too large, you may have bleeding; if it is too small, you could get blood clots.

Do not change your daily dose unless advised to do so by your doctor. To avoid missing any doses, take this medication at the same time that you do something else every day such as eating your dinner. Record each dose on a calender when you take it. *You must continue taking this medication for as long as your doctor tells you to take it.*

If you miss a dose, take it as soon as you remember. If you do not remember until the next day, do not take two doses. Take only the scheduled dose. *Never take a double dose.* If you miss doses for two or more days, call your doctor.

STORAGE

Keep this drug in the container it came in, and keep it out of the reach of children. Do not allow anyone else to take it.

High Blood Cholesterol

Cholesterol and triglycerides are fatty acids found in body tissues and in the blood. People with high blood levels of certain types of fats have a greater risk of heart disease than people with low levels. When large amounts of fatty substances are present in the blood, they can deposit, build up and harden along the walls of the coronary arteries (blood vessels that supply oxygen and nutrients to the heart). This buildup is called atherosclerosis. Atherosclerosis decreases the flow of blood and thus the supply of oxygen to the heart muscle, causing heart disease, angina (heart pain), heart attack or stroke.

There are generally three causes of high cholesterol and triglycerides in the blood: diet (eating too many foods high in cholesterol and fat and drinking too much alcohol), various diseases and heredity.

It is thought that lowering the blood level of cholesterol and triglycerides with drug therapy and diet (restricted intake of fats, cholesterol and alcohol) is helpful in preventing heart disease, angina, heart attack and stroke.

If your doctor has suggested a diet and exercise program, follow this plan carefully. You will also have regular blood tests to determine whether the drugs, diet and exercise are effective. In addition, you may have tests to determine if the drugs are causing any harmful effects.

Drugs used to lower blood levels of fatty acids—cholesterol and triglycerides—are called antilipemics.

ANTILIPEMICS

Cholestyramine
(koe less' tir a meen)

PRODUCT INFORMATION
Brand name: Questran

USES
Cholestyramine is used with diet therapy to reduce the amount of cholesterol in the blood. It has been shown to reduce the risk of developing coronary (heart) disease and myocardial infarction (heart attack) in men with high cholesterol. Cholestyramine is also prescribed to relieve itching caused by certain kinds of jaundice.

UNDESIRED EFFECTS

The most common side effect of cholestyramine is constipation. This is usually mild but, if it persists, contact your doctor.

Other undesired effects are heartburn, nausea, vomiting, stomach pain and bloating. Contact your doctor if these effects are severe or persist.

PRECAUTIONS

Tell your doctor if you have ever had an allergic reaction to aspirin or tartrazine (a yellow dye found in some foods and drugs including cholestyramine).

Tell your doctor if you are constipated or have heart disease, especially angina (heart pain), or stomach, intestinal or gallbladder disease.

Cholestyramine may affect the way your body responds to certain other drugs, including anticoagulants (blood thinners). Before you take cholestyramine, tell your doctor what other prescription and nonprescription drugs you are taking. If you do not know the names of the drugs or what they were prescribed for, take the labeled containers to your doctor or pharmacist.

Cholestyramine may interfere with the absorption of other drugs such as digitalis, iron, tetracycline, thyroid, folic acid, loperamide, phenobarbital, phenylbutazone, oxyphenbutazone, vitamins and thiazide diuretics (water pills). These drugs should be taken one hour before or four hours after cholestyramine is taken.

Your doctor may want you to have laboratory tests to determine your response to cholestyramine. *Be sure to keep your appointments for these tests* because they give your doctor important information about the effectiveness of the drug.

Follow your doctor's advice about diet and drinking alcoholic beverages.

Tell your doctor if you are pregnant or breast-feeding a baby. It is not known whether it is safe to take cholestyramine during pregnancy or while breast-feeding.

DOSAGE

Cholestyramine comes as a dry powder. It is usually taken three or four times a day, before meals and at bedtime. Your prescription label tells you when to take this medication and how much to take at each dose. Follow these instructions carefully. Ask your doctor or pharmacist to explain any part you do not understand.

Cholestyramine powder must be mixed with fluid. *Do not take the powder alone.* To use the powder, follow these steps:

1. Spread the powder on the surface of a glass of water, milk, fruit juice or another noncarbonated beverage.
2. Let the powder stand for one minute, then stir it into the beverage and drink it.
3. Put more of the beverage in the glass and drink the beverage to be sure you are consuming all of the powder.

The powder also may be mixed with soup, applesauce, crushed pineapple or pureed fruit. The powder should be added to the liquid or food just before you consume it.

If you forget to take a dose, take it as soon as you remember. Take the remaining doses for that day at evenly spaced intervals. However, if you remember a missed dose at the time you are scheduled to take another dose, omit the missed dose and take only the scheduled one. *Do not take a double dose.*

STORAGE
Cholestyramine should be kept in the container it came in, tightly closed and away from moisture. Keep it out of the reach of children, and do not allow anyone else to take it.

Colestipol
(koe les' ti pole)

PRODUCT INFORMATION
Brand name: Colestid

USES
Colestipol is used to reduce the amount of cholesterol in the blood.

UNDESIRED EFFECTS
Constipation is the most common side effect of colestipol and can be severe. Usually, it is mild and disappears as your body adjusts to the drug, but, if it persists, contact your doctor. Other side effects that may occur are skin rash, headache, dizziness, muscle and joint pain, loss of appetite, fatigue, shortness of breath and stomach upset. If these effects are bothersome, contact your doctor.

PRECAUTIONS
Tell your doctor if you have a history of unusual bleeding, have an underactive thyroid or are constipated. Colestipol can make constipation worse.

Tell your doctor what prescription and nonprescription drugs you are taking. If you do not know the names of the drugs or what they were prescribed for, take the labeled containers to your doctor or pharmacist.

Colestipol may reduce the effect of other medications, particularly digitalis (heart medication), penicillin G and tetracycline, by binding to them in the stomach or intestine and preventing absorption. Take these drugs at least one hour before or four hours after colestipol.

It may also interfere with the absorption of certain vitamins (A, D, E and K). If you experience unusual bleeding, contact your doctor; this may be a sign of vitamin K deficiency. Your doctor may recommend a vitamin supplement.

Follow your doctor's advice about diet and drinking alcoholic beverages. Do not stop taking colestipol without consulting your doctor. Discontinuation of colestipol may affect your response to other medications (due to greater absorption).

Tell your doctor if you are pregnant, plan to become pregnant or are breast-feeding a baby. It is not known if it is safe to take colestipol during pregnancy or while breast-feeding.

DOSAGE

Colestipol is usually taken two to four times a day. Follow the instructions on your prescription label carefully, and ask your doctor or pharmacist to explain any part you do not understand.

Colestipol comes as a powder to be taken by mouth. The powder should be mixed with food or fluids. *Do not take the powder alone.* Your prescription label tells you how much powder to take at each dose. To use the powder, follow these steps:

1. Spread the powder on the surface of a glass of water, milk, fruit juice or soft drink.
2. Let the powder stand for one minute, then stir it into the beverage and drink it.
3. Rinse the drinking glass with more of the beverage and drink it to be sure you are getting the entire dose.

The powder also may be mixed with cereal, soup, applesauce, crushed pineapple or pureed fruit. The powder should be added to the liquid or food just before you take it.

If you forget to take a dose, take the missed dose as soon as you remember. Take any remaining doses for that day at evenly spaced intervals. However, if it is almost time for your next scheduled dose, omit the missed dose and take only the scheduled dose. *Do not take a double dose.*

Your doctor may want you to take laboratory tests to determine how your body is responding to this medication. Be sure to keep your appointments for these tests because they give your doctor important information about the effectiveness of the medication.

STORAGE

Keep the container tightly closed and away from moisture. Keep this medication out of the reach of children, and do not allow anyone else to take it.

Niacin

(ney' a sin)

PRODUCT INFORMATION

Brand names: Niac, Nico-400, Nicobid, Nicolar, Nicotinex, Nicotym and others

USES

Niacin, also known as nicotinic acid, is one of the B vitamins (B_3). In large doses, niacin reduces the amount of cholesterol and triglycerides in the blood. When given in large doses, niacin also dilates (opens) blood vessels to improve circulation.

Niacin is prescribed for three different conditions. It is used to prevent buildup of fatty deposits inside the blood vessels and, with other vasodilator drugs, to treat conditions caused by poor circulation. It is also used to prevent and treat pellagra (niacin deficiency disease), which can result from an inadequate diet, chronic stomach and intestinal disease or alcoholism.

UNDESIRED EFFECTS

Niacin can cause flushing, itching and a sensation of burning, stinging or tingling of the skin (especially the face and neck), headache, nausea, vomiting and diarrhea. These effects usually go away as you continue to take the medicine, but, if they bother you, take it with antacids or food. Contact your doctor if these effects persist; it may be necessary to reduce your dosage.

Niacin may make you dizzy, especially when moving suddenly from a lying to a sitting position or from a sitting to a standing position. Avoid sudden changes in position.

Other side effects include skin rash, dry skin and mouth, changes in vision and nervousness. Contact your doctor if these effects are bothersome.

PRECAUTIONS

Niacin may affect the way your body responds to certain other drugs, particularly medications prescribed for high blood pressure or diabetes. Niacin may increase your blood glucose level and, if you have diabetes, affect your dosage requirement for insulin or oral diabetes medication. Tell your doctor what prescription and nonprescription drugs you are taking before you take niacin. If you do not know the names of the drugs or what they were prescribed for, take the labeled containers to your doctor or pharmacist.

Before you take niacin, tell your doctor if you have diabetes, gallbladder disease or a history of jaundice or liver disease, gout, peptic ulcer or allergy. Tell your doctor if you ever had an allergic reaction to aspirin or tartrazine (a yellow dye found in certain foods and drugs including some brands of niacin).

Your doctor may want you to have laboratory tests to determine how you are responding to this medication. *Keep your appointments for these tests* because they give your doctor important information about the effectiveness of the drug.

DOSAGE

Niacin comes as oral solution, regular tablets and extended-release tablets and capsules.

Niacin is usually taken two to four times a day. Your prescription label tells you how often to take niacin and how much to take at each dose. Follow the instructions and ask your doctor or pharmacist to explain any part you do not understand.

This drug should be taken with meals or immediately after eating. If you forget to take a dose, take the missed dose as soon as you remember. However, if you remember a missed dose at the time you are scheduled to take another dose, omit the missed dose and take only the scheduled one. *Do not take a double dose.*

STORAGE

This medication should be kept in the container it came in, tightly closed and away from moisture. Keep it out of the reach of children, and do not allow anyone else to take it.

Probucol
(proe' byoo kole)

PRODUCT INFORMATION
Brand name: Lorelco

USES
Probucol is used with diet therapy to reduce the amount of cholesterol circulating in the blood in people with high cholesterol.

UNDESIRED EFFECTS
Common side effects of probucol include diarrhea, nausea, vomiting, abdominal pain and gas. These effects are usually mild and disappear as your body adjusts to the drug. Other less common side effects include excessive sweating, foul-smelling sweat, swelling of the face, hands or feet, itching eyes and increased appetite. If these effects persist or are bothersome, contact your doctor.

PRECAUTIONS
Tell your doctor if you ever had a heart attack or arrhythmias (irregular heartbeat). Contact your doctor if you have fainting spells.

Tell your doctor if you are pregnant, plan to become pregnant or are breast-feeding a baby. Probucol should not be taken by women who are pregnant or are breast-feeding.

Women capable of becoming pregnant should practice birth control while taking this drug. If you plan to become pregnant, you should stop taking probucol six months before trying to become pregnant. Discuss this with your doctor.

DOSAGE
Probucol comes as film-coated tablets. It is usually taken twice a day with the morning and evening meals. Follow the instructions on your prescription label and ask your doctor or pharmacist to explain any part you do not understand. Probucol must be taken regularly to be effective. Do not stop taking this medication until your doctor tells you to.

If you forget to take a dose, take it as soon as you remember. If you do not remember until it is almost time for your next scheduled dose, take only the scheduled dose and omit the missed dose. *Do not take a double dose to make up for a missed dose.*

Follow your doctor's advice about diet and drinking alcoholic beverages.

Your doctor may ask you to have laboratory tests and an electrocardiogram (EKG) done periodically to determine how your body is responding to the medication and whether you should continue to take it. *Keep all appointments with your doctor and the laboratory.*

STORAGE

Keep this medication in the container it came in, and keep it tightly closed. Keep it out of the reach of children. Do not allow anyone else to take your probucol.

Miscellaneous Drugs Used in Treating Heart Diseases and Diseases of the Circulatory System

Potassium Supplements

PRODUCT INFORMATION

Brand names: K-Lor, K-Lyte, Kaochlor, Kaon, K-Tab, Kay Ciel, Kaylixir, Klorvess, Klotrix, Slow-K, Tri-K, Trikates and others

USES

Potassium is essential for the proper function of the heart, kidneys, muscles, nerves and digestive system. Usually the food you eat supplies all of the potassium you need. However, certain diseases (e.g., kidney disease, gastrointestinal disease with vomiting and diarrhea) and drugs, particularly diuretics (water pills), digitalis (heart medication) and steroids (cortisone-type drugs), remove potassium from the body, and it must be replaced. If you are taking a diuretic (water pill) for high blood pressure, your doctor may tell you to eat more potassium-rich foods and take a potassium supplement. (See the monograph titled Thiazide Diuretics for more information.)

Potassium supplements are taken to replace potassium losses and prevent potassium deficiency (and weakness and tiredness). Although several potassium salts (acetate, bicarbonate, chloride, citrate and gluconate) are available, potassium chloride is the most commonly used salt.

UNDESIRED EFFECTS

Nausea, vomiting and diarrhea are the most common undesired effects of potassium supplements. To avoid or diminish these effects, take the medication after eating a meal or a snack, or take it with a full glass of water. Contact your doctor if stomach upset continues to occur.

Taking too much potassium can cause weakness or heaviness of the legs; mental confusion; listlessness; cold, gray skin; irregular heartbeat or a "pins and needles" feeling or tingling of the hands or feet. Stop taking potassium and contact your doctor if you experience any of these effects. *Do not take more than the amount specified on your prescription label.* While taking potassium, keep in touch with your doctor. Your doctor may have your blood level of potassium tested to see if your dosage needs to be adjusted. *Keep all appointments with your doctor and the laboratory.* If you are using a salt substitute, tell your doctor. Many salt substitutes contain potassium. Your doctor will take this into consideration in determining your dosage of potassium supplement.

PRECAUTIONS

Some *tablet* forms of potassium that are swallowed have produced ulceration and obstruction in the small intestine or stomach. If you develop abdominal or stomach pain, persistent indigestion, vomiting or intestinal bleeding or if you have chronic constipation while taking potassium, stop taking it and contact your doctor.

If you are taking another medication with the potassium supplement and stop taking the other medication or start taking another drug, ask your doctor whether you should continue to take the potassium supplement. Do not take potassium if you are taking the drug amiloride, spironolactone or triamterene. Tell your doctor what prescription and nonprescription drugs you are taking, especially corticosteroids and heart medications.

Tell your doctor about any medical conditions you have, particularly heart and kidney disease, before you take this drug.

Do not take potassium if you have muscle cramps or are dehydrated or overheated from too much exposure to the sun or exercise in hot weather; contact your doctor.

Potassium supplements can be taken safely during pregnancy and while breast-feeding a baby. Take the medication exactly as directed.

DOSAGE

Potassium supplements come in four forms—powder, liquid, tablets to be dissolved in water before ingestion and tablets to be swallowed. Your doctor will choose the best form for you and determine how often you should take it and how much you should take at each dose. Follow the instructions on your prescription label carefully and ask your doctor or pharmacist to explain any part you do not understand. Potassium is usually taken two to four times a day.

The liquid should be added to or the powder should be dissolved in water, milk, coffee, tea, soft drinks or fruit juice and mixed well just before you take it. Measure the liquid carefully to be sure you take the proper dose. *Take potassium with or after food or a meal to avoid stomach irritation.*

The tablets to be dissolved in water should be thoroughly dissolved and mixed just before you take them. *The tablets to be swallowed must be swallowed, not chewed or dissolved in the mouth.* Take them with a full glass of water and with food or after meals.

If you forget to take a dose, take it as soon as you remember and take any remaining doses for that day at evenly spaced intervals. *Do not take a double dose to make up for a missed dose.* Be sure you have enough of this medication on hand at all times to permit you to take all of the prescribed doses. Check your supply before holidays, when you plan to be away from home and at any other time when it may be difficult to obtain a refill.

STORAGE
Keep your medication in the container it came in, and keep it out of the reach of children. Do not allow anyone else to take it.

Infections

DRUGS USED TO TREAT INFECTIONS

Anti-infectives

The drugs used to help the body fight infections are called, simply, anti-infectives. Infections may be caused by a wide variety of organisms, including bacteria, protozoa, fungi, rickettsiae, spirochetes and viruses. Each anti-infective drug is effective against only particular organisms. A few anti-infectives have a broad spectrum of activity, fighting infections caused by several different organisms.

Anti-infectives must reach high enough concentrations in body tissues and fluids to "overcome" the infection. Some anti-infectives are absorbed into the bloodstream from the stomach or intestines and are distributed throughout the body. Thus, these *systemic* anti-infectives (primarily antibiotics) are used to treat pneumonia, flu or other respiratory infections, sore throat, skin infections, ear or sinus infections and venereal infections. Other anti-infectives reach sufficient concentrations only in certain areas of the body—in the urine, for example. Still others are most effective when applied directly to the site of the infection, such as the eye or the skin. These drugs are called *topical* or *local* anti-infectives.

Antibiotics are anti-infectives derived from bacteria, molds, fungi or other living substances. Some synthetic and semisynthetically produced antibiotics were originally obtained from microorganisms. Antibiotics can be classified according to their activity against the various classes of microorganisms: gram-positive and gram-negative bacteria, rickettsiae, viruses, spirochetes, fungi and protozoa. Antibiotics that are effective against several strains from different classes of organisms are broad-spectrum antibiotics.

In selecting an anti-infective for you, your doctor must consider the probable infecting organism and the location of the infection in your body. "Culture and sensitivity" laboratory tests identify the causative organism and the best drug for treating your infection. In some instances, the organism causing the infection may be obvious (nail infections usually are caused by fungi) or your doctor may know of a community or family "epidemic" caused by a particular organism. In other situations, a broad-spectrum antibiotic may be prescribed because it is effective against a wide range of organisms.

Many anti-infectives, including antibiotics, do not actually destroy the infecting organism. They only slow down or interrupt its growth and reproduction. Your body then takes over, and your natural defense mechanisms destroy or remove the infecting organism. Thus, when you have a prescription for an anti-infective, it is important that you *take all of the medication prescribed*. Since the drug only controls growth and slows down the infection, you must take the medication long enough to give your body a fair chance to overcome the infecting organism. If you stop taking the drug after a few days because you feel better, the infection may flare up again before your body has completed the fight.

No anti-infectives are effective against the virus that causes the common cold. Antibiotics may be useful in treating other infections, primarily caused by bacteria, that follow a bad cold. In general, however, a cold should *not* be treated with antibiotics. Treat a cold's symptoms as they occur. (See the section Allergies, Colds and Coughs, page 263.)

Many organisms can become resistant to anti-infectives, and the drugs no longer prevent their growth. If you are taking one anti-infective and it doesn't seem to be working, your doctor may prescribe a different drug.

If you have medication remaining when your prescription is changed, do not save it for future use or let anyone else take it.

When taken orally, anti-infectives generally are absorbed from the stomach and intestines. Solid food, milk and some drugs, such as antacids, may interfere with this absorption. Ask your doctor or pharmacist about the problem. If you are told to take the anti-infective on an "empty stomach" (to be certain that enough of the drug is absorbed to treat infection), take it one hour before or two hours after food. Some anti-infectives may cause nausea or vomiting if taken on an empty stomach but can be taken with a light snack to avoid stomach upsets.

Since some anti-infectives can inhibit growth of many different organisms, these anti-infectives can stop the growth of bacteria that normally live in the gastrointestinal or urinary tract. These natural bacteria are needed to maintain certain body functions (for example, the breakdown of waste products), but anti-infectives may destroy them. Then other bacteria, fungi and organisms that are not destroyed by the anti-infectives may flourish. Symptoms may include severe diarrhea, nausea and vomiting, a feeling of abdominal fullness, abdominal pain and weakness. The lining of the mouth and the tongue and gums may be covered with white patches that leave reddened surfaces when removed. The vaginal or rectal area may be affected in the same way. *If these symptoms of "super-infection" or overgrowth of nonsusceptible organisms occur, you should stop taking the anti-infective drug and contact your doctor.*

Antibiotic drugs are easily divided into groups (sometimes called "families") because of their similar chemical structures and uses in treating infections. Thus, the first part of this chapter discusses several groups of antibiotics—cephalosporins, erythromycins, penicillins and tetracyclines. Anti-infectives that do not fit neatly into any large family are described afterwards.

Other groups of anti-infectives are discussed in relation to the kinds of infections against which they are commonly used. These anti-infectives include drugs used primarily to treat tuberculosis, urinary tract infections, vaginal infections, worm infections and eye infections.

Many of the antibiotics discussed in the first part of the chapter are also used to treat infections in the urinary tract, vagina and eyes.

To find the information on the drug you are interested in, use the Index at the back of this book.

CEPHALOSPORINS
Cefaclor
(sef' a klor)

PRODUCT INFORMATION
Brand name: Ceclor

USES
Cefaclor is a cephalosporin antibiotic that is similar to the penicillins in the way it eliminates bacteria. It is used to treat certain infections in the throat, ears, skin and urinary tract.

Cefaclor can be used for infections caused by bacteria that produce penicillinase (a substance that makes some penicillins ineffective). However, penicillins are generally preferred to cefaclor in the treatment of "strep" infections and in the prevention of rheumatic fever.

UNDESIRED EFFECTS
Tell your doctor if you ever had an allergic reaction to any cephalosporin or to any form of penicillin. A serious reaction is more likely in a person with other allergies.

Allergic reactions, although rare, have occurred with cefaclor. If you get a rash, hives or itching or have difficulty breathing, call your doctor or a hospital immediately. You may need emergency treatment.

Some allergic reactions, such as rash and itching all over your body, joint pains, fever or swollen glands, develop only after several days of therapy. Contact your doctor if you experience any of these effects.

The most common side effects of cefaclor are diarrhea, nausea and vomiting. These effects usually are mild and tend to disappear as your body adjusts to the cefaclor. If these side effects are severe or last for more than two days, contact your doctor.

Cefaclor also can upset your stomach or give you stomach cramps. Usually these reactions can be relieved by taking cefaclor with crackers or a light snack. Contact your doctor if these problems continue.

In people who are sensitive to this drug, cefaclor can cause blood problems, such as bone marrow depression or a decrease in one of the blood clotting factors. Contact your doctor if you notice any unusual bleeding or easy bruising, get painful sores in your mouth or throat or develop chills and fever.

Long-term therapy with cefaclor may result in an overgrowth of other organisms in the body. Some symptoms of this condition are itching of the anus, sore mouth or tongue and vaginal infection. If you experience any of these symptoms, stop taking cefaclor and contact your doctor.

PRECAUTIONS
Before you start taking cefaclor, be sure to tell your doctor or pharmacist if you

ever had an allergic reaction to any cephalosporin or to any form of penicillin. Your doctor also should be told if you have kidney disease or a history of allergy.

Some other medications, particularly gout medicines, should not be taken with cefaclor. Tell your doctor what other prescription or nonprescription drugs you are taking. If you do not know the names of the drugs you are taking or what they were prescribed for, bring them in their labeled containers to your doctor or pharmacist.

Even if you feel better in a few days, take *all* of the medication prescribed for you by your doctor. Bacterial infections take several days to weeks to be cured completely. If you stop taking cefaclor, those bacteria still alive can multiply and cause a recurrence of the infection. However, if your symptoms do not improve within a few days or if they become worse, contact your doctor. It may be necessary to change your medication.

Be sure to tell your doctor if you are pregnant or are nursing an infant. Although problems with this medication have not been published, your doctor should have this information.

Diabetics should be aware that cefaclor can cause false results in some tests for urine sugar. Do not change your diet or the dosage of your diabetes medicine until you check with your doctor.

DOSAGE

Your doctor will determine how often you should take cefaclor and how much you should take at each dose. Follow the instructions on your prescription label, and ask your doctor or pharmacist to explain any part you do not understand.

Doses of cefaclor should be taken as far apart as possible during the day. If your doctor tells you to take it four times a day, take a dose every six hours. If you give cefaclor to a child, make sure he or she receives it around the clock, even if you have to wake the child for doses.

Cefaclor is best taken on an "empty stomach," one hour before meals or two hours after eating. However, if cefaclor upsets your stomach, you can take it with meals or a light snack.

Cefaclor comes in capsules and liquid form. The capsules should be taken with a full eight-ounce glass of water.

The liquid should be shaken thoroughly to mix the medication evenly before each dose is poured. Measure the prescribed dose with a specially marked measuring spoon or dropper to be sure the dose is accurate. Contact your pharmacist if you have any questions about measuring the liquid.

If you forget to take a dose, take it as soon as you remember. Take any remaining doses for that day at evenly spaced intervals. If you still have symptoms of the infection after you have taken all of your medicine, contact your doctor.

STORAGE

When your doctor tells you to stop taking cefaclor, throw away any unused portion. Cefaclor may lose its effectiveness and should not be saved to treat another infection. Because this medication was prescribed for your particular condition, do not allow anyone else to take it.

Keep this medication in the container it came in. Keep liquid cefaclor in the refrigerator but *do not freeze it*. On the container, you will find an expiration date. Do not take the medication after that date. Throw it away, and if you need more, get a new supply. If you are not sure of the expiration date or have any questions about a refill, contact your pharmacist.

Keep this medication out of the reach of children.

Cefadroxil
(sef a drox′ ill)

PRODUCT INFORMATION
Brand names: Duricef, Ultracef

USES
Cefadroxil is a cephalosporin antibiotic that is similar to the penicillins in the way it eliminates bacteria. It is used to treat certain infections in the throat, skin and urinary tract.

Cefadroxil can be used for infections caused by bacteria that produce penicillinase (a substance that makes some penicillins ineffective). However, penicillins are generally preferred in the prevention of rheumatic fever.

UNDESIRED EFFECTS
Tell your doctor if you ever had an allergic reaction to any cephalosporin or to any form of penicillin. A serious reaction is more likely in a person with other allergies.

Allergic reactions, although rare, have occurred with cefadroxil. If you get a rash, hives or itching or have difficulty breathing, call your doctor or hospital immediately. You may need emergency treatment.

Some allergic reactions, such as rash and itching all over your body, joint pains, fever or swollen glands, develop only after several days of therapy. Contact your doctor if you have any of these effects.

The most common side effects of cefadroxil are diarrhea, nausea and vomiting. These effects usually are mild and tend to disappear as your body adjusts to the cefadroxil. If these effects are severe or last for more than two days, contact your doctor.

Cefadroxil also can upset your stomach or give you stomach cramps. Usually these reactions can be relieved by taking the medication with food. Contact your doctor if these problems continue.

In people who are sensitive to this drug, cefadroxil can cause blood problems, such as bone marrow depression or a decrease in one of the blood clotting factors. Contact your doctor if you notice any unusual bleeding or easy bruising, get painful sores in the mouth or throat or develop chills and fever.

Long-term therapy with cefadroxil may result in an overgrowth of other organisms in the body. Some symptoms of this condition are itching of the anus, sore mouth or tongue and vaginal infection. If you experience any of these symptoms, stop taking cefadroxil and contact your doctor.

PRECAUTIONS

Before you start taking cefadroxil, be sure to tell your doctor or pharmacist if you ever had an allergic reaction to any cephalosporin or to any form of penicillin. Your doctor also should be told if you have kidney disease or a history of allergy.

Some other medications, particularly gout medicines, should not be taken with cefadroxil. Tell your doctor what other prescription or nonprescription drugs you are taking. If you do not know what drugs you are taking or what they were prescribed for, bring them in their labeled containers to your doctor or pharmacist.

Even if you feel better in a few days, take *all* of the medication prescribed for you by your doctor. Bacterial infections take several days to weeks to be cured completely. If you stop taking cefadroxil, the bacteria still alive can multiply and cause a recurrence of the infection. However, if your symptoms do not improve within a few days or if they become worse, contact your doctor. It may be necessary to change your medication.

Be sure to tell your doctor if you are pregnant or are nursing an infant. Although problems with this medication have not been published, your doctor should have this information.

Diabetics should be aware that cefadroxil can cause false results in some tests for urine sugar. Do not change your diet or the dosage of your diabetes medication until you check with your doctor.

DOSAGE

Your doctor will determine how often you should take cefadroxil and how much you should take at each dose. Follow the instructions on your prescription label, and ask your doctor or pharmacist to explain any part you do not understand.

Cefadroxil is usually taken once or twice a day. It may be taken with food.

Cefadroxil comes in capsules, tablets and liquid form. The tablets and capsules should be taken with a full eight-ounce glass of water.

The liquid should be shaken thoroughly to mix the medication evenly before each dose is poured. Measure the prescribed dose with a specially marked measuring spoon or dropper to be sure the dose is accurate. Contact your pharmacist if you have any questions about measuring the liquid.

If you forget to take a dose, take it as soon as you remember. Take any remaining doses for that day at evenly spaced intervals. If you still have symptoms of the infection after you have taken all of your medicine, contact your doctor.

STORAGE

When your doctor tells you to stop taking cefadroxil, throw away any unused portion. Cefadroxil may lose its effectiveness and should not be saved to treat another infection. Because this medication was prescribed for your particular condition, do not allow anyone else to take it.

Keep cefadroxil in the container it came in. Keep liquid cefadroxil in the refrigerator but *do not freeze it.* On the container, you will find an expiration date. Do not take the medication after that date. Throw it away and, if you need more, get a new supply. If you are not sure of the expiration date or have any questions about a refill, contact your pharmacist.

Keep this medication out of the reach of children.

Cephalexin
(sef a lex' in)

PRODUCT INFORMATION
Brand name: Keflex

USES
Cephalexin is a cephalosporin antibiotic that is similar to the penicillins in the way it eliminates bacteria. It is used to treat certain infections in the throat, ears, skin, urinary tract and bones.

Cephalexin can be used for infections caused by bacteria that produce penicillinase (a substance that makes penicillins ineffective). However, penicillins are generally preferred to cephalexin in the treatment of "strep" infections and in prevention of rheumatic fever.

UNDESIRED EFFECTS
Tell your doctor if you ever had an allergic reaction to any cephalosporin or to any form of penicillin. A serious reaction is more likely in a person with other allergies.

Allergic reactions, although rare, have occurred with cephalexin. If you get a rash, hives or itching or have difficulty breathing, call your doctor or a hospital immediately. You may need emergency treatment.

Some allergic reactions, such as rash and itching all over your body, joint pains, fever or swollen glands, develop only after several days of therapy. Contact your doctor if you have any of these effects.

The most common side effects of cephalexin are diarrhea, nausea and vomiting. These effects usually are mild and tend to disappear as your body adjusts to the cephalexin. If these effects are severe or last for more than two days, contact your doctor.

Cephalexin can also upset your stomach or give you stomach cramps. Usually these reactions can be relieved by taking the medication with crackers or a light snack. Contact your doctor if these problems continue.

In people who are sensitive to this drug, cephalexin can cause blood problems, such as bone marrow depression or a decrease in one of the blood clotting factors. Contact your doctor if you notice any unusual bleeding or easy bruising, get painful sores in the mouth or throat or develop chills and fever.

Long-term therapy with cephalexin may result in an overgrowth of other organisms in the body. Some symptoms of this condition are itching of the anus, sore mouth or tongue and vaginal infection. If you experience any of these symptoms, stop taking cephalexin and contact your doctor.

PRECAUTIONS

Before you start taking cephalexin, be sure to tell your doctor or pharmacist if you ever had an allergic reaction to any cephalosporin or to any form of penicillin. Your doctor also should be told if you have kidney disease or a history of allergy.

Some other medications, particularly gout medicines, should not be taken with cephalexin. Tell your doctor what other prescription or nonprescription drugs you are taking. If you do not know what drugs you are taking or what they were prescribed for, bring them in their labeled containers to your doctor or pharmacist.

Even if you feel better in a few days, take *all* of the medication prescribed for you by your doctor. Bacterial infections take several days to weeks to be cured completely. If you stop taking cephalexin, those bacteria still alive can multiply and cause a recurrence of the infection. However, if your symptoms do not improve within a few days or if they become worse, contact your doctor. It may be necessary to change your medication.

Be sure to tell your doctor if you are pregnant or are nursing an infant. Although problems with this medication have not been published, your doctor should have this information.

Diabetics should be aware that cephalexin can cause false results in some tests for urine sugar. Do not change your diet or the dosage of your diabetes medicine until you check with your doctor.

DOSAGE

Your doctor will determine how often you should take cephalexin and how much you should take at each dose. Follow the instructions on your prescription label, and ask your doctor or pharmacist to explain any part you do not understand.

Doses of cephalexin should be taken as far apart as possible during the day. If your doctor tells you to take it four times a day, take a dose every six hours. If you give cephalexin to a child, make sure he or she receives it around the clock, even if you have to wake the child for doses.

Cephalexin is best taken on an "empty stomach," one hour before meals or two hours after eating. However, if this medication upsets your stomach, you can take it with meals or a light snack.

Cephalexin comes in capsules, tablets and liquid form. The tablets and capsules should be taken with a full eight-ounce glass of water.

The liquid should be shaken thoroughly to mix the medication evenly before each dose is poured. Measure the prescribed dose with a dropper or a specially marked measuring spoon to be sure the dose is accurate. Contact your pharmacist if you have any questions about measuring the liquid.

If you forget to take a dose, take it as soon as you remember. Take any remaining doses for that day at evenly spaced intervals. If you still have symptoms of the infection after you have taken all of your medicine, contact your doctor.

STORAGE

When your doctor tells you to stop taking cephalexin, throw away any unused portion. Cephalexin may lose its effectiveness and should not be saved to treat another infection. Because this medication was prescribed for your particular condition, do not allow anyone else to take it.

Keep cephalexin in the container it came in. Keep liquid cephalexin in the refrigerator but *do not freeze it*. On the container, you will find an expiration date. Do not take the medication after that date. Throw it away, and if you need more, get a new supply. If you are not sure of the expiration date or have any questions about a refill, contact your pharmacist.

Keep this medication out of the reach of children.

Cephradine

(sef′ ra deen)

PRODUCT INFORMATION

Brand names: Anspor, Velosef

USES

Cephradine is a cephalosporin antibiotic that is similar to the penicillins in the way it eliminates bacteria. It is used to treat certain infections including pneumonia and infections of the throat, ears, urinary tract and skin.

Cephradine can be used for infections caused by bacteria that produce penicillinase (a substance that makes some penicillins ineffective). However, penicillins are generally preferred to cephradine in the treatment of "strep" infections and in the prevention of rheumatic fever.

UNDESIRED EFFECTS

Tell your doctor if you ever had an allergic reaction to any cephalosporin or to any form of penicillin. A serious reaction is more likely in a person with other allergies.

Allergic reactions, though rare, have occurred with cephradine. If you get a rash, hives or itching or have difficulty breathing, call your doctor or a hospital immediately. You may need emergency treatment.

Some allergic reactions, such as rash and itching all over your body, joint pains, fever or swollen glands, develop only after several days of therapy. Contact your doctor if you experience any of these effects.

The most common side effects of cephradine are diarrhea, nausea and vomiting. These effects usually are mild and tend to disappear as your body adjusts to the cephradine. If these effects are severe or last for more than two days, contact your doctor.

Cephradine can also upset your stomach or give you stomach cramps. Usually these reactions can be relieved by taking the medication with crackers or a light snack. Contact your doctor if these problems continue.

In people who are sensitive to this drug, cephradine can cause blood problems, such as bone marrow depression or a decrease in one of the blood clotting factors. Contact your doctor if you notice any unusual bleeding or easy bruising, get painful sores in the mouth or throat or develop chills and fever.

Long-term therapy with cephradine may result in an overgrowth of other organisms in the body. Some symptoms of this condition are itching of the anus, sore mouth or tongue and vaginal infection. If you are experiencing any of these symptoms, stop taking cephradine and contact your doctor.

PRECAUTIONS

Before you start taking cephradine, be sure to tell your doctor or pharmacist if you ever had an allergic reaction to any cephalosporin or to any form of penicillin. Your doctor also should be told if you have kidney disease or a history of allergy.

Some other medications, particularly gout medicines, should not be taken with cephradine. Tell your doctor what other prescription or nonprescription drugs you are taking. If you do not know what drugs you are taking or what they were prescribed for, bring them in their labeled containers to your doctor or pharmacist.

Even if you feel better in a few days, take *all* of the medication prescribed for you by your doctor. Bacterial infections take several days to weeks to be cured completely. If you stop taking cephradine, those bacteria still alive can multiply and cause a recurrence of the infection. However, if your symptoms do not improve within a few days or if they become worse, contact your doctor. It may be necessary to change your medication.

Be sure to tell your doctor if you are pregnant or are nursing an infant. Although problems with this medication have not been published, your doctor should have this information.

Diabetics should be aware that cephradine can cause false results in some tests for urine sugar. Do not change your diet or the dosage of your diabetes medicine until you check with your doctor.

DOSAGE

Your doctor will determine how often you should take cephradine and how much you should take at each dose. Follow the instructions on your prescription label, and ask your doctor or pharmacist to explain any part you do not understand.

Doses of cephradine should be taken as far apart as possible during the day. If your doctor tells you to take it four times a day, take a dose every six hours. If you give cephradine to a child, make sure he or she receives it around the clock, even if you have to wake the child for doses.

Cephradine is best taken on an "empty stomach," one hour before meals or two hours after eating. However, if this medication upsets your stomach, you can take it with meals or a light snack.

Cephradine comes in capsules and liquid form. The capsules should be taken with a full eight-ounce glass of water.

The liquid should be shaken thoroughly to mix the medication evenly before each dose is poured. Use a specially marked measuring spoon to be sure the dose is accurate. Contact your pharmacist if you have any questions about measuring the liquid.

If you forget to take a dose, take it as soon as you remember. Take any remaining doses for that day at evenly spaced intervals. If you still have symptoms of the infection after you have taken all of your medicine, contact your doctor.

STORAGE

When your doctor tells you to stop taking cephradine, throw away any unused portion. Cephradine may lose its effectiveness and should not be saved to treat another infection. Because this medication was prescribed for your particular condition, do not allow anyone else to take it.

Keep cephradine in the container it came in. Keep liquid cephradine in the refrigerator but *do not freeze it*. On the container, you will find an expiration date. Do not take the medication after that date. Throw it away and, if you need more, get a new supply. If you are not sure of the expiration date or have any questions about a refill, contact your pharmacist.

Keep this medication out of the reach of children.

ERYTHROMYCINS
(eh rith roe mye′ sins)

PRODUCT INFORMATION

Brand names of erythromycin: E-Mycin, ERYC, Ery-Tab, Erythromycin Base Filmtab, Ilotycin, Robimycin, RP-Mycin

Brand name of erythromycin estolate: Ilosone

Brand names of erythromycin ethylsuccinate: EES, E-Mycin E, EryPed, Pedia-mycin, Wyamycin E

Brand names of erythromycin stearate: Bristamycin, Erypar, Erythrocin Stearate, Ethril, Pfizer-E, SK-Erythromycin, Wintrocin, Wyamycin S

Brand name of a combination product containing erythromycin ethylsuccinate and sulfisoxazole: Pediazole

USES

The erythromycins are available in a number of chemical forms, including e-rythromycin (base), estolate, ethylsuccinate and stearate. All of these forms of erythromycin share the same uses, side effects and precautions except erythromycin *estolate,* which produces liver problems more frequently than other erythromycins (see Undesired Effects and Precautions).

The erythromycins are systemic antibiotics used to treat a wide variety of infections, including throat, ear and skin infections, pneumonia and diphtheria. They are considered good drugs to treat or prevent "strep" infections in people who have a history of rheumatic fever or rheumatic heart disease and who may be sensitive or allergic to penicillins.

The erythromycins are the preferred drugs to eliminate diphtheria-causing bacteria from people who show no signs of the disease but are infecting others. There is some evidence that erythromycins are effective against Legionnaires' disease.

UNDESIRED EFFECTS

A serious side effect of erythromycin *estolate* is inflammation of the liver. Symptoms include severe stomach pain, fever, unusual weakness or tiredness, yellowing of the eyes or skin (jaundice), dark or amber urine and pale stools. If you have any of these symptoms, stop taking the medication and contact your doctor. Liver problems occur more frequently in adults than in children and usually appear after 10 days. The other erythromycins rarely cause inflammation of the liver.

Allergic reactions, ranging from mild rash to hives to a sometimes fatal reaction, are rare. No one who ever had an allergic reaction to any erythromycin should take this medication again.

When you start taking an erythromycin, you may experience nausea, diarrhea or vomiting. These effects tend to go away as your body adjusts to the medicine. Contact your doctor if these problems get worse or last for more than two days.

If an erythromycin upsets your stomach, take the medicine with crackers or a light snack. Contact your doctor if you continue to have stomach upsets.

When you take any erythromycin for a long time, bacteria that it does not eliminate may multiply too rapidly. Some symptoms of this overgrowth are itching of the rectal and genital areas, sore mouth or tongue and vaginal infection. If you have any of these effects, contact your doctor.

PRECAUTIONS

Erythromycin *estolate* should not be taken by people with liver disease.

Before you take an erythromycin, tell your doctor if you have liver disease, if you ever had an allergic reaction to any erythromycin or if you have a history of drug allergy.

Tell your doctor what other prescription or nonprescription drugs you are taking. The erythromycins can affect the way your body responds to other medications, particularly carbamazepine (medicine for seizures), methylprednisolone, nadolol, theophylline and warfarin. If you do not know the names of the drugs or what they were prescribed for, bring them in their labeled containers to your doctor or pharmacist.

Food and beverages that contain acids may also affect the way you respond to these medicines. Do not take these medicines with, or immediately after, fruit juice or carbonated beverages.

Even if you feel better in a few days after taking an erythromycin, take *all* of the medicine your doctor has prescribed, particularly if you have a "strep" infection. Serious heart problems can result later if the infection is not completely cured. Bacterial infections take several days to weeks to be cured completely. However, if your symptoms do not improve in a few days or if they get worse, contact your doctor. It may be necessary to change your medication.

Although no problems have been published concerning the use of erythromycin by pregnant women or nursing mothers, tell your doctor if you are pregnant or nursing your baby. This information will help your doctor select the best treatment for you and your baby.

If you are taking erythromycin *estolate*, your doctor may want to test its effect on your liver function. *Keep all appointments with your doctor and the laboratory.*

DOSAGE

Erythromycin comes in capsules and chewable tablets, coated tablets and suspension form (liquid) to be taken by mouth.

Your doctor will determine how much erythromycin you should take at each dose and how often you should take it. Carefully follow the instructions on your prescription label, and ask your doctor or pharmacist to explain any part you do not understand.

Doses of the erythromycins should be taken as far apart as possible during the day. If your doctor instructs you to take this medication four times a day, take a dose every six hours. If you give an erythromycin to a child, be sure he or she receives it around the clock, even if you have to wake the child for doses.

The erythromycin tablets should be taken with a full eight-ounce glass of water. Some tablets are to be chewed or crushed before they are swallowed, and your prescription label will include instructions. Erythromycins are best taken on an "empty stomach," one hour before meals or two hours after eating. However, some brands of coated tablets and all forms of erythromycin *estolate* and *ethylsuccinate* can be taken without regard to meals. Ask your doctor or pharmacist if you have questions about taking your medication with food.

The liquid should be shaken well before use to mix the medication evenly in each dose. Measure the liquid in a specially marked dropper or measuring spoon to be sure the dose is accurate. (The drops for children are to be taken orally, even though they are in a dropper bottle.)

If you forget a dose, take it as soon as you remember it. However, if it is almost time for the next dose, you may either double it or space the missed dose and the next dose one to two hours apart. Then go back to your regular dosing schedule.

If you still have symptoms of the infection after you have taken all of the medicine prescribed, contact your doctor.

STORAGE

When your doctor tells you to stop taking the medicine, throw away any unused portion. This medication may lose its effectiveness and should not be saved to treat another infection. Because an erythromycin was prescribed for your particular condition, do not allow anyone else to take it.

Keep this medication in the container it came in. Store the tablets at room temperature. The liquid preparations should be kept in the refrigerator but *should not be frozen.* Check the container for an expiration date. Do not take this medication after the expiration date. Throw away the medication and, if you need more, get a new supply. Contact your pharmacist if you are not sure of the expiration date or need information about a refill.

Keep this medication out of the reach of children.

PENICILLINS

USES

Penicillins are antibiotic anti-infective drugs derived originally from a mold called *Penicillium*. Now, a variety of penicillins are produced by chemically modifying the basic chemical from this mold. All penicillins contain the same basic chemical structure, but this structure is modified to produce drugs with different antibacterial characteristics that may make one preferable to another in a given situation.

The penicillins may either kill organisms causing infection or merely slow them down to allow the body's defenses to take over. Some penicillins are active only against a few bacteria, while others are effective against a wide variety. For example, some bacteria produce a substance called penicillinase, which destroys some penicillins, making them ineffective in treating infections caused by those bacteria. Other penicillins, however, are not affected by penicillinase-producing bacteria.

Penicillins are not effective against viruses, fungi, rickettsiae or yeasts.

PRECAUTIONS

Before you begin to take penicillin, tell your doctor if you are taking any other medicine and about any chronic health problems you have.

Inform your doctor if you ever had an allergic reaction to any penicillin product.

Penicillins usually begin to clear up infections within a few days. If you do not begin to feel better after a few days or if your symptoms get worse, contact your doctor.

It is important to use all of the penicillin your doctor has prescribed, even though you begin to feel better before you finish all of the medication. If you stop taking the penicillin too soon, the bacteria still alive may cause a recurrence of the infection. This precaution is particularly important when treating "strep" infections, because heart problems can develop if the infection is not completely cured.

DOSAGE

Penicillins are available in several forms, including tablets, capsules, liquid and injection. Your doctor will choose the form best for you and will give you specific instructions on how to take it.

To kill or immobilize bacteria, it is necessary to keep a certain amount of penicillin in your bloodstream at all times. Therefore, try to take each dose on schedule.

It is best to take penicillins on an "empty stomach," either one hour before meals or two hours after meals.

The liquid should be shaken thoroughly each time a dose is poured. Ask your pharmacist for a special spoon so that you can measure the doses accurately.

STORAGE

If your doctor prescribes a liquid form of penicillin, be sure to read all of the labels on the bottle. Liquid penicillins must be stored in the refrigerator (not in the freezer).

Your prescription bottle will have an expiration date on it. Do not use liquid penicillin after that date—throw it away and get a fresh supply.

Amoxicillin
(a mox' i sill in)

PRODUCT INFORMATION

Brand names: Amoxil, Larotid, Polymox, Sumox, Trimox, Utimox, Wymox

USES

See the general statement titled Penicillins.

Amoxicillin is a penicillin-like antibiotic, very similar in chemical structure and activity to ampicillin. It is a broad-spectrum antibiotic, which means it eliminates a number of different bacteria. It is, however, inactivated by penicillinase and cannot be used against infections caused by penicillinase-producing bacteria.

Amoxicillin is used to treat certain types of pneumonia and infections of the ear, urinary tract and skin. Sometimes it is used to treat gonorrhea.

UNDESIRED EFFECTS

Tell your doctor if you ever had an allergic reaction to amoxicillin or any form of penicillin or cephalosporin.

Allergic reaction is the most common side effect of amoxicillin. Serious and sometimes fatal allergic reactions have occurred, although they are rare. A serious reaction is more likely in a person with other allergies but can happen even if you have taken penicillin before with no problems.

Call your doctor or a hospital immediately if you start wheezing or have difficulty breathing immediately after taking amoxicillin or if you develop a rash, itching or hives. You may need emergency treatment.

Amoxicillin can cause nausea and vomiting, irritation of the mouth and tongue and diarrhea. These effects tend to decrease or disappear as your body adjusts to amoxicillin. Nausea and vomiting may be relieved if you take amoxicillin with food or a light snack. If diarrhea is severe or lasts more than two days, contact your doctor.

Other allergic reactions may take longer to develop, such as rash and itching all over the body and in the mouth, fever, joint pain and swollen glands. Contact your doctor if you experience any of these effects.

In people sensitive to amoxicillin, it can cause blood problems such as bone marrow depression or a decrease in the number of blood platelets. If you experience unusual bleeding, easy bruising, painful sores of the mouth and throat or chills and fever, contact your doctor.

PRECAUTIONS

Before you start taking amoxicillin, be sure to tell your doctor if you ever had an allergic reaction to any form of penicillin, cephalosporin or amoxicillin. Your doctor should be informed if you have ever had any kind of allergy, including asthma and hay fever, and if you have kidney disease.

To help select the best treatment for your problem, tell your doctor what other medicines you are taking, particularly allopurinol and probenecid (gout medication) and tetracyclines (another type of antibiotic). Tetracyclines may decrease the ability of amoxicillin to kill bacteria rapidly. Probenecid can increase the effect of amoxicillin and the possibility of an allergic reaction. If you do not know what drugs you are taking or what they were prescribed for, take the labeled containers to your doctor or pharmacist.

Take *all* of the medication prescribed for you, even if you feel better a few days after you start taking amoxicillin. It takes several days or weeks to cure most infections. If you stop taking amoxicillin before you are cured, the bacteria still alive can multiply and cause a recurrence of the infection. However, if your symptoms do not improve within a few days or if they become worse, contact your doctor. It may be necessary to change the medication.

Although it is not known whether it is safe to take amoxicillin during pregnancy, pregnant women with gonorrhea may be given amoxicillin to protect the child from the infection. This medication can pass through the milk to a nursing infant, so your doctor should be told if you are nursing a baby.

DOSAGE

Your doctor has determined how often you should take amoxicillin and how much you should take at each dose. Follow the instructions on your prescription label carefully, and ask your doctor or pharmacist to explain any part you do not understand. Doses of this medication should be taken as far apart as possible during the day. If your doctor instructs you to take it three times a day, take a dose every eight hours. If you give amoxicillin to a child who sleeps more than eight hours a night, wake the child for the dose when it is scheduled.

Amoxicillin comes in capsules, chewable tablets, liquid form and pediatric drops to be taken orally. The container of liquid or pediatric drops should be shaken well before each use to mix the medication. Measure the dose with the bottle dropper or a specially marked measuring spoon from your pharmacist to be sure the dose is accurate.

The liquid dose may be added to infant formula, milk, fruit juice, water or ginger ale and then taken immediately.

Capsules should be taken with a full eight-ounce glass of water. Chewable tablets should be crushed or chewed thoroughly before swallowing.

If you forget to take a dose, take it as soon as you remember, and take the remaining doses for that day at evenly spaced intervals. Take all of this medication exactly as prescribed. If you still have symptoms of the infection after you have taken all of the medication, contact your doctor.

STORAGE

After your doctor tells you to stop taking amoxicillin, throw away any unused portion. Amoxicillin may lose its effectiveness so it should not be saved to treat another infection. Because this medication was prescribed for your particular condition, do not allow anyone else to take your amoxicillin.

Keep this medication in the container it came in. Keep liquid amoxicillin in the refrigerator, but do not freeze it. You will find an expiration date on the container. Do not take liquid amoxicillin after that date. Throw it away and, if you need more, get a new supply. If you are not sure of the expiration date or have any questions about a refill, contact your pharmacist.

Keep this medication out of the reach of children.

Ampicillin
(am pi sill' in)

PRODUCT INFORMATION

Brand names: Amcap, Amcill, D-Amp, Omnipen, Penamp, Pfizerpen A, Polycillin, Principen, SK-Ampicillin, Supen, Totacillin

USES

See the general statement titled Penicillins.

Ampicillin is a member of the penicillin family of antibiotics and has a broad spectrum of activity against bacteria. It eliminates a number of different bacteria including several of the bacteria against which penicillin G is not effective. Ampicillin is, however, inactivated by penicillinase and cannot be used against infections caused by penicillinase-producing bacteria.

Ampicillin is used to treat many kinds of infections caused by bacteria known to be sensitive to it. These infections include pneumonia and bronchitis and infections in the ears, urinary tract and skin. It is sometimes used as a single-dose treatment for gonorrhea.

UNDESIRED EFFECTS

Tell your doctor if you ever had an allergic reaction to ampicillin or any form of penicillin or cephalosporin.

Allergic reaction is the most common side effect of ampicillin. Serious and sometimes fatal allergic reactions have occurred, although they are rare, particularly when the medication is taken orally. A serious reaction is more likely in a person with other allergies but can happen even if you have taken penicillin before with no problems.

Call your doctor or a hospital immediately if you start wheezing or have difficulty breathing right after you take ampicillin or if you develop a rash, itching or hives. You may need emergency treatment.

Ampicillin can cause diarrhea, especially in children. It also can cause nausea, vomiting and irritation of the mouth and tongue. These effects tend to decrease or disappear as your body adjusts to ampicillin. If these effects are severe or last more than two days, contact your doctor.

Other allergic reactions may take longer to develop, such as rash and itching all over the body and in the mouth, joint pain, fever and swollen glands. Contact your doctor if you experience any of these effects.

In people sensitive to ampicillin, it can cause blood problems such as bone marrow depression or a decrease in the number of blood platelets. If you experience unusual bleeding, easy bruising, painful sores of the mouth and throat or chills and fever, contact your doctor.

PRECAUTIONS

Before you start taking ampicillin, be sure to tell your doctor if you ever had an allergic reaction to any form of penicillin, cephalosporin or ampicillin. Your doctor should be informed if you have kidney disease and if you ever had any kind of allergy, including asthma and hay fever.

Tell your doctor what other prescription and nonprescription drugs you are taking, particularly allopurinol and probenecid (medications for gout), birth-control pills, rifampin and the antibiotic tetracycline. Tetracyclines may decrease the ability of ampicillin to kill bacteria rapidly. If you do not know the names of the drugs you are taking or what they were prescribed for, bring the labeled containers to your doctor or pharmacist.

Take *all* of the medication prescribed for you, even if you feel better after taking it for a few days. Most infections take several days or weeks to cure. If you stop taking ampicillin before you are cured, bacteria still alive can multiply and cause a recurrence of the infection. However, if your symptoms do not improve within a few days or if they become worse, contact your doctor. It may be necessary to change the medication.

Diabetics should know that ampicillin can cause false results for some urine sugar tests. Check with your doctor before changing your diet or the dosage of your diabetes medicine.

Although it is not known whether it is safe to take ampicillin during pregnancy, pregnant women with gonorrhea and urinary tract infections may be given ampicillin to protect the child from the infections. This medication can pass through the milk to a nursing infant, so tell your doctor if you are breast-feeding a baby.

DOSAGE

Your doctor will determine how often you should take ampicillin and how much you should take at each dose. Carefully follow the instructions on your prescription label. Doses of this medication should be taken as far apart as possible during the day. If your doctor instructs you to take it four times a day, take a dose every six hours. If you give ampicillin to a child, make sure the child receives it around the clock, even if you must wake the child for doses.

Ampicillin is best taken on an "empty stomach," one hour before meals or two hours after meals. Ampicillin is available in capsules and in liquid form. Capsules should be taken with a full eight-ounce glass of water.

The container of liquid should be shaken thoroughly before each use to mix the medication evenly. Measure the dose with the bottle dropper or a specially marked measuring spoon from your pharmacist to ensure an accurate dose. The drops are to be taken orally.

If you forget to take a dose, take it as soon as you remember, and take the remaining doses for that day at evenly spaced intervals. Take all of this medication exactly as prescribed. If you still have symptoms of the infection after you have taken all of the medication, contact your doctor.

STORAGE

After your doctor tells you to stop taking ampicillin, throw away any unused portion. Ampicillin may lose its effectiveness so it should not be saved to treat another infection. Because this medication was prescribed for your particular condition, do not allow anyone else to take it.

Keep this medication in the container it came in. Keep liquid ampicillin in the refrigerator, but do not freeze it. You will find an expiration date on the container. Do not take the liquid after that date. Throw away the liquid and, if you need more, get a new supply. If you are not sure of the expiration date or have any questions about a refill, contact your pharmacist.

Keep this medication out of the reach of children.

Cloxacillin

(klox a sill' in)

PRODUCT INFORMATION

Brand names: Cloxapen, Tegopen

USES

See the general statement titled Penicillins.

Cloxacillin is a penicillinase-resistant penicillin. It is used principally to treat infections caused by bacteria that produce penicillinase. These infections include certain types of pneumonia, skin infections and systemic infections.

UNDESIRED EFFECTS

Tell your doctor if you ever had an allergic reaction to any form of penicillin, cephalosporin or cloxacillin.

Allergic reaction is the most common side effect of cloxacillin. Serious and sometimes fatal allergic reactions have occurred, although they are rare. A serious reaction is more likely in a person with other allergies but can occur even if you have taken penicillin before with no problems.

If you start wheezing or have difficulty breathing right after you take cloxacillin or if you develop a rash, hives or itching, call your doctor or a hospital immediately. You may need emergency treatment.

You may also experience diarrhea, nausea or vomiting after you take cloxacillin. These effects tend to decrease or disappear as your body adjusts to cloxacillin. If these effects are severe or last more than two days, contact your doctor.

Other allergic reactions, such as rash and itching all over the body, joint pain, fever and swollen glands, may take longer to develop. If cloxacillin causes any of these effects, contact your doctor.

In people sensitive to this drug, cloxacillin can cause blood problems such as bone marrow depression or a decrease in one of the blood clotting factors. If you experience unusual bleeding, easy bruising, painful sores of the mouth and throat or chills and fever, contact your doctor.

PRECAUTIONS

Before you start to take cloxacillin, be sure to tell your doctor if you ever had an allergic reaction to any form of penicillin, cephalosporin or cloxacillin. Your doctor also needs to know if you have kidney disease and if you ever had any kind of allergy, including hay fever, asthma, hives and rash.

Some other medications, such as probenecid (gout medicine), can increase the effect of cloxacillin and the possibility of allergic reaction. Tell your doctor what other prescription and nonprescription drugs you are taking, particularly probenecid and tetracyclines. Tetracyclines may decrease the ability of cloxacillin to kill bacteria rapidly. If you do not know the names of the drugs or what they were prescribed for, bring the labeled containers to your doctor or pharmacist. Do not start taking any other medication unless you have permission from your doctor.

Even if you feel better a few days after you start taking cloxacillin, continue to take it until you have used *all* that was prescribed. This precaution is particularly important if you have a "strep" infection. Serious heart problems can develop later if the infection is not completely cured. However, if your symptoms do not improve within a few days or if they become worse, contact your doctor. It may be necessary to change your medication.

During long-term therapy, your doctor may want laboratory tests, such as blood counts and tests for kidney and liver function, to determine your response to cloxacillin.

Although the safety of cloxacillin's use during pregnancy has not been established, a pregnant woman with an infection may be given cloxacillin. Your doctor must weigh the benefit against the possible risk. Your doctor should be told if you are nursing a baby, because cloxacillin passes through the milk to the baby.

DOSAGE

Cloxacillin comes in capsules and liquid to be taken by mouth.

Your doctor has determined how often you should take cloxacillin and how much you should take at each dose. Carefully follow the instructions on your prescription label, and ask your doctor or pharmacist to explain any part you do not understand.

Doses of cloxacillin should be taken as far apart as possible during the day. If your doctor instructs you to take it four times a day, take a dose every six hours.

If you give cloxacillin to a child, be sure the child receives it around the clock, even if you have to wake the child for doses.

Cloxacillin is best taken on an "empty stomach," one hour before meals or two hours after eating.

Capsules should be taken with a full eight-ounce glass of water. The container of liquid cloxacillin should be shaken thoroughly before use to mix the medication. Measure doses with a specially marked measuring spoon.

If you forget to take a dose, take it as soon as you remember and take the remaining doses for that day at evenly spaced intervals. However, if it is almost time for another dose, you may either double the next dose or space the missed dose and the next dose one or two hours apart. Then go back to your regular dosing schedule.

Take all of the cloxacillin exactly as prescribed. If you still have symptoms of the infection after you have taken all of the medication, contact your doctor.

STORAGE

After your doctor tells you to stop taking cloxacillin, throw away any unused portion. Cloxacillin may lose its effectiveness so it should not be saved to treat another infection. Because this medication was prescribed for your particular condition, do not allow anyone else to take your cloxacillin.

Keep the cloxacillin in the container it came in. Keep liquid cloxacillin in the refrigerator, but do not freeze it. Check the expiration date on the container, and do not take the liquid after that date. Throw away the liquid and, if you need more, get a new supply. If you are not sure of the expiration date or have any questions about a refill, contact your pharmacist.

Keep this medication out of the reach of children.

Dicloxacillin
(dye klox a sill′ in)

PRODUCT INFORMATION
Brand names: Dycill, Dynapen, Pathocil

USES
See the general statement titled Penicillins.

Dicloxacillin is a penicillinase-resistant penicillin. Dicloxacillin is used principally to treat infections caused by bacteria that produce penicillinase. These infections include certain types of pneumonia, skin infections and systemic infections.

UNDESIRED EFFECTS
Tell your doctor if you ever had an allergic reaction to any form of penicillin, cephalosporin or dicloxacillin.

Allergic reaction is the most common side effect of dicloxacillin. Serious and sometimes fatal allergic reactions have occurred, although they are rare. A serious reaction is more likely in a person with other allergies but can occur even if you have taken penicillin before with no problems.

Call your doctor or a hospital immediately if you start wheezing or have difficulty breathing right after you take dicloxacillin or if you develop a rash, hives or itching. You may need emergency treatment.

You may also experience diarrhea, nausea or vomiting with dicloxacillin. These effects tend to decrease or disappear as your body adjusts to dicloxacillin. If these effects are severe or last more than two days, call your doctor.

Other allergic reactions may take longer to develop. If, after you have been taking dicloxacillin for several days, you get a rash and itching all over your body, joint pain, fever or swollen glands, contact your doctor.

In people sensitive to this drug, dicloxacillin can cause blood problems such as bone marrow depression or a decrease in one of the blood clotting factors. If you experience unusual bleeding, easy bruising, painful sores of the mouth and throat or chills and fever, contact your doctor.

PRECAUTIONS

Before you start to take dicloxacillin, be sure to tell your doctor if you ever had an allergic reaction to any form of penicillin, cephalosporin or dicloxacillin. To select the right medicine for you, your doctor needs to know if you have kidney disease or a history of allergies, including hay fever, asthma, rash and hives.

Some other medications, including probenecid (gout medicine), can increase the effect of dicloxacillin and the possibility of allergic reaction. Tell your doctor what other prescription and nonprescription drugs you are taking, particularly tetracyclines and probenecid. Tetracyclines may decrease the ability of dicloxacillin to kill bacteria rapidly. If you do not know the names of the drugs or what they were prescribed for, bring them in their labeled containers to your doctor or pharmacist. Do not start to take any other medication unless you have permission from your doctor.

Do not stop taking dicloxacillin even if you feel better a few days after taking it. It is important that you take *all* of this medication as prescribed if your infection is to be cured. This precaution is particularly important if you have a "strep" infection. Serious heart problems can develop later if the infection is not completely cured. However, if your symptoms do not improve within a few days or if they become worse, contact your doctor. It may be necessary to change your medication.

During long-term therapy, your doctor may want tests, such as blood counts and tests for kidney and liver function, to determine your response to dicloxacillin.

Dicloxacillin passes through the milk to a breast-fed infant, so tell your doctor if you are nursing a baby. The safe use of dicloxacillin during pregnancy has not been established, but it may be necessary to give it to a pregnant woman with an infection to protect the baby from the infection.

DOSAGE

Dicloxacillin is available in capsules and liquid form. Your doctor will determine how often you should take dicloxacillin and how much you should take at each dose.

Carefully follow the instructions on your prescription label, and ask your doctor or pharmacist to explain any part you do not understand.

Doses of dicloxacillin should be taken as far apart as possible during the day. If your doctor instructs you to take it four times a day, take a dose every six hours. If you give dicloxacillin to a child, be sure the child receives it around the clock, even if you have to wake the child for doses.

Dicloxacillin should be taken on an "empty stomach," one hour before or two hours after meals, unless your doctor gives you different directions.

Dicloxacillin capsules should be taken with a full eight-ounce glass of water. The liquid should be shaken thoroughly before each use to mix the medication. Measure doses with a specially marked measuring spoon.

If you forget to take a dose, take it as soon as you remember and take the remaining doses for that day at evenly spaced intervals. However, if it is almost time for another dose, you may either double the next dose or space the missed dose and the next dose one or two hours apart. Then go back to your regular dosing schedule.

Take all of this medication exactly as prescribed. If you still have symptoms of the infection after you have taken all of the dicloxacillin, contact your doctor.

STORAGE

After your doctor tells you to stop taking dicloxacillin, throw away any unused portion. Dicloxacillin may lose its effectiveness so it should not be saved to treat another infection. Because this medication was prescribed for your particular condition, do not allow anyone else to take your dicloxacillin.

Keep this medication in the container it came in. Keep liquid dicloxacillin in the refrigerator, but do not freeze it. Check the expiration date on the container, and do not take the liquid after that date. Throw away the liquid and, if you need more, get a new supply. Contact your pharmacist if you are not sure of the expiration date or have questions about a refill.

Keep this medication out of the reach of children.

Penicillin G
(pen i sill' in)

PRODUCT INFORMATION
Brand names: Bicillin, Pentids, Pfizerpen G, Wycillin

USES
See the general statement titled Penicillins.

Penicillin G is the most effective penicillin in eliminating bacteria sensitive to penicillin. However, penicillin G is inactivated by penicillinase (a substance produced by bacteria) and cannot be used against infections caused by penicillinase-producing bacteria.

Penicillin G often is the preferred drug in treating certain types of pneumonia, scarlet fever and throat and skin infections. Penicillin G is also used to prevent a recurrence of rheumatic fever. The injectable form of penicillin G is used to treat gonorrhea and syphilis.

UNDESIRED EFFECTS

Tell your doctor if you ever had an allergic reaction to penicillin G or any form of penicillin or cephalosporin.

Allergic reaction is the most common side effect of penicillin G. Serious and sometimes fatal allergic reactions have occurred, although they are rare, particularly when the medication is taken orally. A serious reaction is more likely in a person with other allergies, but it can occur even if you have taken penicillin before with no problems.

If you get a rash, hives or itching, start wheezing or have difficulty breathing right after you take penicillin G, call your doctor or a hospital immediately. You may need emergency treatment.

Penicillin G can cause diarrhea, nausea and vomiting, which tend to decrease or disappear as your body adjusts to penicillin G. If these effects are severe or last more than two days, call your doctor. In some people, penicillin G may cause the tongue to darken or discolor. This effect is temporary and will go away when you stop taking the medication.

Other allergic reactions may develop only after several days of therapy. If you experience a rash and itching all over your body, joint pains, fever or swollen glands, contact your doctor.

In people sensitive to this drug, penicillin G can cause blood problems, such as bone marrow depression or a decrease in one of the blood clotting factors. Some symptoms of such problems are unusual bleeding, easy bruising, painful sores of the mouth and throat and chills and fever. Contact your doctor if you have any of these symptoms.

PRECAUTIONS

Before you start taking penicillin G, be sure to tell your doctor if you ever had an allergic reaction to any form of penicillin, cephalosporin or penicillin G. Your doctor also should be told if you have kidney disease or a history of any kind of allergy, including asthma, hay fever, rash and hives.

Some other medications should not be taken with penicillin G because they increase or decrease its effect. Probenecid (gout medicine) can increase the effect of penicillin G and, therefore, the possibility of allergic reaction. Tetracyclines may decrease the ability of penicillin G to kill bacteria rapidly. Tell your doctor what other prescription and nonprescription drugs you are taking including colestipol, neomycin and medicine for arthritis. If you do not know the names of these drugs or what they were prescribed for, bring them in their labeled containers to your doctor or pharmacist. Do not start to take any other medications, including nonprescription medications, without asking your doctor.

Food and beverages that contain acid may affect the way you respond to penicillin G. Do not take this medication with or immediately after drinking fruit juices or carbonated beverages.

Take *all* of the medication prescribed for you by your doctor, even if you feel better a few days after you start taking it. This precaution is particularly important if you have a "strep" infection. Serious heart problems can result later if the infection is not completely cured.

To help select the treatment best for you, tell your doctor if you are pregnant or are nursing a baby. Penicillin G is passed to an unborn child and to a nursing infant through the mother's milk.

If you have diabetes, penicillin G can cause false results in some tests of sugar in urine. Do not change your diet or the dosage of your diabetes medicine unless you check first with your doctor.

If you get an injection of penicillin G in the doctor's office, stay there for 30 minutes after the injection so you will be close to medical care if you should have a serious allergic reaction to the injection.

DOSAGE
Penicillin G comes in tablets, liquid and a form for injection.

Your doctor will determine how often you should take penicillin G and how much you should take at each dose. Carefully follow the instructions on your prescription label and ask your doctor or pharmacist to explain any part you do not understand. Doses of this medication should be taken as far apart as possible during the day. If your doctor tells you to take it three times a day, take a dose every eight hours. If you give penicillin G to a child, make sure the child receives it around the clock, even if you must wake the child for doses.

Penicillin G should be taken on an "empty stomach," one hour before meals or two hours after eating. The tablets should be taken with a full eight-ounce glass of water. The container of liquid should be shaken thoroughly before each use to mix the medication evenly. Use a specially marked measuring spoon to be sure of an accurate dose.

If you forget to take a dose, take it as soon as you remember. However, if it is almost time for your next dose, you may either double the next dose or space the missed dose and the next dose one to two hours apart. Then go back to your regular dosing schedule. Take all of the penicillin G as prescribed. If you still have symptoms of the infection after you have taken all of the medication, contact your doctor.

STORAGE
After your doctor tells you to stop taking penicillin G, throw away any unused portion of it. Penicillin G may lose its effectiveness so it should not be saved to treat another infection. Because this medication was prescribed for your particular condition, do not allow anyone else to take your penicillin G.

Keep this medication in the container it came in. Keep liquid penicillin G in the refrigerator but do not freeze it. You will find an expiration date on the container. Do not take the medication after that date. Throw it away and, if you need more, get a new supply. If you are not sure of the expiration date or have any questions about a refill, contact your pharmacist.

Keep this medication out of the reach of children.

Penicillin V
(pen i sill′ in)

PRODUCT INFORMATION
Brand names: Beepen VK, Betapen VK, Ledercillin-VK, Pen-Vee K, Pfizerpen VK, Robicillin VK, Uticillin VK, V-Cillin K, Veetids and others

USES
See the general statement titled Penicillins.

Penicillin V is absorbed into the bloodstream faster than penicillin G. However, penicillin V is inactivated by penicillinase (a substance produced by bacteria) and cannot be used against infections caused by penicillinase-producing bacteria.

Penicillin V is used to treat mild to moderate infections of the throat, ears and skin and scarlet fever. Penicillin V is also given to prevent a recurrence of rheumatic fever. Because penicillin V is available in oral form only, it is not used for serious infections that require rapid elimination of bacteria.

UNDESIRED EFFECTS
Tell your doctor if you ever had an allergic reaction to any form of penicillin, cephalosporin or penicillin V.

Allergic reaction is the most common side effect of penicillin V. Serious and sometimes fatal allergic reactions have occurred, although they are rare. A serious reaction is more likely in a person with other allergies but can occur even if you have taken penicillin before with no problems.

If you get a rash, hives or itching, start wheezing or have difficulty breathing right after you take penicillin V, call your doctor or a hospital immediately. You may need emergency treatment.

Penicillin V also can cause diarrhea, nausea and vomiting. These effects tend to decrease or disappear as your body adjusts to penicillin V. Call your doctor if these effects are severe or last more than two days. Penicillin V may cause the tongue to darken or discolor. This effect is temporary and will go away when you stop taking the medication.

Other allergic reactions, such as rash and itching all over the body, joint pains, fever or swollen glands, may develop only after several days of therapy. If you experience any of these effects, contact your doctor.

In people sensitive to this drug, penicillin V can cause blood problems, such as bone marrow depression or a decrease in one of the blood clotting factors. Symptoms of such problems are unusual bleeding, easy bruising, painful sores of the mouth and throat and chills and fever. Contact your doctor if you have any of these symptoms.

PRECAUTIONS
Before you start taking penicillin V, be sure to tell your doctor if you ever had an allergic reaction to any form of penicillin, cephalosporin or penicillin V. Your

doctor should be told if you have kidney disease or a history of any kind of allergy, including asthma, hay fever, rash or hives.

Some medications, such as probenecid (gout medicine), can increase the effect of this drug and, therefore, the possibility of allergic reactions. Tell your doctor what other prescription and nonprescription drugs you are taking, particularly neomycin, colestipol, arthritis medication and tetracyclines. Tetracyclines may decrease the ability of penicillin V to kill bacteria rapidly. Because penicillin V may decrease the effectiveness of birth-control pills, use another method of birth control while taking penicillin V. If you do not know the names of the drugs you are taking or what they are prescribed for, bring them in their labeled containers to your doctor or pharmacist. Do not start taking any other medications while you are taking penicillin V without permission from your doctor.

Even if you feel better a few days after you start taking penicillin V, take *all* of the medication prescribed for you by your doctor. This is particularly important if you have a "strep" infection. Serious heart problems can result later if the infection is not completely cured.

To select the best treatment for you and your baby, tell your doctor if you are pregnant or are breast-feeding a baby. Penicillin V is passed by the mother to her unborn child and to a nursing infant through the mother's milk.

DOSAGE

Your doctor will determine how often you should take penicillin V and how much you should take at each dose. Follow the instructions on your prescription label and ask your doctor or pharmacist to explain any part you do not understand.

Doses of this medication should be taken as far apart as possible during the day. If your doctor tells you to take it four times a day, take a dose every six hours. If you give penicillin V to a child, make sure the child receives it around the clock, even if you have to wake the child for doses.

Penicillin V should be taken on an "empty stomach," one hour before meals or two hours after eating. It comes in tablets and in liquid form. The tablets should be taken with a full eight-ounce glass of water.

The liquid should be shaken thoroughly before each use to mix the medication evenly. Use a specially marked measuring spoon to be sure of an accurate dose.

If you forget to take a dose, take it as soon as you remember. However, if it is almost time for your next dose, you may either double the next dose or space the missed dose and the next dose one to two hours apart. Then go back to your regular dosing schedule.

Take *all* of the penicillin V exactly as prescribed. If you still have symptoms of the infection after you have taken all of the medication, contact your doctor.

STORAGE

After your doctor tells you to stop taking penicillin V, throw away any unused portion. Penicillin V may lose its effectiveness so it should not be saved to treat another infection. Because this medication was prescribed for your particular condition, do not allow anyone else to take your penicillin V.

Keep this medication in the container it came in. Keep liquid penicillin V in the refrigerator, but do not freeze it. You will find an expiration date on the container. Do not take the medication after that date. Throw it away and, if you need more, get a new supply. If you are not sure of the expiration date or have any questions about a refill, contact your pharmacist.

Keep this medication out of the reach of children.

TETRACYCLINES

Tetracyclines are systemic antibiotics commonly described as "broad spectrum" antibiotics. Broad spectrum implies that these drugs have a wide range of activity—that is, they fight infections caused by a variety of different organisms. These drugs are effective in treatment of infections caused by many kinds of bacteria and by some other less common organisms, such as spirochetes and rickettsiae. Tetracyclines are not effective in the treatment of viral infections such as the common cold.

As with many other groups of drugs, there are many tetracyclines, all slight chemical modifications of the basic drug. The names of the individual drugs are demeclocycline, doxycycline, methacycline, minocycline, oxytetracycline and tetracycline.

The tetracyclines are the preferred drugs for treatment of only a few infections—and those infections are relatively uncommon. Because of their broad activity, however, tetracyclines often are used when the infecting organism is unknown. Also, a person may be allergic to the antibiotic that is preferred for treatment of a particular infection (e.g., gonorrhea); a tetracycline might be prescribed as the alternative or "second best" drug.

Tetracyclines are most commonly prescribed for the treatment of infections of the respiratory tract such as pneumonia, tonsillitis, inflammation of the pharynx, bronchitis or whooping cough or for ear or sinus infections. Tetracyclines also are used to treat urinary tract infections, eye infections and infected abscesses, carbuncles, burns or wounds. They may be used following surgery if infection is present. Tetracyclines also are prescribed for the treatment of infections of the digestive tract, such as certain kinds of dysentery and salmonella infections. Rickettsial infections such as Rocky Mountain spotted fever, typhus and Q fever and some infections caused by spirochetal organisms such as yaws and syphilis also are susceptible to treatment with tetracyclines. Tetracycline has also been used investigationally to treat Lyme disease. In addition, tetracyclines have been used in the treatment of acne. Many other infections may be treated successfully if a test of the infecting organism shows that a tetracycline will be effective.

Some organisms become resistant to the tetracyclines, and the drugs no longer effectively prevent their growth. Because the tetracyclines have been used so much over the past several years, many of the more common microorganisms have become resistant to them. The usefulness of these drugs in treatment of "staph" infections, "strep throat" and pneumonia, for example, is limited for this reason.

Demeclocycline
(dem e kloe sye' kleen)

PRODUCT INFORMATION
Brand name: Declomycin

USES
See the general statement titled Tetracyclines.

Demeclocycline is one of the tetracycline antibiotics. It is used to treat a variety of infections, including pneumonia, bladder infections, Rocky Mountain spotted fever and acne. It can be used to treat infections caused by bacteria resistant to penicillin, but it is never the preferred drug for any "staph" infection.

Although penicillin is the preferred drug for treatment of "strep" infections and for the prevention of rheumatic fever, demeclocycline may be used to treat these infections in people who are sensitive or allergic to penicillin if demeclocycline is known to be effective against the infecting strain of "strep."

Demeclocycline has been used investigationally as a diuretic for water retention caused by certain medical conditions.

UNDESIRED EFFECTS
Allergic reactions, ranging from rash and hives to serious and sometimes fatal reactions, can occur especially in persons who have had allergic reactions to other tetracyclines.

Demeclocycline may cause loss of appetite, diarrhea, nausea or vomiting. These effects tend to decrease or disappear as you continue to take it and as your body adjusts to the medication. Contact your doctor if they are severe or last more than two days.

If demeclocycline upsets your stomach or gives you abdominal or stomach cramps, take it with crackers or a light snack (no dairy products). Contact your doctor if these problems continue. This medication may cause a "furry" darkening or black discoloration of the tongue. This change is temporary and will go away when you stop taking demeclocycline.

Demeclocycline can allow an overgrowth of organisms that are not sensitive to tetracyclines. Some symptoms of overgrowth are itching of the rectal or genital area, sore mouth or tongue and vaginal infection. If you have any of these effects, contact your doctor.

Demeclocycline frequently makes people more sensitive to sunlight than they are normally. Limit the amount of time you spend in sunlight. When you are in sunlight, cover your body with clothing, use a sunscreen preparation on exposed parts of your body and wear sunglasses. If you become severely sunburned, contact your doctor or pharmacist. This sensitivity to sunlight may continue for two weeks to several months after you stop taking demeclocycline.

Demeclocycline can have bad effects on the kidneys when taken over a period of time. If you notice excessive thirst, unusual weakness or tiredness or a great increase in the frequency of urination or the amount of urine, stop taking the medication and contact your doctor.

Long-term therapy with demeclocycline may cause blood problems such as bone marrow depression or a decrease in one of the blood clotting factors. Contact your doctor if you notice any unusual bleeding or easy bruising, get painful sores in your mouth or throat or develop chills and fever.

PRECAUTIONS

Demeclocycline should not be taken by children under eight years of age, women past the first trimester of pregnancy or nursing mothers. It can discolor and pit the enamel of children's teeth. Demeclocycline is passed to the unborn child and to the nursing infant and can cause tooth discoloration and retard bone growth. Women who become pregnant while taking demeclocycline should contact their doctors.

Before you start taking demeclocycline, tell your doctor if you have ever had an allergic reaction to any of the tetracyclines. Tell your doctor if you have diabetes insipidus, kidney disease, liver disease or a history of allergies.

Certain medications and foods affect the way your body responds to demeclocycline and should not be taken at the same time. Take demeclocycline one hour before or two hours after you consume antacids, diarrhea medicine, laxatives, baking soda and dairy products such as milk, cheese and ice cream. Do not take iron preparations (many vitamin combinations contain iron) within two hours of the time at which you take demeclocycline.

Tell your doctor what other prescription or nonprescription drugs you are taking, especially antacids, anticoagulants (blood thinners), iron, laxatives or penicillins. If you do not know the names of the drugs or what they were prescribed for, bring them in their labeled containers to your doctor or pharmacist. While you are taking demeclocycline, do not start to take any other medications, including nonprescription medication, unless you first contact your doctor or pharmacist.

Even if you feel better a few days after you start taking demeclocycline, take *all* of the medicine your doctor has prescribed. This is particularly important if you have a "strep" infection. Serious heart problems can result later if the infection is not completely cured. Bacterial infections take several days to weeks to be cured completely. However, if your symptoms do not improve or if they become worse within a few days after you start taking demeclocycline, contact your doctor. It may be necessary to change your medication.

Laboratory tests for liver or kidney function or blood tests may be ordered by your doctor. *Be sure to keep all appointments with your doctor and at the laboratory.*

If you have diabetes, demeclocycline can cause false results in some tests for sugar in your urine. Do not change your diet or the dosage of your diabetes medicine unless you first check with your doctor.

Demeclocycline also can affect the results of several blood tests that indicate kidney and liver function, as well as some urine tests. If you have such tests done, be sure the person responsible for reporting the results knows you have been taking demeclocycline.

Before having surgery with a general anesthetic, including dental surgery, tell the doctor or dentist in charge that you are taking demeclocycline.

DOSAGE

Your doctor has determined how often you should take demeclocycline and how much you should take at each dose. Follow the instructions on your prescription label and ask your doctor or pharmacist to explain any part of the instructions you do not understand.

Doses of demeclocycline should be taken as far apart as possible during the day. If your doctor tells you to take it four times a day, take a dose every six hours *around the clock*.

Demeclocycline comes in capsules and tablets. It should be taken on an "empty stomach," one hour before meals or two hours after eating. However, if this medication upsets your stomach, take it with crackers or a light snack (no dairy products).

The capsules and tablets should be taken with a full eight-ounce glass of water.

If you forget to take a dose, take it as soon as you remember. Then take any remaining doses for that day at evenly spaced intervals. Take all of the demeclocycline exactly as prescribed. If you still have symptoms of the infection after you have taken all of it, contact your doctor.

STORAGE

When your doctor tells you to stop taking demeclocycline, throw away any unused portion of it. This drug may lose its effectiveness over a period of time and should not be saved to treat another infection. Old demeclocycline can cause harmful effects. Do not allow anyone else to take your demeclocycline. It was prescribed for your particular condition.

Keep this medication in the container it came in, tightly closed and in a dry place. Keep it out of the reach of children.

Doxycycline
(dox i sye′ kleen)

PRODUCT INFORMATION
Brand names: Doxy-C, Doxy-Caps, Doxychel, Doxy-Lemmon, Doxy-Tabs, Vibramycin, Vibra-Tabs

USES
See the general statement titled Tetracyclines.

Doxycycline is one of the tetracycline antibiotics. It is used to treat a variety of infections, including pneumonia, Rocky Mountain spotted fever, acne and venereal disease. Doxycycline can be used to treat infections caused by bacteria resistant to penicillin, but it is never the preferred drug for any "staph" infection.

Although penicillin is the preferred drug for "strep" infections and for the prevention of rheumatic fever, doxycycline may be used to treat these infections in people sensitive or allergic to penicillin if doxycycline is known to be effective against the infecting strain of "strep."

Doxycycline has been used investigationally to prevent traveler's diarrhea.

Doxycycline can be given to people with kidney disease with less risk of additional kidney problems than if other tetracyclines are taken. Food does not interfere with the absorption of doxycycline.

UNDESIRED EFFECTS

Allergic reactions, ranging from rash and hives to serious and sometimes fatal reactions, can occur especially in persons who have had an allergic reaction to other tetracyclines.

Doxycycline may cause loss of appetite, diarrhea, nausea or vomiting. These effects tend to decrease or disappear as you continue to take it and as your body adjusts to the medication. Contact your doctor if they are severe or last more than two days.

If doxycycline upsets your stomach or gives you abdominal or stomach cramps, take it with meals, milk or carbonated beverage. Contact your doctor if these problems continue. This medication may cause a "furry" darkening or black discoloration of the tongue. This change is temporary and will go away when you stop taking doxycycline.

Doxycycline can allow an overgrowth of organisms that are not sensitive to tetracyclines. If you experience symptoms of overgrowth such as itching of the rectal or genital area, sore mouth or tongue or vaginal infection, contact your doctor.

Doxycycline can make some people more sensitive to sunlight than they are normally. Limit the amount of time you spend in sunlight until you know how you will react, especially if you sunburn easily. When you are in sunlight, keep your body covered with clothing and use a sunscreen preparation on the exposed parts of your body. If you become severely sunburned, contact your doctor or pharmacist.

Long-term therapy with doxycycline may cause blood problems such as bone marrow depression or a decrease in one of the blood clotting factors. Contact your doctor if you notice any unusual bleeding or easy bruising, get painful sores in your mouth or throat or develop chills and fever.

PRECAUTIONS

Doxycycline should not be taken by children under eight years of age, women past the first trimester of pregnancy or nursing mothers. It can discolor and pit the enamel of children's teeth. Doxycycline is passed to the unborn child and to the nursing infant and can cause tooth discoloration and retard bone growth. Women who become pregnant while taking doxycycline should contact their doctors.

Be sure to tell your doctor if you have ever had an allergic reaction to any of the tetracyclines. Tell your doctor if you have liver disease or a history of allergies before you start taking doxycycline.

Certain medications can affect the way your body responds to doxycycline and should not be taken at the same time. Take doxycycline one hour before or two hours after you consume antacids, laxatives or baking soda. Do not take iron preparations (many vitamin combinations contain iron) within two hours of the time you take doxycycline.

To help select the treatment best for you, tell your doctor what other prescription or nonprescription drugs you are taking, particularly antacids, anticoagulants (blood thinners), barbiturates (e.g., phenobarbital), carbamazepine, iron, laxatives, penicillins, and phenytoin (medicine for seizures). If you do not know the names of the drugs or what they were prescribed for, bring them in their labeled containers to your doctor or pharmacist.

Take *all* of the medicine your doctor has prescribed, even if you feel better a few days after you start taking doxycycline. This is particularly important if you have a "strep" infection. Serious heart problems can result later if the infection is not completely cured. Bacterial infections take several days to weeks to be cured completely. However, if your symptoms do not improve within a few days after you start to take doxycycline or if they become worse, contact your doctor. It may be necessary to change your medication.

If you have diabetes, doxycycline can cause false results in some tests for sugar in your urine. Do not change your diet or the dosage of your diabetes medicine unless you first check with your doctor.

Doxycycline also can affect the results of several blood tests that check liver function, as well as some urine tests. If you have such tests done, be sure the person responsible for reporting the results knows you have been taking doxycycline.

Your doctor may ask you to have laboratory tests to measure the effect of this drug on your blood and liver or kidney function. *Be certain to keep all appointments with your doctor and at the laboratory.*

DOSAGE

Doxycycline comes in capsules, tablets, oral suspension (liquid) and a form for injection. It is usually taken once or twice a day. Your doctor will determine how often you should take this medication and how much you should take at each dose. Follow the instructions on your prescription label and ask your doctor or pharmacist to explain any part you do not understand.

The container of liquid doxycycline should be shaken before each use to mix the medication evenly. Use a specially marked measuring spoon to ensure an accurate dose.

If you forget to take a dose, take it as soon as you remember. Then take any remaining doses for that day at evenly spaced intervals. Take *all* of this medication exactly as prescribed. If you still have symptoms of the infection after you have taken all of your doxycycline, contact your doctor.

STORAGE

When your doctor tells you to stop taking doxycycline, throw away any unused portion of your prescription. This drug may lose its effectiveness over a period of time and should not be saved to treat another infection. Old doxycycline can cause harmful effects. Because this medication was prescribed for your particular condition, do not allow anyone else to take your doxycycline.

Keep this medication in the container it came in and store it at room temperature. You will find an expiration date on the container of liquid. Do not take the liquid after that date. Throw it away and, if you need more, get a new supply. If you are not sure of the expiration date or have any questions about a refill, contact your pharmacist.

Keep this medication out of the reach of children.

Methacycline
(meth a sye′ kleen)

PRODUCT INFORMATION
Brand name: Rondomycin

USES
See the general statement titled Tetracyclines.

Methacycline is one of the tetracycline antibiotics. It is used to treat pneumonia, bladder infections, Rocky Mountain spotted fever and acne. Although it can be used against infections caused by bacteria resistant to penicillin, it is never the preferred drug for any kind of "staph" infection.

Penicillin is the preferred drug for "strep" infections and for the prevention of rheumatic fever, but methacycline may be used to treat these infections in people sensitive or allergic to penicillin if methacycline is known to be effective against the infecting strain of "strep."

UNDESIRED EFFECTS
Allergic reactions, ranging from rash and hives to serious and sometimes fatal reactions, can occur especially in persons who have had allergic reactions to other tetracyclines.

When you start to take methacycline, it may cause loss of appetite, diarrhea, nausea and vomiting. These effects tend to decrease or disappear as you continue to take it and as your body adjusts to the medication. Contact your doctor if they are severe or last more than two days.

If methacycline upsets your stomach or gives you abdominal or stomach cramps, take it with crackers or a light snack (no dairy products). Contact your doctor if these problems continue. Some people get a "furry" darkening or black discoloration of the tongue when they take methacycline. This change is temporary and will go away when you stop taking the medication.

An overgrowth of organisms that are not sensitive to tetracyclines can occur during methacycline therapy. Some symptoms of overgrowth are itching of the rectal or genital area, sore mouth or tongue and vaginal infection. If you experience any of these effects, contact your doctor.

Some people who take methacycline may be more sensitive to sunlight than they are normally. Limit the amount of time you spend in the sunlight until you know how you will react, particularly if you tend to sunburn easily. If you become severely sunburned, contact your doctor or pharmacist.

Long-term therapy with methacycline may cause blood problems such as bone marrow depression or a decrease in one of the blood clotting factors. Contact your doctor if you notice any unusual bleeding or easy bruising, get painful sores in the mouth or throat or develop chills or fever.

PRECAUTIONS

Methacycline should not be taken by children under eight years of age, women past the first trimester of pregnancy and nursing mothers. It can discolor and pit the enamel of children's teeth. Methacycline is passed to the unborn child and to the nursing infant and can cause tooth discoloration and retard bone growth. Women who become pregnant while taking methacycline should contact their doctors.

Before you start taking methacycline, tell your doctor if you have ever had an allergic reaction to another tetracycline. Tell your doctor if you have kidney disease, liver disease or a history of allergies.

Certain medications and foods affect the way your body responds to methacycline and should not be taken at the same time. Take methacycline one hour before or two hours after you consume antacids, laxatives, baking soda and dairy products such as milk, cheese and ice cream. Do not take iron preparations (many vitamin combinations contain iron) within two hours of the time you take methacycline.

Tell your doctor what other prescription or nonprescription drugs you are taking, particularly antacids, anticoagulants (blood thinners), iron, laxatives and penicillins. If you do not know the names of the drugs or what they were prescribed for, bring them in their labeled containers to your doctor or pharmacist. Before you start to take any other medications while you are taking methacycline, contact your doctor or pharmacist.

Even if you feel better a few days after you start to take methacycline, take *all* of the medicine your doctor has prescribed. This is particularly important if you have a "strep" infection. Serious heart problems can result later if a "strep" infection is not completely cured. Bacterial infections take several days to weeks to be cured completely. However, if your symptoms do not improve within a few days or become worse, contact your doctor. It may be necessary to change your medication.

Your doctor may order laboratory tests for liver or kidney function or blood tests. *Be sure to keep all appointments with your doctor and at the laboratory.*

If you have diabetes, methacycline can cause false results in some tests for sugar in your urine. Do not change your diet or the dosage of your diabetes medicine unless you first check with your doctor.

Methacycline can also affect the results of several tests for liver or kidney function. If you have such tests done, be sure the person responsible for reporting the results knows you have been taking methacycline.

If you need surgery with a general anesthetic, including dental surgery, be sure the doctor or dentist knows you are taking methacycline.

DOSAGE

Your doctor has determined how often you should take methacycline and how much you should take at each dose. Follow the instructions on your prescription label and ask your doctor or pharmacist to explain any part of the instructions you do not understand.

Doses of methacycline should be taken as far apart as possible during the day. If your doctor instructs you to take it four times a day, take a dose every six hours *around the clock*.

Methacycline is best taken on an "empty stomach," one hour before meals or two hours after eating. However, if this medication upsets your stomach, take it with crackers or a light snack (no dairy products).

Methacycline comes in capsules. The capsules should be taken with a full eight-ounce glass of water.

Take all of the methacycline exactly as prescribed. If you still have symptoms of the infection after you have taken all of it, contact your doctor.

If you forget to take a dose, take it as soon as you remember and then take any remaining doses for that day at evenly spaced intervals.

STORAGE

When your doctor tells you to stop taking methacycline, throw away any unused portion of it. This drug may lose its effectiveness over a period of time and should not be saved to treat another infection. Old methacycline can cause harmful effects. Because this medication was prescribed for your particular condition, do not allow anyone else to take your methacycline.

Keep this medication in the container it came in and store it, tightly closed, at room temperature. Keep it out of the reach of children.

Minocycline
(mi noe sye' kleen)

PRODUCT INFORMATION
Brand name: Minocin

USES
Refer to the general statement titled Tetracyclines.

Minocycline is one of the tetracycline antibiotics used to treat a variety of infections, including pneumonia, bladder infections, acne (particularly acne that does not respond to tetracycline) and venereal disease. Minocycline is effective in eliminating the bacteria that cause meningitis from the nose and throat of "carriers" who spread the disease. However, it may cause dizziness and unsteadiness. Minocycline is not used to treat meningitis.

Penicillin is the preferred drug for "strep" infections and the prevention of rheumatic fever, but minocycline may be used to treat these infections in people sensitive or allergic to penicillin if minocycline is known to be effective against the infecting strain of "strep."

Food does not interfere with the absorption of minocycline.

UNDESIRED EFFECTS

Allergic reactions, ranging from rash and hives to serious and sometimes fatal reactions, can occur especially in persons who have had an allergic reaction to other tetracyclines.

Minocycline may cause loss of appetite, diarrhea, nausea or vomiting. These effects tend to decrease or disappear as you continue to take minocycline and as your body adjusts to it. Contact your doctor if they are severe or last more than two days.

If minocycline upsets your stomach or gives you abdominal or stomach cramps, take it with meals, milk or carbonated beverage. Contact your doctor if these problems continue. This medication may cause "furry" darkening or black discoloration of the tongue. This change is temporary and will go away when you stop taking the medication.

Minocycline therapy can allow an overgrowth of organisms that are not sensitive to tetracyclines. Contact your doctor if you experience symptoms of overgrowth such as itching of the rectal and genital areas, sore mouth or tongue or vaginal infection.

All tetracyclines can make people more sensitive to sunlight than they are normally. This effect is rare with minocycline, but limit the amount of time you spend in sunlight until you know how you will react, especially if you sunburn easily. If you become severely sunburned, contact your doctor or pharmacist.

Minocycline can make you dizzy, lightheaded or unsteady. Do not drive a car or operate dangerous machinery until you know how you react to this medicine.

Long-term therapy with minocycline may cause blood problems such as bone marrow depression or a decrease in one of the blood clotting factors. Contact your doctor if you notice any unusual bleeding or easy bruising, get painful sores in your mouth or throat or develop chills and fever.

PRECAUTIONS

Minocycline should not be taken by children under eight years of age, women past the first trimester of pregnancy and nursing mothers. It can discolor and pit the enamel of children's teeth. Minocycline is passed to the unborn child and to the nursing infant and can cause tooth discoloration and retard bone growth. Women who become pregnant while taking minocycline should contact their doctors.

Before you start to take minocycline, tell your doctor if you have ever had an allergic reaction to any other tetracycline. Tell your doctor if you have liver disease or a history of allergies.

Certain medications can affect the way your body responds to minocycline and should not be taken at the same time. Take minocycline one hour before or two hours after consuming antacids, laxatives or baking soda. Do not take iron preparations (many vitamin combinations contain iron) within two hours of the time you take minocycline.

To help select the best treatment for you, tell your doctor what other prescription or nonprescription drugs you are taking, especially antacids, anticoagulants (blood thinners), iron, laxatives, and penicillins. If you do not know the names of the drugs or what they were prescribed for, bring them in their labeled containers to your doctor or pharmacist. Do not start to take any other medications, including nonprescription medications, while you are taking minocycline unless you first check with your doctor or pharmacist.

Even if you feel better in a few days, take *all* of the medication your doctor has prescribed. This is particularly important if you have a "strep" infection. Serious heart problems can result later if the infection is not completely cured. Bacterial infections take several days to weeks to be cured completely. However, if your symptoms do not improve within a few days after you start to take minocycline or if they become worse, contact your doctor. It may be necessary to change your medication.

If you plan to have surgery with a general anesthetic, including dental surgery, be sure to tell the doctor or dentist that you are taking minocycline.

Your doctor may ask you to have laboratory tests performed to measure the effect of this drug on your blood or on your kidney function. *Be sure to keep all appointments with your doctor or at the laboratory.*

If you have diabetes, minocycline can cause false results in some tests for sugar in your urine. Do not change your diet or the dosage of your diabetes medicine unless you first check with your doctor.

Minocycline will also affect the results of several blood tests for kidney and liver function. If you have such tests, be sure the person responsible for reporting the results knows you have been taking minocycline.

DOSAGE

Minocycline comes in capsules, tablets, oral suspension (liquid) and in a form for injection. It is usually taken twice a day. Your doctor will determine how often you should take this medication and how much you should take at each dose. Carefully follow the instructions on your prescription label and ask your doctor or pharmacist to explain any part you do not understand.

The container of liquid minocycline should be shaken thoroughly before each use to mix the medication evenly. Use a specially marked measuring spoon to ensure an accurate dose of the liquid or syrup.

If you forget to take a dose, take it as soon as you remember. Then take any remaining doses for that day at evenly spaced intervals. Take *all* of the minocycline exactly as prescribed. If you still have symptoms of the infection after you have taken it all, contact your doctor.

STORAGE

When your doctor tells you to stop taking minocycline, throw away any unused portion of it. This drug may lose its effectiveness over a period of time and should not be saved to treat another infection. Old minocycline can cause harmful effects. Because this medication was prescribed for your particular condition, do not allow anyone else to take your minocycline.

Keep this medication in the container it came in and store it, tightly closed, at room temperature. Keep it out of the reach of children.

Oxytetracycline
(ox i te tra sye′ kleen)

PRODUCT INFORMATION
Brand names: E.P. Mycin, Terramycin, Uri-Tet
Brand name of a combination product containing nystatin: Terrastatin
Brand name of a combination product containing phenazopyridine and sulfa-methizole: Urobiotic

USES
Refer to the general statement titled Tetracyclines.
Oxytetracycline is one of the tetracycline antibiotics. It is used to treat pneumonia, bladder infections, Rocky Mountain spotted fever and acne. Oxytetracycline can be used in infections caused by bacteria resistant to penicillin, but it is never the preferred drug for any kind of "staph" infection.

Although penicillin is the preferred drug for "strep" infections and for the prevention of rheumatic fever, oxytetracycline may be used to treat these infections in people who are sensitive or allergic to penicillin if oxytetracycline is known to be effective against the infecting strain of "strep."

UNDESIRED EFFECTS
Allergic reactions, ranging from rash and hives to serious and sometimes fatal reactions, can occur especially in people who have had allergic reactions to other tetracyclines.

Oxytetracycline may cause loss of appetite, diarrhea, nausea and vomiting. These problems tend to decrease or disappear as you continue to take it and as your body adjusts to the medication. Contact your doctor if they are severe or last more than two days.

If this medication upsets your stomach or gives you abdominal or stomach cramps, take it with crackers or a light snack (no dairy products). Contact your doctor if these problems continue. Some people get a "furry" darkening or black discoloration of the tongue when they take oxytetracycline. These changes are temporary and will go away when you stop taking the medication.

Oxytetracycline can allow an overgrowth of organisms that are not sensitive to tetracyclines. Some symptoms of overgrowth are itching of the rectal or genital area, sore mouth or tongue and vaginal infection. Contact your doctor if you have any of these problems.

Some people who take oxytetracycline may become more sensitive to sunlight than they are normally. Limit the amount of time you spend in sunlight until you know how you will react, particularly if you tend to burn easily. While in sunlight, keep your body covered with clothing, use a sunscreen preparation on the exposed parts of your body and wear sunglasses. Contact your doctor or pharmacist if you become severely sunburned.

Long-term therapy with oxytetracycline may cause blood problems such as bone marrow depression or a decrease in one of the blood clotting factors. If you notice any unusual bleeding or easy bruising, get painful sores in the mouth or throat or develop chills and fever, contact your doctor.

PRECAUTIONS

Oxytetracycline should not be taken by children under eight years of age, women past the first trimester of pregnancy or nursing mothers. It can discolor and pit the enamel of children's teeth. Oxytetracycline given to an expectant mother or nursing mother is passed to the baby and can discolor the teeth and retard bone growth. Women who become pregnant while taking oxytetracycline should contact their doctors.

Before you start taking oxytetracycline, tell your doctor if you have ever had an allergic reaction to another tetracycline. To help select the best treatment for you, tell your doctor if you have kidney disease, liver disease or a history of drug allergy.

Certain medications and foods affect the way your body responds to oxytetracycline and should not be taken at the same time. Take oxytetracycline one hour before or two hours after you consume antacids, laxatives, baking soda and dairy products such as milk, cheese and ice cream. Do not take iron preparations (many vitamin combinations contain iron) within two hours of the time you take oxytetracycline.

Tell your doctor what other prescription or nonprescription drugs you are taking, especially antacids, anticoagulants (blood thinners), iron, laxatives and penicillin. If you do not know the names of the drugs or what they were prescribed for, bring them in their labeled containers to your doctor or pharmacist.

Take *all* of the medicine your doctor has prescribed, even if you feel better after you have taken oxytetracycline for a few days. This is particularly important if you have a "strep" infection. Serious heart problems can result later if a "strep" infection is not completely cured. Bacterial infections take several days to weeks to be cured completely. However, if your symptoms do not improve within a few days after you start taking oxytetracycline or if they become worse, contact your doctor. It may be necessary to change your medication.

Laboratory tests of your blood or for kidney or liver function may be ordered by your doctor. *Be certain to keep all appointments with your doctor or at the laboratory.*

If you have diabetes, oxytetracycline can cause false results in some tests for sugar in your urine. Do not change your diet or the dosage of your diabetes medicine unless you first check with your doctor.

Oxytetracycline can also affect the results of several tests for liver and kidney function. If you have such tests done, be sure the person responsible for reporting the results knows you have been taking oxytetracycline.

Before you have surgery with a general anesthetic, including dental surgery, tell the doctor or dentist that you are taking oxytetracycline.

DOSAGE

Your doctor will determine how often you should take oxytetracycline and how much to take at each dose. Carefully follow the instructions on your prescription label and ask your doctor or pharmacist to explain any part of the instructions you do not understand.

Doses of oxytetracycline should be taken as far apart as possible during the day. If your doctor instructs you to take it four times a day, take a dose every six hours *around the clock.*

Oxytetracycline should be taken on an "empty stomach." However, if this medication upsets your stomach, take it with crackers or a light snack (no dairy products).

Oxytetracycline comes in capsules, tablets and an injectable form. The capsules and tablets should be taken with a full eight-ounce glass of water.

If you forget to take a dose, take it as soon as you remember it. Take any remaining doses for that day at evenly space intervals.

Take *all* of the oxytetracycline exactly as prescribed. If you still have symptoms of the infection after you have taken all of it, contact your doctor.

STORAGE

When your doctor tells you to stop taking oxytetracycline, throw away any unused portion of it. This drug may lose its effectiveness over a period of time and should not be saved to treat another infection. Old oxytetracycline can cause serious problems. Because this medication was prescribed for your particular condition, do not allow anyone else to take your oxytetracycline.

Keep this medication in the container it came in and store it, tightly closed, at room temperature. Keep it out of the reach of children.

Tetracycline
(te tra sye′ kleen)

PRODUCT INFORMATION

Brand names: Achromycin V, Brodspec, Cyclopar, Panmycin, Robitet, SK-Tetracycline, Sumycin, Tetracyn, Tetralan and others

USES

See the general statement titled Tetracyclines.

Tetracycline is used to treat a variety of infections, including pneumonia, bladder infections, Rocky Mountain spotted fever, venereal disease and acne. Although tetracycline can be used against infections caused by bacteria resistant to penicillin, tetracycline is never the preferred drug for any kind of "staph" infection.

Penicillin is the preferred drug for treatment of "strep" infections and for the prevention of rheumatic fever, but tetracycline may be used to treat these infections in people sensitive or allergic to penicillin if tetracycline is known to be effective against the infecting strain of "strep."

Tetracycline has been used investigationally to treat Lyme disease, a spirochetal infection usually transmitted by ticks and characterized by a raised red skin rash.

UNDESIRED EFFECTS

Allergic reactions, ranging from rash and hives to serious and sometimes fatal reactions, can occur especially in people who have had allergic reactions to other tetracyclines.

Tetracycline may cause loss of appetite, diarrhea, nausea and vomiting. These effects tend to decrease or disappear as you continue to take it and as your body adjusts to the medication. Contact your doctor if they are severe or last more than two days.

If tetracycline upsets your stomach or gives you abdominal or stomach cramps, take it with crackers or a light snack (no dairy products). Contact your doctor if these problems continue. Some people get a "furry" darkening or black discoloration of the tongue when they take this medication. These changes are temporary and will go away when you stop taking tetracycline.

An overgrowth of organisms that are not sensitive to this drug can occur during tetracycline therapy. Some symptoms of overgrowth are itching of the rectal or genital area, sore mouth or tongue and vaginal infection. Contact your doctor if you have any of these problems.

Some people who take tetracycline may become more sensitive to sunlight than they are normally. When you start taking this medicine, limit the amount of time you spend in sunlight until you know how you will react, particularly if you tend to burn easily. When you are in sunlight, keep your body covered with clothing, use a sunscreen preparation on the exposed parts of your body and wear sunglasses. If you get severely sunburned, contact your doctor or pharmacist.

Long-term therapy with tetracycline may cause blood problems such as bone marrow depression or a decrease in one of the blood clotting factors. Contact your doctor if you notice unusual bleeding or easy bruising, get painful sores in the mouth or throat or develop chills or fever. Problems of liver or kidney function can also occur.

PRECAUTIONS

Tetracycline should not be taken by children under eight years of age, women past the first trimester of pregnancy or nursing mothers. It can discolor and pit the enamel of children's teeth. Tetracycline is passed to the unborn child or nursing baby and can discolor teeth and retard bone growth. Women who become pregnant while taking tetracycline should contact their doctors.

Before you start taking tetracycline, tell your doctor if you have ever had an allergic reaction to another tetracycline. Tell your doctor if you have kidney disease, liver disease or a history of drug allergy.

Certain medications and foods affect the way your body responds to tetracycline and should not be taken at the same time. Take tetracycline one hour before or two hours after you consume antacids, laxatives, baking soda and dairy products such as milk, cheese and ice cream. Do not take iron preparations (many vitamin combinations contain iron) within two hours of the time you take tetracycline.

Tell your doctor what other prescription or nonprescription drugs you are taking, especially antacids, anticoagulants (blood thinners), birth-control pills, iron, laxatives, lithium and penicillin. If you do not know the names of the drugs or what they were prescribed for, bring them in their labeled containers to your doctor or pharmacist. Before you start taking any other medications while you are taking tetracycline, contact your doctor or pharmacist.

There have been two case reports, one of a pregnancy and one of breakthrough bleeding, in women taking birth-control pills containing estrogen while taking tetracycline. Although it is uncertain whether tetracycline reduces the effectiveness of birth-control pills, it may be advisable to use another method of birth control while taking tetracycline. Discuss this with your doctor.

Even if you feel better a few days after you start taking tetracycline, take *all* of the medicine your doctor has prescribed. This is particularly important if you have a "strep" infection. Serious heart problems can result later if a "strep" infection is not completely cured. Bacterial infections take several days to weeks to be cured completely. However, if your symptoms do not improve within a few days or become worse, contact your doctor. It may be necessary to change your medication.

Your doctor may order laboratory tests for liver or kidney function or blood tests. *Keep all appointments with your doctor or at the laboratory.*

If you have diabetes, tetracycline can cause false results in some tests for sugar in your urine. Do not change your diet or the dosage of your diabetes medicine unless you first check with your doctor.

Tetracycline can also affect the results of several tests for liver and kidney function. If you have such tests done, be sure the person responsible for reporting the results knows that you have been taking tetracycline.

Before surgery with a general anesthetic, including dental surgery, tell the doctor or dentist that you are taking tetracycline.

DOSAGE

Your doctor has determined how often you should take tetracycline and how much to take at each dose. Carefully follow the instructions on your prescription label and ask your doctor or pharmacist to explain any part you do not understand.

Doses of tetracycline should be taken as far apart as possible during the day. If your doctor instructs you to take it four times a day, take a dose every six hours *around the clock.*

Tetracycline should be taken on an "empty stomach," one hour before meals or two hours after eating. However, if this medication upsets your stomach, take it with crackers or a light snack (no dairy products).

Tetracycline comes in capsules, tablets, liquid form and in a form for injection. The capsules and tablets should be taken with a full eight-ounce glass of water. The container of liquid should be shaken thoroughly before each use to mix the medication evenly. Use a specially marked measuring spoon to ensure an accurate dose.

If you forget to take a dose, take it as soon as you remember it. Take any remaining doses for that day at evenly spaced intervals.

STORAGE

When your doctor tells you to stop taking tetracycline, throw away any unused portion of it. This drug may lose its effectiveness over a period of time and should not be saved to treat another infection. Taking old tetracycline can be dangerous. Because this medication was prescribed for your particular condition, do not allow anyone else to take your tetracycline.

Keep this medication in the container it came in and store it, tightly closed, at room temperature. Keep it out of the reach of children.

OTHER ANTI-INFECTIVES

Ketoconazole
(kee toe koe′ na zole)

PRODUCT INFORMATION
Brand name: Nizoral

USES

Ketoconazole is an antifungal agent that is used to treat systemic fungal infections and infections of the mouth, especially candida (thrush), skin (ringworm) and lungs.

UNDESIRED EFFECTS

The most common side effects of ketoconazole are nausea and vomiting. These effects are usually mild and go away as your body adjusts to the drug. Take ketoconazole with food if you experience stomach problems. Contact your doctor if stomach upset persists; it may be necessary to decrease your dose.

Although very rare, ketoconazole can cause severe and sometimes fatal liver damage. Signs of liver damage include yellowing of the skin and eyes, nausea, vomiting, fatigue, dark urine and pale stools. If you experience any of these effects, stop taking this medication and contact your doctor.

PRECAUTIONS

Certain medications, particularly antacids, belladonna, cimetidine, glycopyrrolate, isopropamide, propantheline, and ranitidine, decrease stomach acidity and reduce the absorption of ketoconazole. Tell your doctor what prescription and nonprescription drugs you are taking. If you do not know the names of the drugs or what they were prescribed for, take them in their labeled containers to your doctor or pharmacist.

Tell your doctor if you have a history of liver disease. Your doctor may order liver function tests to be sure ketoconazole is not having a bad effect on your liver. *Keep all appointments with your doctor and the laboratory.*

It may take up to 12 months to cure an infection. Do not stop taking ketoconazole until your doctor tells you to do so. If you still have signs of infection after taking all of the medication, contact your doctor.

If you have a fungal skin infection, good health habits can help cure the infection and prevent reinfection. Wash all towels, sheets and clothing each day after they have come in contact with the infected area.

Tell your doctor if you are pregnant, plan to become pregnant or are breast-feeding a baby. It is not known if it is safe to take ketoconazole during pregnancy or while breast-feeding.

DOSAGE
Ketoconazole comes in tablets to be taken by mouth. Follow the instructions on your prescription label and ask your doctor or pharmacist to explain any part you do not understand. Ketoconazole is usually taken once a day. It is important that you do not miss any doses of this medicine. Take it at the same time as you perform some other regular activity such as brushing your teeth. Take ketoconazole with food if it upsets your stomach.

If you are taking an antacid, belladonna, cimetidine, glycopyrrolate, isopropamide, propantheline or ranitidine, take it at least two hours after you take ketoconazole.

If you are taking ketoconazole once a day and forget a dose, take it as soon as you remember. If it is almost time for the next dose, take the missed dose and the scheduled dose 12 hours apart. Then return to your regular schedule.

STORAGE
Keep this medication in the container it came in. Keep it out of the reach of children.

Neomycin
(nee oh mye' sin)

PRODUCT INFORMATION
Brand names: Mycifradin, Neobiotic

USES
Neomycin is an antibiotic used to treat bowel infections and to help lessen the symptoms of coma resulting from liver disease. It may be given before bowel surgery to help prevent infection.

UNDESIRED EFFECTS
The most common side effects of neomycin taken orally are nausea, vomiting and irritation or soreness of the mouth or rectal area. These effects tend to lessen or disappear as your body adjusts to the medication. If they continue or become bothersome, contact your doctor.

Neomycin may also cause diarrhea, excessive gas and light-colored, frothy, fatty-appearing stools. If these effects are severe or last more than a few days, contact your doctor.

Although serious side effects with oral neomycin are rare, long-term therapy can result in damage to the inner ear or kidneys. Symptoms of ear problems are loss of hearing; a ringing, buzzing sound or feeling of fullness in the ears; clumsiness; and dizziness or unsteadiness. Stop taking the medicine if you develop any of these symptoms, and contact your doctor immediately.

If you are very thirsty or experience a greatly decreased frequency of urination or amount of urine, neomycin may be causing kidney problems. Stop taking the medication and contact your doctor.

Allergic reactions, including rash, hives, itching and fever, occur occasionally. If you have had an allergic reaction to neomycin or to similar antibiotics (amikacin, gentamicin, kanamycin, streptomycin and tobramycin), do not take neomycin.

As in therapy with other antibiotics, neomycin may result in an overgrowth of organisms against which it is not effective. Contact your doctor if you have itching in the rectal or genital area, sore mouth or tongue or vaginal infection.

PRECAUTIONS

Before you start taking neomycin, tell your doctor if you have any of the following medical problems: obstruction of the bowel, eighth-cranial-nerve disease (loss of hearing and/or balance), kidney disease, myasthenia gravis, Parkinson's disease or ulcers of the bowels.

Certain medications should not be taken with neomycin because they increase the possibility of serious ear and kidney problems. These drugs are the other amino-glycosides (amikacin, gentamicin, kanamycin, streptomycin and tobramycin), capreomycin, cephaloridine, cephalothin, cisplatin, polymyxin, vancomycin, viomy-cin and the diuretics (water pills) ethacrynic acid and furosemide.

Tell your doctor what other prescription and nonprescription drugs you are taking, including the above-mentioned drugs, anticoagulants (blood thinners) and digoxin. It may be necessary to adjust the doses of the medications so they will work well together. If you do not know the names of the drugs you are taking or what they were prescribed for, bring them in their labeled containers to your doctor or pharma-cist.

Even if you feel better a few days after you start taking neomycin, take *all* of the medicine your doctor has prescribed. A bacterial infection must be completely cured before you stop taking the medicine. This can require several days to weeks. However, if symptoms do not improve in a few days or get worse, contact your doctor. It may be necessary to change your medication or adjust the dosage.

Tell your doctor if you are pregnant or nursing a baby. This information will help your doctor select the best treatment for you and your baby. Safe use of neomycin for pregnant women has not been established.

Your doctor will want to check regularly the way you are responding to neomycin and may want tests for hearing and kidney function. *Be sure to keep all your appointments with your doctor and at the laboratory.*

Before having surgery with a general anesthetic, including dental surgery, tell the doctor or dentist that you are taking neomycin.

DOSAGE

Your doctor will determine how much neomycin you should take and how often you should take it. Carefully follow the instructions on your prescription label, and ask your doctor or pharmacist to explain any part of the instructions you do not understand. If you are taking neomycin to prepare for surgery, follow your doctor's instructions for diet and the instructions on your prescription label for when to take each dose. Your doctor may instruct you to take a dose every hour for four doses and then every four hours for five more doses.

Neomycin comes in tablets and in liquid form. It can be taken without regard to meals. The tablets should be taken with a full eight-ounce glass of water. The liquid should be measured with a specially marked measuring spoon to be sure of an accurate dose.

If you forget to take a dose, take it as soon as you remember it and take the remaining doses for that day at evenly spaced intervals. If you remember a missed dose when it is close to the time for another, you may double the dose. If you are taking neomycin every hour in preparation for surgery and forget to take a dose, you may take the doses 30 minutes apart until you are back on schedule. Call your doctor if you have questions about your dosage schedule or difficulty following it.

If you have been taking neomycin for an infection and still have symptoms after you have taken all of the neomycin prescribed, contact your doctor.

STORAGE

When your doctor tells you to stop taking neomycin, throw away any unused portion. Neomycin may lose its effectiveness so it should not be saved to treat another infection. Do not allow anyone else to take your neomycin.

Keep neomycin in the container it came in, and store it at room temperature. Keep neomycin out of the reach of children.

Quinine

(kwye' nine)

PRODUCT INFORMATION

Brand names: QM-260, Quinamm, Quine, Quinidan, Quinite, Quiphile

USES

Quinine is used to treat malaria. It also is used to keep leg muscles from cramping, especially during the sleeping hours.

UNDESIRED EFFECTS

Quinine may cause nausea, stomach pain, vomiting and diarrhea. These side effects can be avoided by taking quinine with food or milk. If these problems continue, contact your doctor.

If you experience skin rash, a sudden increase in temperature to over 100°F, sore throat, flushed skin and excessive sweating, stop taking this drug and call your doctor.

Other side effects that require prompt medical attention include changes in vision, dizziness, changes in hearing, ringing in the ear, yellow discoloration of the skin or eyes, heart palpitations, bruising of the skin and bleeding of the gums. Contact your doctor immediately if any of these side effects occur.

PRECAUTIONS

Tell your doctor if you ever had a bad reaction to quinine or quinidine (a medicine for irregular heartbeat) or if you have G6PD deficiency (an inherited blood disease).

Quinine can affect the way your body responds to certain drugs, especially digoxin, digitoxin and anticoagulants (blood thinners). Tell your doctor or pharmacist what other prescription and nonprescription drugs you are taking, especially acetazolamide, antacids, quinidine and sodium bicarbonate. If you do not know the names of your medications or what they were prescribed for, bring them in their labeled containers to your doctor or pharmacist. Do not take any other drugs, including nonprescription drugs, until you tell your doctor or pharmacist that you are taking quinine. Keep in touch with your doctor while taking quinine.

Tell your doctor if you are pregnant or are breast-feeding a baby. Contact your doctor immediately if you become pregnant while taking quinine. Quinine is harmful to unborn children and should not be taken during pregnancy.

Quinine is passed to a breast-fed baby through the milk and may be harmful.

DOSAGE

Quinine comes in capsules and tablets. Quinine should be taken with meals, a snack or a glass of milk so that it does not upset your stomach. Since quinine is very bitter, do not chew a tablet or capsule before swallowing it.

Your doctor has determined how often you should take this medication and how much you should take at each dose. Follow the instructions on your prescription label carefully, and ask your doctor or pharmacist to explain any part you do not understand.

To be effective in treating malaria, quinine must be taken every day. If you are taking quinine for malaria, try to take the medication at the same time you do some other regular activity, such as brushing your teeth in the morning or eating dinner.

If you forget to take a dose, take the missed dose as soon as you remember it. Take any remaining doses for that day at evenly spaced intervals. If you take only one dose a day and remember a missed dose the next day when you are scheduled to take another dose, omit the missed dose and take only the regularly scheduled one. *Do not take a double dose.*

STORAGE

Keep this medication in the container it came in; store the container at room temperature and out of direct sunlight. If the tablets or capsules turn brown in color, throw them away and obtain a new prescription. The brown color indicates that the medication has been exposed to too much sunlight, which will make it ineffective. Keep this medication out of the reach of children.

Tuberculosis

Tuberculosis (TB) is an infection caused by mycobacteria (a type of bacteria). In the past, people with tuberculosis were isolated from the rest of society, usually in a sanatorium, to prevent the spread of TB. Now that health professionals have learned more about the causes and methods of transmitting infections (particularly TB infections), sanatoriums for tuberculosis patients have all but disappeared. Patients with TB rarely need to be hospitalized for treatment.

The bacteria that cause TB can be present in the body for months or years without causing any health problems. This stage is called *asymptomatic*. If not treated, the bacteria can become active and cause *clinical* disease symptoms. Active disease usually involves the lungs (pulmonary tuberculosis) but can also appear in other parts of the body.

The aims of treatment are to prevent the disease from advancing and to prevent it from spreading to other people.

The TB bacteria in the body can be in a harmless resting state or can be active and growing. To cure TB, treatment must be aimed at both resting and active bacteria. Tests must be done to determine the drugs that will be effective in destroying the bacteria.

Usually, more than one drug is used to treat TB and prevent relapse, especially if the disease is active. Tuberculosis can almost always be cured by drug therapy but, as with the use of any anti-infective drug, high enough doses must be taken for a long enough time. The time it takes to cure a patient is variable and depends on many factors, such as age and the duration of the disease before therapy was begun. Usually, 18 to 24 months of treatment are required.

Household members and personal contacts of a person with active TB must also receive drug therapy. The assumption is that they probably have some inactive TB bacteria in their bodies and should be treated to prevent the inactive bacteria from becoming active. A positive sputum test, positive TB skin test or abnormal chest X-ray confirms the need for preventive drug therapy.

Any child younger than six years of age who has a positive TB skin test should receive preventive drugs for one year, even if it is not known whether the child has been in contact with someone with an active TB infection.

Specimens (sputum and blood) must be taken before and during therapy to determine which drugs to use and to check the patient's response to the drugs.

It is very important to take the drugs exactly as prescribed for as long as prescribed.

ANTITUBERCULOSIS DRUGS

Ethambutol

(e tham′ byoo tole)

PRODUCT INFORMATION
Brand name: Myambutol

USES
Ethambutol is an anti-infective drug used to treat tuberculosis (TB). It is prescribed with one or two other antituberculosis drugs to make the infected person unable to spread the infection to others. Usually, ethambutol must be taken for six months to a year to eradicate the infection completely.

UNDESIRED EFFECTS
Ethambutol may cause nausea, vomiting or loss of appetite when you start to take it. These effects tend to disappear as your body adjusts to it. If they continue over a long period or bother you greatly, contact your doctor.

The most serious side effect of ethambutol is inflammation of an important nerve in the eye, the optic nerve. *This problem requires immediate medical attention.* Contact your doctor if you experience blurred vision, loss of vision, eye pain or inability to see the colors red and green.

Other undesired effects of ethambutol are allergic reactions, nerve problems and gout. Contact your doctor if you develop a rash or itching (allergic reaction); numbness, tingling, burning pain or weakness in the hands or feet (nerve problems); chills; or swelling of the big toe, ankle or knee or hot skin over these joints (gout).

PRECAUTIONS
Because ethambutol can worsen certain medical problems, be sure to tell your doctor if you have gout, kidney disease, damage to nerves in the eyes or any eye problems such as cataracts or recurring inflammations.

It is important that you take this medicine exactly as prescribed and continue to take it until your doctor tells you to stop. Even if you begin to feel better, your TB may not be completely cured. It may take a year or more to cure it.

If your symptoms do not improve within three weeks, contact your doctor. It may be necessary to change your medication.

While you are taking ethambutol, your doctor may want to examine your eyes every three to six months to make sure the medicine is not having a bad effect on them. You may also have periodic blood counts and tests for kidney and liver functions. *Keep all appointments with your doctor and at the laboratory.*

Before you start to take ethambutol, tell your doctor if you are pregnant or intend to become pregnant while you are taking this medicine. Although safe use of ethambutol in pregnant women has not definitely been established, a combination of isoniazid and ethambutol usually is used to treat TB in pregnant women.

DOSAGE

Ethambutol comes in tablets. It is usually taken once a day in the morning. Your doctor will determine when you should take this medicine and how much you should take at each dose. Carefully follow the instructions on your prescription label, and ask your doctor or pharmacist to explain any part of the instructions you do not understand.

It is important that you do not miss any doses of this medicine. It may help you to remember to take your daily dose if you take ethambutol at the same time as you perform some other regular activity, such as brushing your teeth or eating your breakfast. Ethambutol can be taken with food if this drug upsets your stomach.

If you forget to take a dose, take it as soon as you remember. If you remember a missed dose when it is time to take the next one, omit the missed dose and take only the regularly scheduled dose. *Do not take a double dose.*

STORAGE

Keep ethambutol in the container it came in, and keep it out of the reach of children. Do not allow anyone else to take your ethambutol.

Isoniazid

(eye soe nye' a zid)

PRODUCT INFORMATION

Brand names: Laniazid, Niconyl, Nydrazid, Panazid, Teebaconin
Brand name of a combination product containing rifampin: Rifamate

USES

Isoniazid is an anti-infective drug used to treat or prevent tuberculosis (TB). Isoniazid is considered one of the most effective antituberculosis drugs and is almost always included in the combination of medications used to treat active disease. Isoniazid may be used alone to prevent TB in people who have been exposed to active disease or who have inactive TB bacteria in their bodies.

Isoniazid eliminates only bacteria that are actively growing. Since many resting (nongrowing) bacteria may persist, therapy with this and other drugs must be continued for a long time (usually six months to two years) to make sure the disease is cured.

UNDESIRED EFFECTS

When you start to take isoniazid, it may make you dizzy, upset your stomach or cause your breasts to enlarge. These effects tend to disappear as your body adjusts to isoniazid. However, if they continue to cause you great discomfort, contact your doctor.

Isoniazid can also decrease the level of vitamin B_6 in your body. If you experience clumsiness, unsteadiness or numbness, tingling or burning in your hands or feet, contact your doctor. You may have to take pyridoxine (vitamin B_6) to counteract these effects.

Liver problems can result from isoniazid therapy. Stop taking the medicine and contact your doctor if you are unusually tired or weak or have a loss of appetite, nausea, vomiting or yellowing of the eyes or skin.

Contact your doctor if you get a skin rash, fever, swollen glands or other signs of allergy or if you experience blurred vision or loss of vision, with or without eye pain.

PRECAUTIONS

To help select the treatment best for you, tell your doctor if you ever had an allergic reaction to isoniazid, an alcohol problem, seizures, diabetes, lupus erythematosus, liver disease or kidney disease.

Before you start taking isoniazid, tell your doctor what other prescription or nonprescription drugs you are taking, including antacids, anticoagulants (blood thinners), drugs to treat diabetes or high blood pressure, disulfiram (medicine to treat alcoholism), phenytoin (medicine for seizures), sleeping medicines, stimulant drugs and rifampin (another antituberculosis drug). If you do not know the names of the drugs you are taking or what they were prescribed for, bring them in their labeled containers to your doctor or pharmacist.

It is very important that you take this medicine exactly as your doctor has prescribed and continue to take it until your doctor says you may stop. You may have to take it for as long as two years.

If your symptoms do not improve within three weeks or if they become worse, contact your doctor. It may be necessay to change your medication.

Do not drink alcoholic beverages while you are taking isoniazid. Regular use of alcohol can increase the possibility of liver problems and may make isoniazid less effective.

If you have diabetes, isoniazid can cause false results with some tests for urine sugar. Do not change your diet or the dosage of your diabetes medicine unless you first check with your doctor.

Tell your doctor if you are pregnant or plan to become pregnant while taking this medicine or if you are nursing a baby. Your doctor will need this information to select the treatment best for you.

Your doctor will want to check on your progress while you are taking isoniazid and may order laboratory tests or eye examinations. *Be sure to keep all appointments with your doctor and at the laboratory.*

DOSAGE

Isoniazid is usually taken once a day, in the morning. To avoid missing a dose, try to take this medicine at the same time you do something else every morning, such as brushing your teeth.

Isoniazid comes in liquid, powder and tablets to be taken orally. Your doctor will choose the best form for you and determine how often you should take isoniazid and how much to take at each dose. Follow the instructions on your prescription label carefully, and ask your doctor or pharmacist to explain any part of the instructions you do not understand.

The container of liquid isoniazid should be shaken well before each use to distribute the medication evenly. Measure each dose with a specially marked measuring spoon to be sure of an accurate dose.

If you forget to take a dose, take it as soon as you remember. If you remember a missed dose at the time you are to take another one, take only the regularly scheduled dose. *Do not take a double dose.*

If your doctor prescribes pyridoxine (vitamin B_6) to prevent or lessen the side effects of isoniazid, take pyridoxine at the same time you take isoniazid. If you forget to take a dose of pyridoxine, take it as soon as possible and then go back to your regular dosing schedule.

STORAGE
Keep isoniazid in the container it came in, and store it at room temperature. Keep it out of the reach of children. Do not allow anyone else to take your isoniazid.

Rifampin
(rif′ am pin)

PRODUCT INFORMATION
Brand names: Rifadin, Rimactane
Brand name of a combination product containing isoniazid: Rifamate

USES
Rifampin is an antibiotic used to treat tuberculosis (TB). Rifampin is usually prescribed with one or two other antituberculosis drugs and often must be taken for three months to two years.

Rifampin also is used to eliminate meningitis bacteria from people who are carriers of the bacteria and are contagious, even if they are not ill.

UNDESIRED EFFECTS
The most frequent side effects of rifampin are stomach and bowel problems (loss of appetite, nausea, vomiting, stomach cramps or diarrhea), headache and muscle pain. These effects tend to lessen or disappear as your body adjusts to the medicine. If they continue or bother you, contact your doctor.

While you are taking rifampin, your urine, stools, saliva, sputum, sweat or tears may have a red-orange color. This effect is harmless, although soft contact lenses may be permanently stained. If rifampin causes a yellow discoloration of your skin, contact your doctor.

Rifampin can cause allergic reactions such as itching, hives, rash or sores on the skin or in the mouth. Contact your doctor if you have these effects. A more serious allergic reaction is a flu-like illness with chills, fever, difficult breathing, dizziness, headache, shivering and muscle and bone pain. If you get these flu-like symptoms, stop taking the medicine and contact your doctor immediately.

Rifampin may cause disturbance of vision or impaired hearing. Rifampin rarely causes kidney, liver or blood problems. Stop taking the medication and contact your doctor if you notice greatly decreased frequency of urination or amount of urine (kidney problem), unusual tiredness or weakness, vomiting or bleeding or sore throat (blood problem).

Some people get drowsy or dizzy when they take rifampin. Do not drive a car or operate dangerous machinery until you know how this drug affects you.

PRECAUTIONS

Before you start to take rifampin, tell your doctor if you have liver disease or an alcohol problem.

Several medications can make rifampin less effective or can be made less effective by rifampin. Some of these medications are aminosalicylic acid (PAS) (another antituberculosis medicine), corticosteroids (e.g., hydrocortisone), digitalis (e.g., digoxin), estrogens, quinidine (heart medicine), methadone, oral anticoagulants (blood thinners), birth-control pills, probenecid (gout medicine) and oral diabetes medicines. Tell your doctor what other prescription or nonprescription drugs you are taking. If you do not know the names of the drugs or what they were prescribed for, bring them in their labeled containers to your doctor or pharmacist.

Birth-control pills may not work well while you are taking rifampin. Unplanned pregnancies, spotting and breakthrough bleeding can occur. You should use a different means of birth control while taking rifampin. Check with your doctor or pharmacist if you have any questions.

It is important that you take rifampin exactly as prescribed and continue to take it until your doctor tells you to stop. It may take from three months to two years to clear up your TB completely.

If your symptoms do not improve within three weeks, contact your doctor. It is important that your doctor check your progress while you are taking rifampin. You may need laboratory tests for liver and kidney function, blood tests or eye or ear examinations. *Be sure to keep all your appointments with your doctor and at the laboratory.*

Do not drink alcoholic beverages while you are taking rifampin. Regular consumption of alcohol increases the possibility of liver problems and may make rifampin less effective.

To help select the best treatment for you, tell your doctor if you are nursing a baby, are pregnant or intend to become pregnant while taking this medicine. If you become pregnant during treatment, contact your doctor.

DOSAGE

Rifampin comes in capsules. It is usually taken once a day. Carefully follow the instructions on your prescription label, and ask your doctor or pharmacist to explain any part of the instructions you do not understand.

Rifampin works best if it is taken on an "empty stomach," one hour before meals or two hours after eating. However, if you become nauseated when you take it on an empty stomach, you may take it with a light snack.

If you are taking the drug PAS in addition to rifampin, take these two drugs at least eight hours apart.

You may find it easier to remember to take your daily dose of rifampin if you take it at the same time you do something else every day, such as brushing your teeth in the morning or going to bed at night. If you forget a dose, take it as soon as you remember. If you remember a missed dose at the time you are to take the next one, omit the missed dose and take only the regularly scheduled dose. *Do not take a double dose.*

STORAGE

Keep this medicine in the container it came in. Keep it out of the reach of children.

Urinary Tract Infections

The specific drug used to treat an infection of the urinary tract depends on the infecting organism and the location of the infection. Precise diagnosis is essential for relief and permanent cure. Depending on the results of laboratory sensitivity testing, the drug used may be a sulfonamide (sulfa drug), an antibiotic or another urinary anti-infective (antibiotics are discussed in the section beginning on page 83; sulfonamides and other urinary tract anti-infectives are described in this section).

Resistance to drugs used to treat urinary tract infections develops frequently, and more than one drug may be necessary to cure a urinary tract infection. A urinary tract infection is cured when a microscopic examination of laboratory culture tests shows urine samples to be normal (infection-free) for three consecutive weeks after medication has been stopped.

URINARY TRACT ANTI-INFECTIVES

Co-trimoxazole
(koe trye mox' a zole)

PRODUCT INFORMATION
Brand names: Bactrim, Septa

USES
Co-trimoxazole is trimethoprim combined with sulfamethoxazole, one of the sulfonamide or sulfa drugs. This combination is used to treat infections of the lungs, ears, urinary tract and bowels. Together, trimethoprim and sulfamethoxazole seem to be more effective than either drug given separately.

This combination of drugs should not be used for "strep throat," since the sulfa drugs may not eliminate the bacteria and rheumatic fever might occur later.

UNDESIRED EFFECTS
Co-trimoxazole can cause nausea, vomiting, diarrhea and skin rash. These effects are more likely to occur with large doses or long-term therapy.

Some of the more serious side effects are caused by the sulfamethoxazole in co-trimoxazole. These effects include allergic reactions, blood problems, kidney problems, liver problems, thyroid problems and an unusual sensitivity to sunlight. (See the monograph on Sulfamethoxazole for the symptoms of these problems and what to do about them.)

PRECAUTIONS

Before you start taking co-trimoxazole, tell your doctor if you ever had an allergic reaction to any sulfa drug, a diuretic (water pill), oral diabetes medicine or oral medicine for glaucoma. Your doctor will need to know if you have G6PD deficiency (an inherited blood disease), porphyria, kidney disease or liver disease.

To help select the best treatment for you, tell your doctor what other prescription or nonprescription drugs you are taking, including oral anticoagulants (blood thinners), oral diabetes medicine, penicillins, PABA (one of the B complex vitamins), isoniazid (antitubercular drug), methenamine (a urinary antiseptic), methotrexate (psoriasis or antitumor medicine), phenytoin (medicine for seizures), phenylbutazone or oxyphenbutazone (for arthritis), medicine for gout or any medicine to make your urine more alkaline, such as sodium bicarbonate and sodium citrate. If you do not know the names of the drugs or what they were prescribed for, bring them in their labeled containers to your doctor or pharmacist.

Co-trimoxazole should not be taken by infants under two months of age, pregnant women or nursing mothers. Tell your doctor if you are nursing a baby, are pregnant or intend to become pregnant while taking this medicine.

Before having any surgery with a general anesthetic, including dental surgery, tell the doctor or dentist that you are taking co-trimoxazole.

Take *all* of the medicine prescribed. Even if you feel better in a few days, the infection will not be completely cured and can return. Bacterial infections take several days to weeks to be cured completely. However, if your symptoms do not improve after a few days, contact your doctor. Your medication may have to be changed or adjusted.

It is important that you keep all appointments with your doctor so your response to this medicine can be checked with blood counts and urine tests.

DOSAGE

Your doctor will determine how much of this medicine you should take and how often you should take it. Carefully follow the instructions on your prescription label, and ask your doctor or pharmacist to explain any part of the instructions you do not understand.

Co-trimoxazole comes in tablets and in liquid form. It should be taken on an "empty stomach," one hour before meals or two hours after eating. While you are taking this medicine, drink at least eight full eight-ounce glasses of water or other liquids every day.

Both the tablets and the liquid should be taken with a full eight-ounce glass of water. The container of liquid should be shaken well before each use to distribute the medication evenly. Measure doses of liquid with a specially marked measuring spoon to be sure of an accurate dose.

If you forget to take a dose, take it as soon as you remember. However, if you remember a missed dose when it is close to the time for another, you may either double the next dose or space the missed dose and the next dose one or two hours apart. Then go back to your regular dosing schedule.

If you still have symptoms of the infection after you have taken all of the medicine prescribed, contact your doctor.

STORAGE
When your doctor tells you to stop taking the medicine, throw away any unused portion. This medicine should not be saved to treat another infection. Do not allow anyone else to take your co-trimoxazole, which was prescribed for your particular condition.

Keep this medicine in the container it came in, and store it at room temperature. Keep it out of the reach of children.

Methenamine
(meth en′ a meen)

PRODUCT INFORMATION
Brand names: Hiprex, Mandelamine, Mandelamine Forte, Mandelets, Prov-U-Sep, Urex and others

USES
Methenamine is an anti-infective drug used to treat kidney and bladder infections. It works properly only when the urine is very acidic. The action of the acid on methenamine releases formaldehyde, which then eliminates bacteria from the urine.

Methenamine is never used alone against severe or "hot" infections. Its value against such infections is to keep the urinary tract free of bacteria after they have been eliminated by other antibacterial drugs. It is also used to prevent infection when instruments are used to examine parts of the urinary tract such as the bladder.

UNDESIRED EFFECTS
Nausea and upset stomach are common side effects of methenamine. Taking the medicine with meals or a snack should relieve these problems, but contact your doctor if they continue or are severe.

A skin rash, hives or itching may indicate that you are allergic to this medicine. Contact your doctor if you experience these effects.

Methenamine may cause kidney problems. Stop taking the medicine and contact your doctor if you notice blood in your urine, have pain in your lower back or experience pain or burning while urinating.

PRECAUTIONS
To help select the best treatment for you, tell your doctor if you have kidney or liver disease.

Before you start taking methenamine, tell your doctor what other prescription or nonprescription drugs you are taking, particularly antacids, oral medicine for glaucoma, sulfa drugs, thiazide diuretics (water pills), vitamin C or any medicine to make your urine more alkaline such as sodium bicarbonate and sodium citrate. If you do not know the names of these drugs or what they were prescribed for, bring them in their labeled containers to your doctor or pharmacist. Do not take any other medications unless you first check with your doctor or pharmacist.

Your urine must be acid for this medicine to work well. Before you start taking methenamine, ask your doctor what you can do to maintain an acid urine and how to test your urine with special paper for the purpose.

Some changes in your diet may help keep your urine acid. However, check first with your doctor if you are already on a special diet, such as a diet for diabetes. Do not drink milk or eat cheese or other dairy products. Do not take antacids. Try to eat more protein and foods such as cranberries (especially cranberry juice with added vitamin C), plums and prunes. If you have any questions about diet, check with your doctor.

To help cure your infection completely, take *all* of the methenamine your doctor has prescribed. Symptoms of the infection may disappear before the infection is cured. Therefore, do not stop taking this medicine until your doctor tells you to do so.

Your doctor may conduct tests to determine if the infection is cured. Be sure to keep all appointments so that your doctor can decide when you may stop taking methenamine.

DOSAGE

Your doctor will determine how much methenamine you should take and how often you should take it. Carefully follow the instructions on your prescription label, and ask your doctor or pharmacist to explain any part of the instructions you do not understand.

Doses of methenamine should be taken as far apart as possible during the day. If your doctor instructs you to take this medicine twice a day, take one dose in the morning and another dose 12 hours later, in the evening. If you are to take it four times a day, take a dose every six hours.

While you are taking methenamine, drink at least eight full eight-ounce glasses of water or cranberry juice every day. This practice will help the medicine work better and prevent side effects.

Methenamine comes in tablets, liquid and powder. It should be taken with a full glass of water or food. The tablets should be swallowed whole. *Do not break or crush them or take them if they are chipped.* The container of liquid should be shaken well before each use to distribute the medication evenly. Measure doses with a specially marked measuring spoon to be sure of an accurate dose.

The powder should be dissolved in two to four ounces of water. Stir it well and take it immediately. To get the full dose of medicine, be sure to drink all of the liquid.

If you forget a dose, take it as soon as you remember. However, if it is almost time for your next dose, you may either double the dose or space the missed dose and the next dose one or two hours apart. Then go back to your regular dosing schedule.

If you still have symptoms of the infection after you have taken all of the medicine prescribed, contact your doctor.

STORAGE

When your doctor tells you to stop taking methenamine, throw away any unused portion. This medication should not be saved to treat another infection because it loses its effectiveness with time.

Keep methenamine in the container it came in, and store it out of the reach of children. Do not let anyone else take your methenamine.

Nalidixic Acid
(nal i dix′ ik ass′ id)

PRODUCT INFORMATION
Brand name: NegGram

USES

Nalidixic acid is an anti-infective drug that eliminates many kinds of bacteria from the urinary tract. Nalidixic acid is used to treat infections of the bladder and kidneys. However, its usefulness is limited by the tendency of infecting bacteria to become resistant to the drug.

UNDESIRED EFFECTS

Nausea, vomiting and diarrhea may be avoided by taking this medicine with meals or milk. If these effects continue or get worse in spite of your precautions, contact your doctor. If you develop rash, hives or itching or experience joint pain or swelling, you may be having an allergic reaction to nalidixic acid; stop taking the drug and contact your doctor.

Nalidixic acid can cause eye, liver and blood problems that require medical attention. If you experience blurred or decreased vision, double vision, changes in color vision, overbrightness of lights or halos around lights, contact your doctor. Symptoms of blood problems are unusual bleeding or bruising, unusual weakness or tiredness, fever, pale skin and sore throat. If you experience any of these effects or yellowing of the skin or eyes (liver problem), contact your doctor.

Other side effects are dark or amber urine, pale stools and severe stomach pain. Contact your doctor if you have any of these symptoms.

Nalidixic acid causes some people to become drowsy or dizzy. Do not drive a car or operate dangerous machinery until you know how this medicine affects you.

Some people who take nalidixic acid become more sensitive to sunlight than they normally are. Limit the time you spend in sunlight until you know how you react to this medicine, especially if you burn easily. You may be sensitive to sunlight or sunlamps for up to a year after you stop taking this medicine. If you get severely sunburned, contact your doctor.

PRECAUTIONS

Before you start taking nalidixic acid, tell your doctor if you have kidney or liver disease, a history of seizures, Parkinson's disease, severe hardening of the arteries of the brain or any central nervous system (brain and spinal cord) damage.

To help select the best treatment for you, tell your doctor what other prescription or nonprescription drugs you are taking, particularly oral anticoagulants (blood thinners), antacids, vitamin C and nitrofurantoin. If you do not know the names of the drugs or what they were prescribed for, take them in their labeled containers to your doctor or pharmacist.

Take *all* of the medicine your doctor prescribes, even after you begin to feel better. If the infection is not completely cured, it can return. Bacterial infections take several days to weeks to be cured completely, and tests are required to determine whether the infection is cured.

If your symptoms do not improve after a few days, contact your doctor. Your doctor may adjust the dosage or do tests to find out whether the infecting bacteria are still sensitive to nalidixic acid.

If you will be taking this medicine for more than two weeks, your doctor should check your progress with regular blood counts and tests for liver and kidney function. *Be sure to keep all appointments with your doctor and at the laboratory.*

Nalidixic acid should not be taken by infants under three months of age, pregnant women in the first three months of pregnancy or nursing mothers. Tell your doctor if you are nursing a baby, are in the first trimester of a pregnancy or intend to get pregnant while taking the drug.

Diabetics who use Clinitest, Benedict's Qualitative Reagent or Fehling's solution to test their urine for sugar should be aware that nalidixic acid can affect test results. If you use one of these tests, ask your doctor if you should switch to some other type of test.

DOSAGE

Your doctor will determine how much nalidixic acid you should take and how often you should take it. Carefully follow the instructions on your prescription label, and ask your doctor or pharmacist to explain any part you do not understand.

Doses of nalidixic acid should be taken as far apart as possible during the day. If your doctor instructs you to take it four times a day, take a dose every six hours.

Nalidixic acid comes in tablets and in liquid form. It is best taken on an "empty stomach," one hour before meals or two hours after eating. While you are taking this medicine, drink at least eight full eight-ounce glasses of water or other liquids every day. This practice will help prevent undesired effects.

Both the tablets and the liquid should be taken with a full eight-ounce glass of water. The container of liquid should be shaken before each use to distribute the medication evenly. Measure doses of liquid with a specially marked measuring spoon to be sure of an accurate dose.

If you forget to take a dose of nalidixic acid, take it as soon as you remember. Take any remaining doses for the day at evenly spaced intervals.

If you still have symptoms of the infection after you have taken all of the medicine prescribed, contact your doctor.

STORAGE

When your doctor tells you to stop taking nalidixic acid, throw away any unused portion of it. Nalidixic acid should not be saved to treat another infection because it loses its effectiveness with time. This medicine was prescribed for your particular condition; do not allow anyone else to take it.

Keep this medicine in the container it came in, and store it at room temperature. Keep it out of the reach of children.

Nitrofurantoin
(nye troe fyoor an' toyn)

PRODUCT INFORMATION

Brand names: Furadantin, Furalan, Furan, Furatoin, Furaton, Macrodantin, Nitrex

USES

Nitrofurantoin is an anti-infective drug effective against bacteria in the urinary tract. Nitrofurantoin is used to treat infections of the kidneys and the bladder.

UNDESIRED EFFECTS

The most common side effects of nitrofurantoin are diarrhea, loss of appetite, nausea and vomiting. These effects tend to disappear as your body adjusts to this medicine. If they do not disappear or if they grow worse, contact your doctor. If diarrhea persists for longer than 24 hours, stop taking the drug and contact your doctor. To avoid stomach upsets, take nitrofurantoin with food or a glass of milk.

This medicine may turn your urine rust-yellow or brown. This effect is harmless.

Nitrofurantoin can cause a severe allergic reaction with chest pain, chills, fever and cough or difficult breathing. If you have these symptoms, stop taking the medicine and contact your doctor. Less frequently, nitrofurantoin will cause headache, dizziness or drowsiness, weakness and tiredness. Stop taking the medicine and contact your doctor if you have these problems.

Nerve, liver and blood problems can result from nitrofurantoin therapy. If you experience numbness, tingling or burning of the face, mouth, fingers or toes (nerve problem), unusual weakness or tiredness, pale skin (blood problem) or yellowing of the eyes or skin (liver problem), stop taking the medicine and contact your doctor.

PRECAUTIONS

Before you start taking nitrofurantoin, tell your doctor if you ever had an allergic reaction to this drug or to any related drug such as furazolidone and nitrofurazone.

To help select the best treatment for you, tell your doctor if you have G6PD deficiency (an inherited blood disease), lung disease, nerve damage or kidney disease.

Tell your doctor what other prescription or nonprescription drugs you are taking, particularly nalidixic acid (another anti-infective drug) or gout medicines such as probenecid or sulfinpyrazone. If you do not know the names of the drugs or what they were prescribed for, bring them in their labeled containers to your doctor or pharmacist.

Avoid consuming alcoholic beverages while taking nitrofurantoin.

Nitrofurantoin should not be taken by infants under one month of age, pregnant women who are a few weeks away from delivery or nursing mothers. This medicine can cause anemia in newborn babies when given directly or passed to them through the mother. Tell your doctor if you are nursing a baby, are pregnant or intend to get pregnant while taking nitrofurantoin.

Be sure to take *all* of the nitrofurantoin your doctor prescribes. Symptoms of the infection may disappear before it is cured, but bacterial infections take several days to weeks to be cured completely.

Blood tests, laboratory tests for liver function or chest X-rays may be ordered by your doctor while you are taking nitrofurantoin. *Be sure to keep all appointments with your doctor and the laboratory* so tests can be done to determine when the infection is cured and you may stop taking nitrofurantoin.

If your symptoms do not improve within a few days or get worse, contact your doctor. It may be necessary to change your medication, adjust the dosage or treat an overgrowth of bacteria against which this drug is not effective.

If you have diabetes, nitrofurantoin can cause false results of urine sugar tests. Do not change your diet or the dosage of your diabetes medicine unless you first check with your doctor.

DOSAGE

Your doctor will determine how much nitrofurantoin you should take and how often you should take it. Carefully follow the instructions on your prescription label, and ask your doctor or pharmacist to explain any part of the instructions you do not understand.

Doses of nitrofurantoin should be taken as far apart as possible. If your doctor instructs you to take it four times a day, take a dose every six hours.

Nitrofurantoin comes in tablets and in liquid form. It should be taken with meals or with a full eight-ounce glass of water or milk. While taking this medicine, drink at least eight full eight-ounce glasses of water or other liquids (coffee, tea, soft drinks, milk and fruit juice) every day. This practice will prevent side effects.

Shake the container of the liquid form before each use to distribute the medication evenly. Measure the dose of the liquid with a specially marked measuring spoon to ensure an accurate dose. The liquid form may cause a temporary yellow discoloration of the teeth and may be mixed with water, milk, fruit juice or baby formula to lessen this problem. The liquid should be taken immediately after mixing.

If you forget to take a dose of nitrofurantoin, take it as soon as you remember. However, if you remember a missed dose when it is close to the time for another, you may either double the next dose or space the missed dose and the next dose one or two hours apart. Then go back to your regular dosing schedule.

If you still have symptoms of the infection after you have taken all of the nitrofurantoin prescribed, contact your doctor.

STORAGE

When your doctor tells you to stop taking nitrofurantoin, throw away any unused portion of it. Nitrofurantoin should not be saved to treat another infection because it loses its effectiveness with time.

Keep this medicine in the container it came in and store it in a dark place. Do not let anyone else take your nitrofurantoin, and keep it out of the reach of children.

Phenazopyridine
(fen az oh peer′ i deen)

PRODUCT INFORMATION

Brand names: Aqua-Ton, Azo-100, Azodine, Azo-Standard, Di-Azo, Phenazodine, Phenylazo, Pyridiate, Pyridium, Urodine and others

USES

Phenazopyridine is a urinary analgesic used to relieve pain, burning, pressure and other discomfort caused by infection or irritation of the urinary tract. It is not an anti-infective drug and will not cure the infection itself. It is used frequently with anti-infective medicines to treat urinary tract infections.

UNDESIRED EFFECTS

Phenazopyridine can cause dizziness, headache, indigestion and stomach or abdominal pain or cramps. These effects may go away as your body adjusts to the drug. Check with your doctor if these effects continue or bother you.

Stop taking the medicine and contact your doctor if you notice yellowing of the eyes or skin.

Phenazopyridine will color your urine red or orange and may stain clothing. This effect is harmless.

PRECAUTIONS

Before taking phenazopyridine, tell your doctor if you have hepatitis (inflammation of the liver) or kidney disease or if you ever had an allergic reaction to phenazopyridine in the past.

If you have diabetes, phenazopyridine may cause false results of tests for sugar and ketones in your urine. Phenazopyridine also may interfere with tests for kidney and liver functions. If you have any questions, check with your doctor.

If you take phenazopyridine for a long time, your doctor may order laboratory tests for liver function or blood tests.

Tell your doctor if you are pregnant or are nursing a baby so you will receive the best treatment for you and your baby.

DOSAGE

Your doctor will determine how much phenazopyridine you should take and how often you should take it. Carefully follow the instructions on your prescription label, and ask your doctor or pharmacist to explain any part of the instructions you do not understand.

Phenazopyridine comes in tablets. They should be taken with a glass of water during or after meals to lessen stomach upset. *Do not chew or crush the tablets before swallowing them.*

If you forget to take a dose, take it as soon as you remember. If it is almost time for your next dose, do not take the missed dose at all and *do not double the next one.* Instead, go back to your regular dosing schedule.

STORAGE

When your doctor tells you to stop taking phenazopyridine, throw away any unused portion. It should not be saved to treat other urinary tract problems.

Keep this medication in the container it came in, and store it out of the reach of children. Do not allow anyone else to take your phenazopyridine.

Sulfamethoxazole
(sul fa meth ox′ a zole)

PRODUCT INFORMATION
Brand names: Gantanol, Gantanol DS, Methoxanol, Urobak
Brand name of a combination product containing phenazopyridine: Azo Gantanol

USES
Sulfamethoxazole is one of the sulfonamide anti-infectives or sulfa drugs that is used primarily to treat urinary tract infections and to prevent "strep" infections in people with a history of rheumatic fever. Sulfamethoxazole also can be used with penicillin or erythromycins for middle ear infections in children.

UNDESIRED EFFECTS
Sulfamethoxazole, like all sulfa drugs, can cause undesired effects, including allergic reactions and blood, kidney, liver or thyroid problems.

Early signs of allergic reaction are itching, rash and hives. Stop taking the medicine and contact your doctor if any of these effects occurs. Less frequently, sulfamethoxazole will cause fever, aching of the joints and muscles, difficulty in swallowing or redness, blistering, peeling or loosening of the skin. If you experience any of these allergic reactions, stop taking the medicine and contact your doctor.

Symptoms of blood problems are unusual bleeding or bruising, unusual weakness or tiredness, fever, pale skin or sore throat. If you experience any of these symptoms, stop taking the medicine and contact your doctor. Also contact your doctor if you have yellowing of the eyes or skin (liver problems), and stop taking sulfamethox-azole.

Although kidney and thyroid problems are rarely caused by sulfamethoxazole, it can cause blood in the urine, lower back pain, pain or burning while urinating or swelling of the front part of the neck (goiter). If any of these problems occur, stop taking the medicine and contact your doctor.

Some people who take sulfamethoxazole become more sensitive to sunlight than they normally are. Limit the amount of time you spend in the sunlight until you know how you react to sulfamethoxazole, especially if you sunburn easily. You may be sensitive to sunlight and sunlamps for many months after you stop taking sulfamethoxazole. If you become severely sunburned, contact your doctor.

When you start to take this medication, you may develop headache, loss of balance, ringing in the ears, dizziness, loss of appetite, nausea or vomiting or diarrhea. These effects tend to lessen or disappear as your body adjusts to the medication. If they continue or become bothersome, contact your doctor. If sulfamethoxazole upsets your stomach, take it after a meal or with a snack.

PRECAUTIONS

Before you start taking sulfamethoxazole, tell your doctor if you ever had an allergic reaction to any sulfa drug, a diuretic (water pill), oral diabetes medicine or oral medicine for glaucoma. Tell your doctor if you have a history of allergy, hay fever or asthma.

If you have G6PD deficiency (an inherited blood disease), porphyria, kidney disease or liver disease, tell your doctor.

To help select the best treatment for you, tell your doctor what other prescription or nonprescription drugs you are taking, including oral anticoagulants (blood thinners), oral diabetes medicine, penicillins, PABA (one of the B complex vitamins), isoniazid (an antitubercular drug), methenamine (a urinary antiseptic), methotrexate (a psoriasis or antitumor medicine), phenytoin (a medicine for seizures), probenecid or sulfinpyrazone (gout medicines), phenylbutazone or oxyphenbutazone (for arthritis) or any medicine to make your urine more alkaline, such as sodium bicarbonate or sodium citrate. If you do not know the names of the drugs you are taking or what they were prescribed for, bring them in their labeled containers to your doctor or pharmacist.

Sulfamethoxazole should not be taken by an infant under one month of age, pregnant women who are at term (ninth month) or nursing mothers. If you are nursing a baby, are pregnant or intend to become pregnant while taking this medicine, tell your doctor.

Alcoholic beverages should be consumed with caution while you are taking sulfamethoxazole, since the effects of alcohol may be increased by sulfa drugs.

Take *all* of this medication exactly as prescribed. Even if you feel better in a few days, the infection will not be completely cured and can return. Bacterial infections take several days or weeks to cure completely. However, if your symptoms do not improve after a few days, contact your doctor. It may be necessary to change your medication or dose.

It is important that you keep all appointments with your doctor so your response to sulfamethoxazole can be checked with regular blood counts, urine tests and tests for thyroid, liver and kidney function.

Before having any surgery with a general anesthetic, including dental surgery, tell the doctor or dentist that you are taking sulfamethoxazole.

DOSAGE

Your doctor will determine how much sulfamethoxazole you should take and how often you should take it. Follow the instructions on your prescription label carefully, and ask your doctor or pharmacist to explain any part of the instructions you do not understand.

Sulfamethoxazole comes in tablets and in liquid form. It should be taken with a full eight-ounce glass of water on an "empty stomach," one hour before meals or two hours after eating. While you are taking the drug, drink at least eight full eight-ounce glasses of water or other liquids (coffee, tea, soft drinks, milk and fruit juice) every day.

The container of liquid should be shaken before each use to distribute the medication evenly. Measure doses of liquid with a specially marked measuring spoon to ensure an accurate dose.

If you forget to take a dose, take it as soon as you remember. However, if you remember a missed dose when it is close to the time for another, you may either double the dose or space the missed dose and the next dose one or two hours apart. Then go back to your regular dosing schedule.

If you still have symptoms of the infection after you have taken all of the sulfamethoxazole prescribed, contact your doctor.

STORAGE

When your doctor tells you to stop taking sulfamethoxazole, throw away any unused portion of it. This medication should not be saved to treat another infection because it loses its effectiveness with time. Do not allow anyone else to take your sulfamethoxazole, which was prescribed for your particular condition.

Keep this medicine in the container it came in, and store it at room temperature. Keep it out of the reach of children.

Sulfisoxazole

(sul fi sox′ a zole)

PRODUCT INFORMATION

Brand names: Gantrisin, Lipo Gantrisin, SK-Soxazole, Sulfizin and others
Brand names of combination products containing phenazopyridine: Aqua-Ton-S, Azo-Gantrisin, Azo-Sulfisocon, Suldiazo, Uridium

USES

Sulfisoxazole is one of the sulfonamide anti-infectives or sulfa drugs. Because it is rapidly absorbed and quickly eliminated from the body, it often is the preferred sulfa for treating urinary tract infections and other infections. It can also be used to prevent "strep" infections in people with a history of rheumatic fever and, along with penicillin or erythromycins, to treat middle ear infections in children.

UNDESIRED EFFECTS

Allergic reactions are the most common side effects of sulfisoxazole. Stop taking this medicine and contact your doctor if you develop a rash, hives and itching, which are early signs of allergic reaction. Less frequently, sulfisoxazole will cause more serious allergic reactions. If you get fever, aching of the joints or muscles, difficulty in swallowing or skin problems (redness, blistering, peeling or loosening of the skin), stop taking the medicine and contact your doctor.

When you start to take sulfisoxazole, you may experience diarrhea, loss of appetite, abdominal pain, nausea or vomiting, dizziness and headache, loss of balance or ringing in the ears. These effects tend to lessen or disappear as your body adjusts to the drug. If they continue or are bothersome, contact your doctor. If this medication upsets your stomach, take it with a meal or a snack.

Sulfisoxazole also can cause blood problems and liver problems. Stop taking the medicine and contact your doctor if you experience unusual bleeding or bruising, unusual weakness and tiredness, fever, pale skin or sore throat (symptoms of blood problems) or yellowing of the eyes or skin (symptoms of liver problems).

Sulfisoxazole may cause a brownish discoloration of the urine; this is harmless. Sulfisoxazole rarely will cause kidney or thyroid problems. If you notice blood in your urine, lower back pain, pain or burning while urinating or a swelling of the front part of the neck (goiter), stop taking the medicine and contact your doctor.

Some people who take sulfisoxazole may become more sensitive to sunlight than they are normally. Limit the amount of time you spend in sunlight until you know how you react to sulfisoxazole, especially if you tend to sunburn easily. You may still be more sensitive than you are normally to sunlight and sunlamps for many months after you stop taking sulfisoxazole. If you become severely sunburned, contact your doctor.

PRECAUTIONS

Before you start taking sulfisoxazole, tell your doctor if you ever had an allergic reaction to any sulfa drug, a diuretic (water pill), oral diabetes medicine or oral medicine for glaucoma. Your doctor should also know if you have a history of allergy, hay fever or asthma.

To select the best treatment for you, your doctor needs to know if you have G6PD deficiency (an inherited blood disease), porphyria, kidney disease or liver disease or if you ever had anemia produced by a drug.

Certain other medicines, when taken with sulfisoxazole, will affect the way your body responds to this drug. Tell your doctor what other prescription or nonprescription drugs you are taking, including oral anticoagulants (blood thinners), oral diabetes medicines, penicillins, PABA (one of the B complex vitamins), isoniazid (an antituberculosis drug), methenamine (a urinary antiseptic), methotrexate (a psoriasis or antitumor medicine), phenylbutazone or oxyphenbutazone (for arthritis), phenytoin (a medicine for seizures), probenecid or sulfinpyrazone (gout medicines) or any medicine to make your urine more alkaline, such as sodium bicarbonate or sodium citrate. If you do not know the names of the drugs you are taking or what they were prescribed for, bring them in their labeled containers to your doctor or pharmacist.

Alcoholic beverages should be taken with caution while you are using sulfisoxazole, since the effects of alcohol may be increased by sulfa drugs.

Take *all* of the sulfisoxazole your doctor prescribes, even after you feel better. If the infection is not completely cured, it can return. Bacterial infections take several days or weeks to cure completely. However, if your symptoms do not improve after a few days, contact your doctor. Your doctor may want to change your medication or dose.

Sulfisoxazole should not be taken by infants under one month of age, pregnant women who are at term (ninth month) or nursing mothers. Tell your doctor if you are nursing a baby, are pregnant or intend to become pregnant while taking this medicine.

It is important that you keep all appointments with your doctor so your response to this medicine can be checked with regular blood counts, urine tests and tests for thyroid, liver and kidney function.

Before having any surgery with a general anesthetic, including dental surgery, be sure to tell the doctor or dentist that you are taking sulfisoxazole.

DOSAGE

Your doctor has determined how much sulfisoxazole you should take and how often you should take it. Carefully follow the instructions on your prescription label, and ask your doctor or pharmacist to explain any part of the instructions you do not understand.

Sulfisoxazole comes in tablets and in liquid form. It should be taken on an "empty stomach," one hour before meals or two hours after eating. While you are taking this medicine, drink at least eight full eight-ounce glasses of water or other liquids (coffee, tea, soft drinks, milk and fruit juice) every day. This practice will help protect your kidneys from problems caused by sulfisoxazole.

Both the tablets and the liquid should be taken with a full eight-ounce glass of water. The container of liquid should be shaken before each use to distribute the medication evenly. Measure doses of liquid with a specially marked measuring spoon to ensure an accurate dose.

If you forget to take a dose of sulfisoxazole, take it as soon as you remember. However, if you remember a missed dose when it is close to the time for another, you may either double the next dose or space the missed dose and the next dose one to two hours apart. Then go back to your regular dosing schedule.

If you still have symptoms of the infection after you have taken all of the medicine prescribed, contact your doctor.

STORAGE

When your doctor tells you to stop taking sulfisoxazole, throw away any unused portion of it. Sulfisoxazole should not be saved to treat another infection because it loses its effectiveness with time. Because this medicine was prescribed for your particular condition, you should not allow anyone else to take your sulfisoxazole.

Keep this medicine in the container it came in, and store it at room temperature. Keep it out of the reach of children.

Vaginal Infections

Drugs discussed in this section are used to treat vaginitis—an inflammation of the vagina characterized by an itching or burning sensation and excessive vaginal discharge. The more common types of vaginitis, named for the organisms causing infection, are trichomonal vaginitis and monilial vaginitis. Trichomonal vaginitis is caused by an organism known as a protozoa, and monilial vaginitis is caused by a fungus. Bacteria such as a hemophilus, "staph" or "strep" organisms cause what is commonly referred to as nonspecific vaginitis.

VAGINAL ANTI-INFECTIVES
Metronidazole
(me troe ni′ da zole)

PRODUCT INFORMATION
Brand names: Flagyl, Metryl, Protostat, Sātric

USES
   Metronidazole is an anti-infective drug which eliminates protozoa (tiny one-celled organisms) that cause infection. Metronidazole is used most often to treat intestinal and genital infections, particularly vaginal infections.
   To cure a vaginal infection completely and to prevent it from recurring, the woman and her male sexual partner are treated at the same time with metronidazole. Metronidazole is given by injection to treat serious abdominal and gynecologic infections.

UNDESIRED EFFECTS
   The most common side effects of metronidazole are diarrhea, loss of appetite, nausea, vomiting and stomach pain. If stomach discomfort occurs, take this medicine with food. Usually, these effects will lessen as your body adjusts to metronidazole. If they continue or are troublesome, contact your doctor.
   Metronidazole may give you constipation, headache, dizziness or lightheadedness, dryness of the mouth or unusual tiredness or weakness. If these effects are severe, contact your doctor.
   Another side effect of this medicine is an unpleasant or sharp metallic taste in your mouth. Chew gum or suck mints to overcome this problem. This medicine can also cause a darkening of the urine. This effect is harmless and will go away when you stop taking the medicine.

If you experience any irritation, discharge or dryness of the vagina not present before you started taking this medicine, or if you notice a white, furry growth on your tongue, metronidazole may not be working as it should or you may have an overgrowth of fungus. Contact your doctor. It may be necessary to change your medication or treat the fungal overgrowth.

More serious side effects of metronidazole, although they do not occur frequently, are allergic reactions, blood problems and nerve problems. Skin rash, hives and itching are signs of an allergic reaction. Contact your doctor if you experience these effects.

If you get a numbness, tingling, pain or weakness in the hands and feet or notice clumsiness or unsteadiness, mood or mental changes or seizures, contact your doctor. Metronidazole may be having a bad effect on your nerves.

Contact your doctor if you get a sore throat or fever, which can indicate blood problems. Your doctor may ask you to have some blood tests or other laboratory tests while taking metronidazole.

Drinking alcoholic beverages while you are taking this medicine may cause stomach pain, nausea, vomiting, headache, flushing or redness of the face. *Do not drink alcoholic beverages while taking metronidazole.* If you have any questions, ask your doctor or pharmacist.

PRECAUTIONS

Metronidazole has been shown to cause cancer in animals. Before you start taking this medicine, discuss the use of this drug with your doctor.

Before you start taking metronidazole, tell your doctor if you have a history of blood disease or if you have central nervous system disease.

Tell your doctor what other prescription or nonprescription drugs you are taking, including anticoagulants (blood thinners) and disulfiram (a drug to help curb drinking of alcohol). If you do not know the names of the drugs you are taking or what they were prescribed for, bring them in their labeled containers to your doctor or pharmacist.

When you are taking metronidazole, you should not douche unless your doctor specifically tells you to do so. Wear only clean, freshly laundered panties of cotton or panties and pantyhose with cotton crotches until the infection is cured. Do not wear panties made of silk, nylon, Dacron or other synthetic fabrics; these garments do not allow air to flow freely around the vagina so they create conditions favorable to the growth of infecting organisms in the vagina.

Be sure to take *all* of the doses of metronidazole your doctor prescribes. Do not stop taking the medicine even though the symptoms of the infection disappear. You must take metronidazole for as long as your doctor tells you to or the infection may return. However, if your symptoms do not improve in a few days or become worse, contact your doctor.

If you are taking this medicine for a genital infection, your sexual partner should be treated at the same time; the infection may spread to another person during sexual intercourse. If you have any questions, check with your doctor.

Metronidazole should not be taken by pregnant women in the first three months of pregnancy and should be used with caution by nursing mothers and children under two years of age. Tell your doctor if you are pregnant or intend to become pregnant while taking this medicine or if you are nursing a baby.

DOSAGE
Metronidazole comes in tablets to be swallowed and in a form for injection. Your doctor will decide how often you should take metronidazole and how much you should take at each dose. Follow the instructions on your prescription label, and ask your doctor or pharmacist to explain any part you do not understand.

Metronidazole tablets may be taken with meals or a light snack to avoid stomach upset.

If you miss a dose of metronidazole, take it as soon as you remember it. Take any remaining doses for that day at evenly spaced intervals. *Do not take a double dose to make up for a missed one.*

STORAGE
Keep this medication in the container it came in, and keep it out of the reach of children.

Miconazole
(mi kon′ a zole)

PRODUCT INFORMATION
Brand names: Monistat-Derm, Monistat 7

USES
Miconazole is an antifungal agent used to treat infections of the vagina and skin infections such as athlete's foot and jock itch. It is available as cream and lotion for topical use and as cream and suppositories for intravaginal use.

UNDESIRED EFFECTS
Side effects of miconazole are irritation and allergic reactions. If you experience vaginal itching, burning or irritation not present before using the vaginal cream or suppositories, contact your doctor.

Stop using miconazole and contact your doctor if you get pelvic cramps, skin rash, hives or headache (signs of an allergic reaction). Your doctor may want to change your medication.

PRECAUTIONS
Before you start using the vaginal cream or suppositories, tell your doctor if you are pregnant or are breast-feeding a baby. A small amount of miconazole is absorbed from the vagina and may affect the health of the developing baby. If you become pregnant while using miconazole, contact your doctor immediately. It is not known if miconazole is transferred to a breast-fed baby through the milk.

Use *all* of the miconazole prescribed by your doctor, even though you may think the infection has disappeared. Failure to use all of the medicine prescribed can allow the infection to return. Continue to use miconazole vaginal cream and suppositories as prescribed, even if you begin to menstruate during the time of treatment. It may be necessary to use this medication for one month to prevent athlete's foot from recurring.

Keep miconazole cream and lotion away from the eyes.

Tell your doctor if you are using a diaphragm for birth control and are being treated for a vaginal infection. If you are using a diaphragm, you should not use miconazole vaginal suppositories because the suppository base may interact with the latex diaphragm. You should select another method of birth control or use vaginal cream instead of suppositories.

To help cure vaginal infections and prevent reinfection, wear only clean, freshly laundered panties of cotton or panties and pantyhose with cotton crotches. Do not wear panties made of nylon, rayon or other synthetic fabrics. These garments do not allow air to flow freely around the vagina so they help create the conditions favorable to growth of fungus in the vagina.

While you are using miconazole vaginal cream or suppositories, do not douche unless your doctor tells you to do so. You may wish to wear a sanitary napkin while using this medicine to protect your clothing from stains.

DOSAGE

Your doctor will determine how often you should use miconazole and how much to use at each dose. Carefully follow the instructions on your prescription label, and ask your doctor or pharmacist to explain any part of the instructions you do not understand.

Miconazole cream and lotion for topical use are applied sparingly and rubbed gently into the skin once or twice a day.

Miconazole vaginal cream and suppositories are usually used once a day at bedtime for at least seven days. The vaginal cream and suppositories come with a special applicator and written instructions:

1. Fill the special applicator with cream to the level indicated, or unwrap a suppository and place it on the applicator as shown in the accompanying instructions.
2. Lie on your back with your knees drawn upward and spread apart (similar to the position for a vaginal examination).
3. Gently insert the applicator into the vagina, and push the plunger to release the medication.
4. Discard the applicator if it is disposable. If not, clean it thoroughly with soap and warm water after each use.

If you forget a dose, take it as soon as you remember. If you remember a missed dose at the time you are scheduled to apply the next one, omit the missed dose completely and use only the regularly scheduled dose.

STORAGE

Keep this medicine in the container it came in. Keep it out of reach of children. Do not allow anyone else to use your miconazole.

Nystatin
(nye stat′ in)

PRODUCT INFORMATION

Brand names: Candex, Korostatin, Mycostatin, Nilstat, Nystex, O-V Statin

USES

Nystatin is an antifungal antibiotic. Nystatin vaginal tablets are inserted in the vagina to treat fungal infections. The vaginal tablets are sometimes used by pregnant women with vaginal infections to prevent fungal infections in the baby's mouth.

Nystatin oral tablets may be swallowed for intestinal infections. The oral tablets also have been used investigationally to treat mouth infections (dissolved in the mouth three or four times daily).

Other forms of nystatin include an oral suspension for mouth infections (thrush) and cream, powder, lotion and ointment for skin infections, such as diaper rash and infections of the fingernails.

UNDESIRED EFFECTS

Side effects with nystatin vaginal tablets are rare. However, if you develop irritation of the vagina not present before using this medicine, contact your doctor. Side effects with oral nystatin suspension and tablets are mild and decrease as you continue to take the drug. These effects include nausea, vomiting and diarrhea. Contact your doctor if these effects persist or are bothersome.

PRECAUTIONS

Use all of the nystatin your doctor has prescribed, even if you think the infection has disappeared. Failure to use all of the medicine prescribed can allow the infection to return. Continue to use vaginal tablets as prescribed even if you begin to menstruate.

Be sure to tell your doctor if you ever had a bad reaction to nystatin. You should not use this drug if you are allergic to it.

Discuss with your doctor any questions you have about douching or sexual intercourse during treatment with nystatin vaginal tablets. You may wish to wear a sanitary napkin while using the vaginal tablets to protect your clothing from stains. You can help cure the infection and prevent reinfection if you wear only clean, freshly laundered cotton panties or panties and pantyhose with cotton crotches. Do not wear panties made of nylon, rayon or other synthetic fabrics. These garments do not allow air to flow freely around the vagina so they create the conditions favorable to growth of fungus in the vagina.

DOSAGE

Nystatin comes as oral suspension, oral tablets, vaginal tablets, cream, powder, lotion and ointment.

Your doctor will determine how often you should use nystatin and how much to use at each dose. Carefully follow the instructions on your prescription label, and ask your doctor or pharmacist to explain any part you do not understand.

Nystatin vaginal tablets usually are inserted high in the vagina once or twice daily for two weeks. They come with a special applicator, instructions and diagram showing how to insert them. Unwrap nystatin vaginal tablets just before inserting. Wash the applicator with soap and warm water after each use.

Nystatin oral suspension is usually taken four times daily for mouth infections. The container of suspension should be shaken well before each use to mix the medication evenly. Measure doses with a special calibrated measure from your pharmacist to ensure an accurate dose. Place one-half of the dose in each side of the mouth and hold it there for several minutes before swallowing.

Nystatin cream, lotion, ointment and powder are usually applied several times daily. If you are using powder for infected feet, dust your shoes and stockings as well as your feet with the powder.

If you forget to take a dose, take it as soon as you remember and take the rest of the doses for that day at evenly spaced intervals. *Do not take a double dose.*

STORAGE

Keep nystatin vaginal tablets in the container they came in and store them in the refrigerator. Keep nystatin oral suspension and tablets in the containers they came in, and store them at room temperature. Do not allow nystatin suspension to freeze. Keep this medicine out of the reach of children.

Worm Infections

ANTHELMINTICS

Pyrantel
(pi ran′ tel)

PRODUCT INFORMATION
Brand names: Antiminth, Banminth, Combantrin

USES
Pyrantel is an anthelmintic (antiworm medicine) and is used to treat worm infections. Pyrantel acts by killing the parasitic worm in the intestinal tract so it can be eliminated from the body in the stool. Pyrantel is commonly prescribed for the treatment of pinworms and roundworms. It has also been used investigationally for the treatment of hookworms.

UNDESIRED EFFECTS
Occasionally, mild stomach upset and diarrhea may occur after taking pyrantel. If these effects persist, contact your doctor.

PRECAUTIONS
Tell your doctor if you ever had a bad reaction to pyrantel.

Because pyrantel can make some medical conditions worse, tell your doctor if you have liver disease, anemia or malnutrition.

Pyrantel should not be taken while taking piperazine, another drug used to treat roundworms and pinworms.

It is not known if pyrantel is safe for children younger than two years old. Ask your doctor to recommend treatment for children in this age group.

Tell your doctor if you are pregnant. It is not known if it is safe to take pyrantel during pregnancy.

DOSAGE
Pyrantel is available as a caramel-flavored liquid. It may be taken at any time of day, without regard to food intake. The dosage depends on your body weight and has been determined by your doctor. Pyrantel liquid must be shaken well to ensure even distribution of the medicine in each dose. Pyrantel may be taken with milk or fruit juices. Follow the instructions on the prescription label carefully. Ask your doctor or pharmacist if you have any questions.

To eradicate pinworms, every person in your household must receive a dose of pyrantel. If one person is infected, the worm is easily transmitted by bed clothing, food, undergarments and even air to other family members and contacts.

Usually, only one dose is required. If evidence of the worm infection is still present after two to three weeks, a second dose should be administered.

In addition to treatment with pyrantel, follow these steps to get rid of pinworms:
1. Keep fingernails trimmed short.
2. Scrub hands and nails often, especially after using the toilet and before eating.
3. Take a shower or stand-up bath every day.
4. Wear snug-fitting undergarments and change daily.
5. Launder all night clothes and bed linen in hot water daily.
6. Air bedroom daily.
7. Scrub bathroom floors and toilet seat with disinfectant solution.
8. Vacuum (do not sweep) all floors and upholstered furniture every day to remove pinworm eggs.

In addition to treatment with pyrantel, follow these steps to get rid of round-worms:
1. Avoid placing fingers or hands in mouth, especially when playing or working out-of-doors in the dirt.
2. Scrub hands and nails often, especially after using the toilet and before eating.
3. Wash all fruit and vegetables before eating.

STORAGE

Keep pyrantel liquid in the container it came in, and store it at room temperature. Keep this medication out of the reach of children.

Pyrvinium
(peer vin' ee um)

PRODUCT INFORMATION
Brand name: Povan

USES

Pyrvinium is an anthelmintic (antiworm medicine) and is used to treat worm infections. Pyrvinium acts by killing the parasitic worm in the intestinal tract so it can be eliminated from the body in the stool. Pyrvinium is commonly prescribed for the treatment of pinworms.

UNDESIRED EFFECTS

Occasionally, stomach upset, diarrhea, vomiting and dizziness may occur after taking pyrvinium. If these effects persist, contact your doctor.

Although allergic reactions are rare, contact your doctor if you experience a skin rash, itching or hives.

PRECAUTIONS

Tell your doctor if you ever had a bad reaction to pyrvinium or have inflammatory bowel disease. Tell your doctor if you are pregnant. It is not known if it is safe to take pyrvinium during pregnancy.

DOSAGE

Pyrvinium is available in tablets and liquid. Your doctor has chosen the best form for you. The dosage depends on your body weight and has been determined by your doctor.

Pyrvinium liquid must be shaken well to ensure even distribution of the medicine in each dose. To avoid staining the teeth, do not chew or crush the tablets; swallow them whole.

Pyrvinium may be taken at any time of day, without regard to food intake. Follow carefully the instructions on your prescription label, and ask your doctor or pharmacist to explain any part you do not understand.

Pyrvinium liquid is a dye and may stain anything it contacts. To avoid accidental staining of clothing, sheets, fingers, or countertops, handle this medication with care. Also, due to this staining property, your stools may appear red as may your vomitus if you vomit. This effect is harmless, however, and should not cause you concern.

To eradicate pinworms, every person in your household must receive a dose of pyrvinium. If one person is infected, the worm is easily transmitted by bed clothing, food, undergarments and even air to other family members and contacts.

Usually, only one dose is required. If evidence of the worm infection is still present after two to three weeks, a second dose should be administered.

In addition to treatment with pyrvinium, follow these steps to get rid of pinworms:
1. Keep fingernails trimmed short.
2. Scrub hands and nails often, especially after using the toilet and before eating.
3. Take a shower or stand-up bath every day.
4. Wear snug-fitting undergarments and change daily.
5. Launder all night clothes and bed linen in hot water daily.
6. Air bedroom daily.
7. Scrub bathroom floors and toilet seat with disinfectant solution.
8. Vacuum (do not sweep) all floors and upholstered furniture every day to remove pinworm eggs.

In addition to treatment with pyrvinium, follow these steps to get rid of roundworms:
1. Avoid placing fingers or hands in mouth, especially when playing or working out-of-doors in the dirt.
2. Scrub hands and nails often, especially after using the toilet and before eating.
3. Wash all fruit and vegetables before eating.

STORAGE

Keep this medication in the container it came in. Store pyrvinium liquid at room temperature. Keep this medication out of the reach of children.

Eye Infections

Drugs applied to the eye are called ophthalmic drugs.

Apply an ophthalmic *ointment* to your eye in the following way:

1. Use a mirror or have someone else apply the ointment.
2. Before applying the ointment, wash your hands thoroughly with soap and water.
3. Avoid touching the tip of the tube against the eye or against anything else.
4. Holding the tube between your thumb and index finger, place it as near as possible to your eyelid without touching it.
5. Brace the remaining fingers of that hand against your cheek or nose to steady your hand.
6. Tilt your head back
7. With your index finger of your other hand, pull the lower lid of the eye down to form a pocket.
8. Place the proper amount of ointment into the pocket made by the lower lid and the eye.
9. Blink your eye gently.
10. Wipe off any excess ointment from the eyelid and lashes with a clean tissue.
11. Replace and tighten the cap right away.
12. Wash your hands again to remove any medicine.

Apply eye *drops* in the following way:

1. Use a mirror or have someone else put the drops in your eye.
2. Before using the drops, wash your hands thoroughly with soap and water.
3. Make sure there are no chips or cracks at the end of the dropper.
4. Avoid touching the dropper against the eye or against anything else.
5. Hold the dropper tip down at all times. This position prevents the drops from flowing back into the bulb, where they may become contaminated.
6. Lie down or tilt your head back.
7. Holding the bulb of the dropper between your thumb and index finger, place the dropper as near as possible to your eyelid without touching it.
8. Brace the remaining fingers of that hand against your cheek or nose to steady your hand.
9. With the index finger of your other hand, pull the lower lid of the eye down to form a pocket.
10. Drop the prescribed number of drops into the pocket made by the lower lid and the eye. Placing drops on the surface of the eyeball can cause stinging.
11. Replace and tighten the cap or dropper right away. Do not wipe or rinse it off.

12. Press your finger against the inner corner of your eye for one minute to prevent medication from entering the tear duct.
13. Close your eye gently and wipe off any excess liquid with a clean tissue.
14. Wash your hands again to remove any medicine.

Do not use eye makeup when you have an infection in one or both eyes. Eye makeup is a frequent source of cross-contamination, spreading the infection from one eye to the other or from one person to another when eye makeup is shared.

Infections in the *outer* ear also can be treated with ophthalmic preparations. In some cases, an ophthalmic ointment or solution is used in the ear; for others, a special otic (ear) product is used. You can put drops in your ear yourself or have someone do it for you.

Apply eardrops in the following way:
1. Before using the drops, wash your hands thoroughly with soap and water.
2. Make sure there are no chips or cracks at the end of the dropper.
3. Avoid touching the dropper against the ear or against anything else.
4. Hold the dropper tip down at all times. This position prevents the drops from flowing back into the bulb, where they may become contaminated.
5. Lie down on your side with the affected ear up, or tilt your head to the side.
6. To allow the drops to run in, hold the earlobe up and back.
7. Drop the prescribed number of drops in the ear.
8. Replace and tighten the cap or dropper right away. Do not wipe or rinse it off.
9. Keep the ear tilted up for a few minutes or insert a soft cotton plug, whichever has been recommended by your doctor or pharmacist.
10. Wash your hands again to remove any medicine.

OPHTHALMIC ANTI-INFECTIVES

Bacitracin
(bass i tray′ sin)

PRODUCT INFORMATION
Brand name: Baciguent Ophthalmic
Brand name of a combination product containing polymyxin: Polysporin
Brand names of a combination product containing polymyxin and neomycin:
Mycitracin, Neosporin

USES
Bacitracin is an antibiotic that eliminates bacteria causing certain eye infections. In addition to being used alone to treat eye problems, bacitracin is combined with the antibiotics neomycin and polymyxin to treat eye infections.

UNDESIRED EFFECTS
When used to treat the eyes, bacitracin has few side effects. However, allergic

reactions have occurred. If this medicine causes itching, burning or redness of the skin, stop using it and contact your doctor.

A more serious allergic reaction also can occur. Stop using this medicine and contact your doctor immediately if you experience itching all over your body, swelling of the lips and face or difficulty breathing. You may need emergency treatment.

PRECAUTIONS
Before you start to use bacitracin, tell your doctor if you have any history of allergies such as asthma, hay fever or hives and if you ever had an allergic reaction to bacitracin.

Do not apply bacitracin to areas of the body other than those indicated by your doctor. Do not apply it more frequently than stated on your prescription label, and do not cover the medication with any dressing not recommended by your doctor.

If your eye infection appears to be worse after you start using bacitracin, contact your doctor. It may be necessary to change your medication.

DOSAGE
Bacitracin comes as an ointment. Your doctor will determine how often you should use bacitracin and how much to use at each application. Carefully follow the instructions on your prescription label, and ask your doctor or pharmacist to explain any part of the instructions you do not understand.

Refer to the general statement titled Eye Infections for instructions on how to apply bacitracin ointment to your eye.

If you forget to apply a dose, apply the ointment as soon as you remember it. Then go back to your regular dosing schedule. *Do not apply a double dose to make up for a missed dose.*

STORAGE
When your doctor tells you to stop using bacitracin, throw away any ointment you have left. Do not save it for another infection, and do not allow anyone else to use it.

Keep bacitracin in the container it came in, and keep it out of the reach of children.

Chloramphenicol
(klor am fen′ i kole)

PRODUCT INFORMATION
Brand names: AntiBiOpto, Chloromycetin, Chloroptic, Chloroptic S.O.P., Econochlor, Ophthochlor

Brand name of a combination product containing polymyxin: Chloromyxin

USES
In addition to oral and injectable forms used to treat serious infections within the body, chloramphenicol is available in solution and ointment forms that are applied

directly to the eye or outer ear to treat infections. However, chloramphenicol should only be used for infections caused by bacteria against which it is known to be effective when safer antibiotics have not worked.

UNDESIRED EFFECTS
The most common side effects of chloramphenicol eye or ear medicines are allergic reactions. If you experience burning, itching, rash, redness, swelling or any other sign of irritation not present before you began to use this medicine, stop using it and contact your doctor.

When chloramphenicol is used over a long time or for repeated short periods, it can interfere with proper development of the bone marrow. Chloramphenicol also can be absorbed into the body from the eye or ear and cause some of the serious blood problems associated with its use when it is taken by mouth or by injection. Symptoms of these blood problems include unusual bleeding or bruising, unusual weakness or tiredness, fever, pale skin and sore throat.

As with other antibiotics, use of chloramphenicol for the eyes and ears may cause overgrowth of organisms against which it is not effective. If your infection does not improve in a few days or if it worsens, stop using chloramphenicol and contact your doctor.

PRECAUTIONS
Before you use this medicine, tell your doctor if you ever had any problem with chloramphenicol.

Use *all* of the medicine your doctor has prescribed, even though your symptoms improve in a few days. However, do not use chloramphenicol more often or for a longer period than your doctor has ordered because it may increase the chance of side effects.

Tell your doctor if you are pregnant or are breast-feeding a baby. Although problems are not likely, your doctor should have this information to select the best treatment for you and your baby.

DOSAGE
Your doctor will determine how often you should use chloramphenicol and how much you should use with each application. Carefully follow the instructions on your prescription label, and ask your doctor or pharmacist to explain any part of the instructions you do not understand.

Chloramphenicol comes in drops and ointment for the eyes and in drops for the ears. If the eyedrops or eardrops look cloudy, shake the bottle for about 10 seconds. Warm the eardrops to near body temperature by holding the bottle in your hand for a few minutes.

See the general statement titled Eye Infections for instructions on how to administer eyedrops, eye ointment and eardrops.

If you miss a dose of this medicine, apply it as soon as you remember. However, if it is almost time for another application, use only the regularly scheduled dose. Skip the missed dose entirely. *Do not apply a double dose.*

STORAGE

Keep chloramphenicol in the container it came in, and keep it out of the reach of children.

Erythromycin

(eh rith roe mye' sin)

PRODUCT INFORMATION

Brand name: Ilotycin Ophthalmic

USES

Erythromycin, an antibiotic used to treat general systemic infections when given by mouth or injection, is also available as an ointment to treat bacterial infections of the eyes. See the general statement titled Erythromycins.

UNDESIRED EFFECTS

If you ever had an allergic reaction to any erythromycin, you should not use erythromycin eye ointment. Although allergic reactions to the eye medication are rare, they can occur in people who are sensitive to it.

The use of erythromycin can result in an overgrowth of organisms against which it does not work. If your eye infection does not improve in a few days or if it worsens, contact your doctor.

PRECAUTIONS

Before you use this medicine, tell your doctor if you ever had problems with erythromycin.

Use all of the medicine your doctor has prescribed, even though your symptoms improve in a few days. It takes time for a bacterial infection to be cured completely. If it is not cured, it can return.

DOSAGE

Your doctor will determine how often you should use erythromycin and how much you should use with each application. Carefully follow the instructions on your prescription label, and ask your doctor or pharmacist to explain any part of the instructions you do not understand.

Erythromycin comes in ointment that is applied to the eye. Refer to the general statement titled Eye Infections for instructions on how to apply eye ointments.

If you miss a dose, apply the ointment as soon as you remember. If it is almost time for another dose, use only the regularly scheduled dose and skip the missed dose entirely. Then go back to your regular dosing schedule. *Do not apply a double dose.*

STORAGE

Keep erythromycin ointment in the container it came in. Keep it out of the reach of children, and do not allow anyone else to use it.

Gentamicin

(jen ta mye' sin)

PRODUCT INFORMATION

Brand names: Garamycin Ophthalmic, Genoptic, Genoptic S.O.P., Gentacidin, Gentafair

USES

Gentamicin is an antibiotic available in injectable form to treat serious systemic infections. It is also available as eyedrops and ointment to be applied directly to the eye to treat some bacterial infections.

UNDESIRED EFFECTS

When applied to the eye, gentamicin eyedrops and ophthalmic ointment may cause a temporary burning or stinging sensation.

Occasionally, gentamicin will cause increased redness or tearing of the eye. If you experience these effects or any sign of irritation (redness, swelling or itching) you did not have before using this medicine, stop using it and contact your doctor.

The use of gentamicin can result in an overgrowth of organisms against which it does not work. Stop using gentamicin and contact your doctor if your symptoms do not improve in a few days or if they get worse.

PRECAUTIONS

Before you start using gentamicin, tell your doctor if you ever had any problems with gentamicin.

Use all of the medicine your doctor has prescribed, even if your symptoms disappear after a few days. Bacterial infections often take many days to cure completely. If they are not completely cured, they can return.

DOSAGE

Your doctor will determine how often you should use gentamicin and how much you should use at each dose. Carefully follow the instructions on your prescription label, and ask your doctor or pharmacist to explain any part of the instructions you do not understand.

Gentamicin comes in eyedrops and in ointment to be placed in the eye. Refer to the general statement titled Eye Infections for instructions on how to apply these medicines.

STORAGE

Keep gentamicin eyedrops and ointment in the containers they came in. Keep both forms of this eye medicine out of the reach of children.

Idoxuridine
(eye dox yoor' i deen)

PRODUCT INFORMATION
Brand names: Herplex, Stoxil

USES
Idoxuridine is used to treat viral infections of the eye. It is considerably more effective against first infections than against recurrent or chronic infections. Idoxuridine has been used investigationally to treat herpes skin infections.

UNDESIRED EFFECTS
Idoxuridine can cause pain, itching or swelling of the eye. If you experience these effects and they are mild, continue to use the medicine. Contact your doctor if these problems become severe.

While you are using idoxuridine, your eyes may be more sensitive to light. Avoid exposing your eyes to bright lights; when you are in sunlight, wear sunglasses or a sunshade.

PRECAUTIONS
Before you use idoxuridine, tell your doctor if you ever had problems with this medicine. If you ever had an allergic reaction to idoxuridine, do not use it.

Follow the treatment schedule prescribed by your doctor as closely as possible. If your eye infection has not improved within one week, contact your doctor. It may be necessary to change your medication.

When the infected eye appears to be healed, continue to use the medicine for one more week, unless your doctor specifically tells you to stop using it.

Do not use any other eye medications while using idoxuridine. If you have questions, ask your doctor or pharmacist.

DOSAGE
Your doctor will determine how often you should use idoxuridine and how much you should use at each dose. It is important that the medication be applied frequently. Carefully follow the instructions on your prescription label, and ask your doctor or pharmacist to explain any part of the instructions you do not understand.

Idoxuridine comes as drops and as ointment to be used in the eyes. Refer to the general statement titled Eye Infections for instructions on how to apply the drops and the ointment.

If you forget a dose, apply it when you remember. Apply any remaining doses for that day at regularly spaced intervals. If you remember a missed dose at the time you are to apply another, omit the missed dose entirely and apply only the regularly scheduled dose. *Do not apply a double dose*. Then continue to follow your regular medication schedule.

STORAGE
When your doctor tells you to stop using idoxuridine, throw away any unused

portion. Do not save it for use against another infection, and do not allow anyone else to use it.

Keep idoxuridine eyedrops in the container they came in and store the container in the refrigerator. The ointment may be refrigerated or stored at room temperature. Keep these medicines out of the reach of children.

Neomycin
(nee oh mye' sin)

PRODUCT INFORMATION
Brand names of a combination product containing bacitracin and polymyxin: Ak-Sporin, Biotic-O, Mycitracin, Neosporin, Neotal
Brand name of a combination product containing hydrocortisone and polymyxin: Cortisporin
Brand name of a combination product containing polymyxin: Statrol

USES
Neomycin is an antibiotic that eliminates certain bacteria that cause infections of the eye and outer ear. It is used alone or in combination with other antibiotics (e.g., bacitracin and polymyxin) or hydrocortisone to treat eye infections. Neomycin is used in combination with other drugs to treat outer ear infections. However, there is no substantial evidence that these combinations are effective against outer ear infections, and they may cause skin irritation.

UNDESIRED EFFECTS
The application of neomycin to the eyes and ears frequently causes allergic reactions. If you get swelling, burning, itching or redness from this medicine, stop using it and contact your doctor.

Neomycin ointment can also cause ear and kidney problems. Stop using the medicine and contact your doctor if you have any loss of hearing; a ringing, buzzing sound or a feeling of fullness in the ears; or clumsiness, dizziness or unsteadiness.

If you notice excessive thirst or a greatly decreased frequency of urination or amount of urine, neomycin may be giving you kidney problems. Stop using the medicine and contact your doctor.

PRECAUTIONS
Before you use neomycin, tell your doctor if you ever had an allergic reaction to neomycin or to other similar antibiotics (amikacin, gentamicin, kanamycin, streptomycin or tobramycin). If you ever had an allergic reaction to these drugs, you should not use neomycin.

To help select the treatment best for you, tell your doctor if you have inner ear disease, kidney disease, myasthenia gravis or Parkinson's disease.

Tell your doctor what prescription or nonprescription drugs you are taking, including amikacin, anticoagulants (blood thinners), capreomycin, cephaloridine, cephalothin, digoxin (heart medicine), ethacrynic acid, furosemide, gentamicin, kanamycin, polymyxin, streptomycin, tobramycin, vancomycin and viomycin. If you do not know the names of the drugs or what they were prescribed for, bring them in their labeled containers to your doctor or pharmacist.

If your symptoms do not improve within a few days or if they get worse, contact your doctor. The neomycin may not be effective against the bacteria causing your infection, or an overgrowth of bacteria against which it does not work has caused a second infection.

Tell your doctor if you are pregnant or think you may become pregnant while you are using neomycin. Safe use of this medicine in pregnant women has not been established.

DOSAGE

Neomycin comes in eardrops, eyedrops and eye ointment. Your doctor will determine how much neomycin you should use and how much you should apply at each dose. Carefully follow the instructions on your prescription label, and ask your doctor or pharmacist to explain any part of the instructions you do not understand.

Do not apply this medication to areas of your body other than those indicated by your doctor. Do not apply neomycin more frequently than stated on the prescription label. Refer to the general statement titled Eye Infections for instructions on applying eye ointment, eardrops and eyedrops.

If you forget a dose, apply it as soon as you remember. Then go back to your regular dosing schedule. *Do not apply a double dose to make up for a missed dose.*

STORAGE

When your doctor tells you to stop using neomycin, throw away any unused portion. Do not save it for use against another infection, and do not allow anyone else to use it.

Keep neomycin in the container it came in, and keep it out of the reach of children.

Sulfacetamide
(sul fa see' ta mide)

PRODUCT INFORMATION
Brand names: Ak-Sulf, Ak-Sulf Forte, Bleph-10 Liquifilm, Bleph-10 S.O.P., Cetamide, Isopto Cetamide, Sulamyd Sodium, Sulf-10, Sulfacel-15, Sulfair, Sulfair Forte, Sulfair 10, Sulfair 15, Sulten-10

USES
Sulfacetamide is a sulfonamide (sulfa-type) antibacterial drug that stops the growth of bacteria causing certain eye infections. It is also used to prevent infection after injury to the eyes. For serious infections, it may be necessary to take an oral antibacterial agent along with sulfacetamide eyedrops or ointment.

Sulfacetamide is also combined with cortisone-like drugs (e.g., hydrocortisone) and with drugs that narrow the blood vessels (e.g., phenylephrine) to treat certain eye problems.

UNDESIRED EFFECTS

Sulfacetamide may make your eyes red, sore or watery. Contact your doctor if you have any of these effects.

Although very little sulfacetamide is absorbed into the body when it is applied to the eye, an allergic reaction can occur in a person who is very sensitive to sulfa drugs. If you develop itching, rash, fever, aching of the joints and muscles, difficulty in swallowing or redness, blistering, peeling or loosening of the skin, you may be having an allergic reaction. Stop using this medicine and contact your doctor immediately.

PRECAUTIONS

Before you use sulfacetamide, tell your doctor if you ever had an allergic reaction to any sulfa drug, thiazide diuretic (water pill), oral diabetes medicine or oral medicine for glaucoma.

Tell your doctor what prescription or nonprescription drugs you are taking. If you do not know the names of the drugs or what they were prescribed for, bring them in their labeled containers to your doctor or pharmacist.

If your infection has not improved within two to three days after you start using sulfacetamide, contact your doctor. It may be necessary to change your medication or add another drug. The lack of improvement also might indicate an overgrowth of bacteria against which sulfacetamide does not work.

DOSAGE

Your doctor will determine how often you should use sulfacetamide and how much you should use at each application. Carefully follow the instructions on your prescription label, and ask your doctor or pharmacist to explain any part of the instructions you do not understand.

Sulfacetamide comes in drops and ointment for the eyes. If the solution looks cloudy, shake the bottle for about 10 seconds. Refer to the general statement titled Eye Infections for instructions on using the eyedrops and the ointment.

If you forget a dose, apply it when you remember. Apply any remaining doses for that day at evenly spaced intervals. If you remember a missed dose at the time you are scheduled for the next one, omit the missed dose completely and apply only the scheduled one. *Do not apply a double dose.* Then return to your regular dosing schedule.

STORAGE

When your doctor tells you to stop using sulfacetamide, throw away any of the medicine that is left. Do not save it for use against another infection, and do not allow anyone else to use it.

Keep sulfacetamide in the container it came in, and store it away from excess heat. Keep it out of the reach of children.

Vidarabine

(vye dare' a been)

PRODUCT INFORMATION
Brand name: Vira-A

USES
Vidarabine is an antiviral agent used to treat certain viral eye infections, including those caused by herpes and hepatitis viruses. It is used by people who are resistant to idoxuridine (another antiviral drug) and who suffer from recurrent infections.

UNDESIRED EFFECTS
The most common side effects of vidarabine are a temporary visual haze and burning, itching and mild irritation of the affected eye. Your eye may also be more sensitive to light while using this medication, so wear sunglasses for protection.

PRECAUTIONS
Keep all appointments with your doctor while using this medication. Tell your doctor if you are pregnant or breast-feeding a baby. Although little drug is absorbed through the eye, it is not known whether vidarabine is safe to use during pregnancy or while breast-feeding.

DOSAGE
Your doctor will determine how often you should use vidarabine ointment and how much you should use for each application. Carefully follow the instructions on your prescription label, and ask your doctor or pharmacist to explain any part of the instructions you do not understand.

Do not apply this medication to areas of your body other than those indicated by your doctor. Do not apply the ointment more frequently than stated on the prescription label.

Refer to the general statement titled Eye Infections for instructions on applying an eye ointment.

Vidarabine is usually applied frequently to maintain a high concentration of drug at the surface of the eye. If you forget a dose, apply it as soon as you remember. Then go back to your regular dosing schedule.

If your symptoms do not improve within a few days or if they get worse, contact your doctor. Up to three weeks of treatment may be necessary. If the symptoms of infection are still present after the prescribed treatment period, contact your doctor. Do not stop using this medication as soon as the infection heals. Continue using it for five to seven days after healing to prevent recurrence. Contact your doctor if you have any questions about how long to use vidarabine.

STORAGE
Do not allow anyone else to use your vidarabine ointment, because it may become

contaminated and spread the infection. Check the expiration date on the crimp of the ointment tube and discard it if this date has passed.

Store the ointment at room temperature away from excessive heat. Keep it out of the reach of children.

Skin Problems

DRUGS USED TO TREAT SKIN PROBLEMS

Skin Infections

This section describes a few of the many medicines used to treat skin infections. Skin infections can be treated with *systemic* drugs (drugs that act throughout your body) or with drugs applied directly to the skin. Drugs applied directly to the skin are called "topical," and the drugs are said to be applied "topically."

Proper washing and care of the skin are extremely important in combating any skin disease. Ask your doctor about proper hygienic practice for your particular condition. Follow your doctor's advice about what kind of soaps (if any) to use and other precautions to follow in caring for your skin.

Before beginning to use any medicine on your skin, discuss with your doctor or pharmacist the way to apply it (for example, rub it in or lay it on), the methods of "dressing" the infected area (for example, leave it open or cover it, and what to use to cover it) and the way to remove the medicine, if necessary.

Although many antibiotic creams, lotions and ointments are available to treat bacterial skin infections, most health professionals question the use of topical antibiotics except for infected burns. Minor skin infections usually heal without drug treatment if proper hygienic measures are followed. Serious or extensive bacterial skin infections require *systemic* anti-infective therapy. (Some examples of bacterial infections are erysipelas, impetigo, carbuncles and abscesses.) Casual use of topical antibiotics should be avoided because it can lead to the development of strains of bacteria that are resistant to the antibiotic used and to similar antibiotics.

Culture and sensitivity tests should be done before any antibiotic is prescribed. Among the systemic antibiotics useful in treating bacterial infections of the skin are erythromycin, penicillins and tetracyclines.

Fungal infections of the skin or nails are treated with topical medicines and medicines taken orally that have a particular affinity for skin or nail tissue.

Specific parasiticides are available for topical application in the treatment of scabies, a scaly and itchy skin disease caused by the itch mite, and in the treatment of pediculosis, caused by lice.

ANTIBACTERIAL ANTI-INFECTIVES (TOPICAL)

Nitrofurazone

(nye troe fyoor′ a zone)

PRODUCT INFORMATION

Brand names: Furacin, Nisept, Nitrazone, Nitrofurastan, Nitrozone

USES

Nitrofurazone is an antibacterial agent that is effective against a wide variety of bacteria, including some that are resistant to sulfa drugs and other antibiotics. Nitrofurazone is used to prevent and treat infections of second- and third-degree burns when such an infection might be caused by resistant bacteria.

This medication is also used on skin grafts when bacteria on the grafts or at the donor site might cause graft rejection, particularly when the bacteria are resistant to other anti-infectives.

UNDESIRED EFFECTS

Allergic skin reactions are the most common problem when you use nitrofurazone. Stop using this medication and contact your doctor immediately if you experience redness, itching or burning of the skin, swelling, blisters or ulcers.

Nitrofurazone also can cause hives, peeling of the skin and a serious and sometimes fatal allergic reaction. If you have any of these symptoms, stop using the medication and contact your doctor immediately—you may need emergency treatment.

During nitrofurazone therapy, bacteria and fungi against which this medicine is not effective may overgrow. If your condition does not improve within a few days, stop using nitrofurazone and contact your doctor.

PRECAUTIONS

Before using nitrofurazone, tell your doctor if you ever had an allergic reaction to it.

Tell your doctor if you are pregnant or think you may be. Safe use of nitrofurazone in pregnant women has not been established.

DOSAGE

Your doctor will determine how often you should apply nitrofurazone and how much to use at each application. Carefully follow the instructions on your prescription label, and ask your doctor or pharmacist to explain any part of the instructions you do not understand.

Nitrofurazone comes in powder, liquid spray, ointment, cream and wet dressings. Your doctor will determine which form is best for you.

Nitrofurazone powder comes in a shaker-top vial and can be applied directly to the area to be treated. The liquid spray also can be applied directly to a burned area. If you are using the ointment or cream, you may put it directly on the area to be treated or apply it to the dressings to cover the area.

The wet dressings that already contain nitrofurazone ointment or liquid are put directly on the area to be treated and then covered with dry gauze or a blanket to prevent drying or evaporation.

The frequency of application of nitrofurazone depends on your condition and the form used. If you are treating second- or third-degree burns, it usually is best to change the dressing every day. With second-degree burns that are oozing very little, the dressing may be left in place for four or five days. If you have any questions about the way to treat your burn or how long to leave dressings in place, contact your doctor.

STORAGE
Keep nitrofurazone in the container it came in, and store it in a cool, dry place. Keep nitrofurazone out of the reach of children.

Silver Sulfadiazine
(sul fa dye′ a zeen)

PRODUCT INFORMATION
Brand name: Silvadene

USES
Silver sulfadiazine is a combination of silver nitrate and sulfadiazine (a sulfa drug) that is effective against a wide variety of bacteria. This cream is used to prevent and treat infections of second- and third-degree burns. It is usually used in a hospital.

UNDESIRED EFFECTS
Occasionally, application of silver sulfadiazine will cause burning, rash or itching. It is necessary to stop using the medicine only if these effects are severe.

Because significant amounts of silver sulfadiazine are absorbed into the body, side effects caused by all sulfa drugs can occur. These effects include allergic reactions, blood problems and kidney and liver problems. Contact your doctor if you experience fever, aching of the joints or difficulty swallowing (symptoms of allergic reaction); unusual bleeding or bruising, unusual weakness or tiredness, fever, pale skin or sore throat (symptoms of blood problems); yellowing of the eyes or skin (symptoms of liver problems); or blood in the urine, low back pain or pain or burning while urinating (symptoms of kidney problems).

PRECAUTIONS
To select the best treatment, tell your doctor if you ever had an allergic reaction to silver sulfadiazine, methylparaben or any sulfa drug and if you have G6PD deficiency (an inherited blood disease) or kidney or liver disease.

Tell your doctor what other prescription or nonprescription drugs you are taking. If you do not know the names of the drugs or what they were prescribed for, bring them in their labeled containers to your doctor or pharmacist.

Tell your doctor if you are pregnant or think you may be. Silver sulfadiazine should not be used by pregnant women unless the burned area covers more than 20 percent of their bodies or the potential benefit to the mother would be greater than the possible risk to the baby. This medicine should not be used by pregnant women within two to three weeks of delivery or by premature babies or infants under one month of age. It can cause harmful jaundice in newborn babies.

Do not stop using silver sulfadiazine without your doctor's permission. Your burn must be sufficiently healed that the possibility of infection is no longer a problem.

DOSAGE
Your doctor will determine how often you should apply silver sulfadiazine and how much to use at each application. Carefully follow the instructions on your prescription label, and ask your doctor or pharmacist to explain any part of the instructions you do not understand.

Silver sulfadiazine cream usually is applied to the cleaned area of a burn once or twice a day. First put on a sterile, disposable glove. Then cover the burned area with a one-sixteenth-inch thickness of cream. *The burned area should be covered at all times.* If necessary, reapply the cream to any area that becomes uncovered. Dressings usually are not required but may be used.

STORAGE
Keep silver sulfadiazine in the container it came in, and store it at room temperature. Keep it out of the reach of children.

ANTIFUNGAL ANTIBIOTICS (TOPICAL)

Econazole
(e kone′ a zole)

PRODUCT INFORMATION
Brand name: Spectazole

USES
Econazole is an antifungal agent that is applied to the skin to treat fungal infections including athlete's foot, jock itch and body ringworm. It has also been used investigationally for some vaginal and ear infections.

UNDESIRED EFFECTS
Econazole may cause a burning or stinging sensation, itching and redness when

applied to the skin. These symptoms usually disappear as you continue to use this medication. If they persist, contact your doctor.

PRECAUTIONS
Keep econazole away from your eyes.

Do not stop using this medication until your doctor tells you to, even if your symptoms improve. If your infection has not cleared up after using econazole as instructed, contact your doctor. Although most infections disappear after one or two weeks, athlete's foot may require up to six weeks of treatment.

If you ever had a bad reaction to econazole, particularly skin irritation, you should not use this medication.

Good health habits can help cure your skin infection and prevent reinfection. Wash all towels, sheets and clothing each day after they have come in contact with the affected area.

Tell your doctor if you are pregnant, plan to become pregnant or are breast-feeding a baby. It is not known if the use of econazole during pregnancy or while breast-feeding is safe for the baby.

DOSAGE
Econazole comes in cream for topical use. Follow the instructions on your prescription label, and ask your doctor or pharmacist to explain any part you do not understand.

Econazole cream is usually applied once or twice a day, in the morning and evening.

Wash the affected area with mild soap and warm water, and dry it thoroughly before applying the cream. Rub the cream gently into the affected area.

STORAGE
Keep econazole out of the reach of children.

Griseofulvin
(gri see oh ful' vin)

PRODUCT INFORMATION
Brand names: Fulvicin P/G, Fulvicin-U/F, Grifulvin V, Grisactin, Gris-PEG

USES
Griseofulvin is an antifungal antibiotic that is taken orally to treat ringworm infections of the skin, hair, fingernails and toenails. Griseofulvin keeps the fungus infection from spreading to new skin or nails as they develop. It takes from several weeks to several months to cure the infection completely.

UNDESIRED EFFECTS
Headache is the most common side effect when you first start to take this medicine

but tends to disappear as your body adjusts to griseofulvin. Contact your doctor if you continue to have headaches.

Upset stomach, diarrhea, nausea and vomiting can occur when you take griseofulvin; these problems may be controlled if you take it after meals. If this medicine makes your mouth dry, you can suck lozenges or hard candies, chew gum or drink liquids to relieve it.

Griseofulvin also can cause dizziness, insomnia and tiredness. Contact your doctor if these effects bother you.

More serious side effects of griseofulvin are allergic reactions, blood problems and infection of the mouth by fungi against which griseofulvin is not effective. Contact your doctor if you develop skin rash, hives or itching; mental confusion; soreness or irritation of the mouth; numbness, tingling, pain or weakness in the hands or feet; or sore throat or fever.

Some people who take griseofulvin become more sensitive to sunlight. Until you know how you will react to this medicine, avoid exposure to sunlight and sunlamps, particularly if you sunburn easily. When you are in sunlight, keep your body well covered with clothing, use a sunscreen preparation and wear sunglasses. If you become severely sunburned, contact your doctor.

PRECAUTIONS

Before you start taking griseofulvin, tell your doctor if you ever had an allergic reaction to any penicillin. People who are sensitive to penicillin also may be sensitive to griseofulvin. Your doctor also will need to know if you have liver disease, porphyria or lupus erythematosus.

Tell your doctor what other prescription or nonprescription drugs you are taking, particularly sleeping pills and anticoagulants (blood thinners). If you do not know the names of the drugs or what they were prescribed for, bring them in their labeled containers to your doctor or pharmacist.

Do not drink alcoholic beverages while taking griseofulvin. The combination of alcohol and griseofulvin can make your heartbeat unusually fast and cause a flushing or redness of your face.

Be sure to take all doses of this medicine prescribed by your doctor, and continue to take it until your doctor tells you to stop. It may be some time before your infection is completely cured—from two to six weeks for infections of the scalp or the skin on most parts of the body, from four to eight weeks for infections of the palms of the hands and the soles of the feet, from four to six months for fingernail infections and from six to 12 months for toenail infections. *Do not stop taking griseofulvin because you see signs of improvement. You must take it until the infection is completely gone.*

Your doctor will want to check your progress while you are taking griseofulvin, particularly if treatment will continue for a long period. *Be sure to keep all appointments with your doctor and the laboratory for blood counts and tests for liver and kidney function.*

Griseofulvin should not be taken by pregnant women or by children under two years of age. Before taking this medicine, tell your doctor if you are pregnant or intend to become pregnant while taking griseofulvin. If you become pregnant while taking griseofulvin, contact your doctor.

DOSAGE

Your doctor will determine how often you should take griseofulvin and how much you should take at each dose. Carefully follow the instructions on your prescription label, and ask your doctor or pharmacist to explain any part of the instructions you do not understand.

Griseofulvin comes in tablets and in liquid form. It should be taken with, or right after, meals to lessen stomach upset. This medicine works better if you eat high-fat meals, so be sure to include fats such as butter and vegetable oil in your diet every day. Your doctor can give you more information about diet.

If you forget to take a dose of this medicine, take it as soon as you remember. Take the remaining doses for that day at evenly spaced intervals. *Do not take a double dose to make up for a missed one.*

If you take the liquid form of griseofulvin, be sure to shake the container well to distribute the medication evenly before removing each dose. Measure each dose with a specially marked measuring spoon to assure an accurate dose.

STORAGE

Keep griseofulvin in the container it came in, and keep it out of the reach of children. Do not allow anyone else to take it.

Haloprogin
(ha loe proe' jin)

PRODUCT INFORMATION
Brand name: Halotex

USES

Haloprogin is an antifungal agent used to treat athlete's foot, jock itch and other fungal infections of the skin, especially the hands.

UNDESIRED EFFECTS

Haloprogin may cause irritation, burning, itching or blistering of the skin. If irritation or symptoms of allergy (itching, rash, hives and wheezing) occur, stop using this medication and contact your doctor.

PRECAUTIONS

Do not allow this medication to come in contact with the eyes. If you ever had an allergic reaction to this drug, do not use it again.

Good health habits can help cure your skin infection and prevent reinfection. Wash all towels, sheets and clothing each day after they have come in contact with the infected area.

DOSAGE

Haloprogin is available as a cream and as a solution to be applied to the skin. *Haloprogin must be used regularly to be effective.* Follow the instructions on your prescription label, and ask your doctor or pharmacist to explain any part you do not understand. This medication is usually used twice a day for two to three weeks.

Do not stop using this medication until your doctor tells you to do so. It may take up to four weeks for complete healing of infections between the fingers. Contact your doctor if symptoms persist after using haloprogin as directed.

Wash the affected area with mild soap and warm water and dry thoroughly before applying the cream or solution. Apply plenty of the medication to the affected area. The infection will heal faster if kept uncovered and exposed to fresh air. If you have athlete's foot, wear clean white cotton socks rather than colored socks.

STORAGE

Keep this medication out of the reach of children.

Tolnaftate
(tole naf' tate)

PRODUCT INFORMATION
Brand names: Aftate, Tinactin

USES

Tolnaftate is an antifungal agent that is applied to the skin to treat such fungal infections as athlete's foot, jock itch and body ringworm. This medicine is available without a prescription.

UNDESIRED EFFECTS

Tolnaftate rarely causes undesired effects. However, if you get a skin irritation that was not present before using this medicine, contact your doctor.

When you apply the spray liquid form of tolnaftate, you may notice a mild stinging sensation, which quickly goes away.

PRECAUTIONS

Tolnaftate preparations should not come in contact with the eyes.

Contact your doctor if your skin infection has not improved after you have used tolnaftate for four weeks. Your doctor may want to change your medication or supplement it with oral antifungal medicine.

Unless instructed otherwise by your doctor, continue to use tolnaftate for two weeks *after* the symptoms (burning, itching, etc.) disappear to be sure that your infection is cured completely.

Good health habits can help cure your skin infection and prevent reinfection. Wash all towels, sheets and clothing each day after they have come in contact with the infected area. After treatment with tolnaftate, you may continue to use it to *prevent* reinfection. Apply the powder or aerosol powder form each day after you have bathed and dried carefully.

If you ever had an allergic reaction to this drug, do not use it.

DOSAGE

Tolnaftate comes in cream, liquid, powder, gel, aerosol powder, aerosol liquid and spray liquid forms. Your doctor or pharmacist can help you choose the form best for your problem.

Tolnaftate must be used regularly to be effective. It should be applied twice a day until the infection is gone and continued for another two weeks. Before applying tolnaftate, wash and dry the area to be treated carefully. Put on enough medicine to cover the area.

When you use the powder to treat your feet, sprinkle it between your toes, on the rest of the foot and in your socks and shoes.

Shake the aerosol powder well before each use. Then spray the affected area from a distance of six to 10 inches. To treat your feet, spray the powder between your toes, on the rest of the foot and in your shoes and socks. Do not inhale the powder, and do not use it near heat, near an open flame or while smoking.

If tolnaftate liquid becomes solid, warming will melt it. To melt it, place the closed container in warm water.

If you are using the aerosol liquid, shake it well before each use. Then spray the infected area from a distance of six inches. To treat your feet, spray between your toes and over the rest of the foot. Do not inhale the vapors from the aerosol liquid. Do not use it near heat, near an open flame or while smoking.

If you use the spray liquid, spray the infected area from a distance of four to six inches. As with other spray forms, do not use near heat, near an open flame or while smoking.

STORAGE

Keep all forms of tolnaftate in a cool, dry place. Keep tolnaftate out of the reach of children.

PARASITICIDE

Lindane
(lin' dane)

PRODUCT INFORMATION
Brand name: Kwell

USES

Lindane, formerly known as gamma benzene hexachloride, is applied to the skin or scalp to treat infections of lice and scabies. One application usually will kill these parasites and their eggs.

UNDESIRED EFFECTS

When you apply lindane, it may make your skin itch. This itching should ease, but contact your doctor if it continues or grows worse.

Lindane can cause allergic reactions. Contact your doctor if you develop a skin irritation or a rash that was not present before using this medicine.

Lindane is absorbed through the skin, and there is a chance that you may experience symptoms such as clumsiness or unsteadiness; convulsions or seizures; muscle cramps; unusual nervousness, restlessness or irritability; unusually fast heartbeat; and vomiting. If you experience any of these side effects, contact your doctor.

If your skin has become sensitive to mites, itching may continue one to two weeks after treatment. This does not mean that the treatment was a failure and is not necessarily a reason for further treatment. If you have any questions, contact your doctor.

PRECAUTIONS

Before taking this medicine, tell your doctor if you have ever had an allergic reaction to lindane (gamma benzene hexachloride). Your doctor should also know if you are presently using any skin preparations such as lotions, ointments or oils. Use of other skin preparations along with lindane increases the chance of absorption of lindane through the skin and the chance of undesired effects.

Use lindane only as directed by your doctor. Do not use more of it, do not use it for a longer time and do not use it more often than your doctor has instructed. Using lindane exactly as prescribed will lessen the chance of serious side effects.

Do not put this medicine on your face, and be sure to keep it away from your eyes. If you accidentally get lindane in your eyes, flush them thoroughly with water.

Because lindane is absorbed through the skin, it should be used with caution by pregnant women and infants. To help select the best treatment for you, tell your doctor if you are pregnant or think you may be. If you are treating a small child with lindane, be careful to prevent the child from getting any of the medicine in the mouth, as by thumb-sucking.

Take precautions to prevent reinfection or spreading of the infection to other people. Boil or dryclean any clothing, bedding, towels or other things in which the parasites that caused the problem may be living. Thoroughly clean all bathtubs, showers and toilets in your home with a solution of 70 percent alcohol. When the problem is head lice, combs and brushes can be cleaned with lindane shampoo, but they must be rinsed thoroughly with water to remove all of the drug.

DOSAGE

Lindane comes in lotion, cream and shampoo form. Your doctor will determine which form is best for you. Carefully follow the instructions on your prescription label, and ask your doctor or pharmacist to explain any part of the instructions you do not understand.

If your doctor has prescribed cream or lotion for scabies, do the following:

1. Take a hot, soapy bath or shower.
2. Dry yourself well.

3. Apply the lotion or cream to all parts of your body from the neck down. Do not apply it to the face or head. Rub it in well.
4. Leave the cream or lotion on your body for 12 hours. Do not take a bath during this 12-hour period. Do not wash off any of the cream or lotion.
5. Dress in clean clothes. Do not change your clothes during the 12-hour period that the medicine is left on your skin.
6. When the 12-hour period is over, take another hot, soapy bath or shower.
7. Dry yourself well with a clean, dry towel.
8. Dress in freshly laundered or drycleaned clothing.

If your doctor has prescribed cream or lotion for lice, do the following:
1. Apply enough medicine to cover only the affected areas, and rub it well into the hair and skin.
2. Leave the cream or lotion on for 12 hours. Do not wash off any of the medicine.
3. When the 12-hour period is over, remove the cream or lotion in a hot, soapy bath or shower.
4. Put on freshly laundered or drycleaned clothing.

If your doctor has prescribed the shampoo, do the following:
1. Take a hot, soapy bath or shower. Shampoo your hair with your regular shampoo.
2. While your hair is still wet, apply one ounce (two tablespoonfuls) of the lindane shampoo. Lather the shampoo into your hair for a full five minutes.
3. Rinse your hair thoroughly with water. Dry it with a clean towel.
4. Comb through your hair with a fine-tooth comb.

STORAGE
Keep lindane at room temperature. Keep it out of the reach of children.

ANTIVIRAL ANTI-INFECTIVE (TOPICAL)

Acyclovir
(ay sye′ kloe ver)

PRODUCT INFORMATION
Brand name: Zovirax

USES
Acyclovir is an antiviral agent. Acyclovir topical ointment controls the symptoms but does not cure lip and genital herpes infections. It decreases the duration of shedding of the virus, the duration of pain and itching and the time required for healing of sores. It is more effective for first time than recurrent sores. *Acyclovir*

ointment will not prevent spread of infection to other people or prevent infections from recurring.

UNDESIRED EFFECTS
You may experience mild pain, burning or stinging after applying the ointment to open sores. This may be due to direct irritation (touch); try to rub the ointment in gently. Contact your doctor if these symptoms are severe.

If a rash and itching occur, contact your doctor immediately; these may be symptoms of an allergic reaction.

PRECAUTIONS
Acyclovir ointment does not prevent the spread of infection or the recurrence of sores. Do not use this medication to prevent the recurrence of sores, because this may lead to the development of strains of the virus that are resistant to acyclovir. Do not use more of the ointment or use it more often or for longer than your doctor tells you.

Do not apply acyclovir ointment to your eyes unless your doctor directs you to do so.

Tell your doctor if you are pregnant or are breast-feeding a baby. It is not known if it is safe to use acyclovir during pregnancy or while breast-feeding.

DOSAGE
Your doctor will decide how much acyclovir you should use and how often you should apply it. It is usually used every three hours six times daily for seven days. Contact your doctor if your symptoms do not improve after seven days. Follow the instructions on your prescription label carefully and ask your doctor or pharmacist to explain any part you do not understand.

Wash and dry the skin area thoroughly before applying the medication. Use rubber gloves when applying the ointment to prevent spread of the infection. Use enough ointment to cover each sore. Rub the ointment into the affected area gently.

For best results, start using the ointment as soon as symptoms of infection appear. Try to keep the infected area clean and dry, and wear loose-fitting clothing to avoid irritating the sores.

If you forget a dose, apply the missed dose as soon as you remember it. Apply any remaining doses for that day at evenly spaced intervals. *Do not apply a double dose* to make up for the missed one.

STORAGE
Keep this medication in the container it came in, and store it at room temperature in a dry place. Keep it out of the reach of children. Do not allow anyone else to use this medication.

Inflammation of the Skin

The drugs described in this section are used to treat inflammation of the skin. Inflammation may be a symptom of an allergic reaction or the result of other skin conditions such as eczema or psoriasis.

Steroids are used to treat various inflammatory skin problems. In some cases, steroids are taken orally and used topically at the same time. Usually, minor skin problems are treated with topical ointments and creams, which help relieve redness and itching.

The topical steroids come in cream, ointment and aerosol forms. Your doctor will choose the form best suited to your condition and will give you specific instructions on how to use it.

TOPICAL STEROIDS

Betamethasone
(bay ta meth' a sone)

PRODUCT INFORMATION
Brand names: Benisone, Beta-Val, Celestone, Diprolene, Diprosone, Uticort, Valisone

USES
Betamethasone is a steroid or cortisone-like medicine that relieves the redness, itching and discomfort of many skin problems. Like all drugs of this type, betamethasone helps control the skin disease but does not cure it.

UNDESIRED EFFECTS
When you apply this medicine, a mild temporary stinging can be expected. Betamethasone can cause burning, itching, blistering or peeling of the skin not present before its use. If you experience any skin reactions or signs of irritation or infection when you use betamethasone, contact your doctor.

PRECAUTIONS
Before you start to use betamethasone, tell your doctor if you have an infection. This medicine can hide the symptoms of infection or make it worse.

If you are using this medicine on a baby's diaper area, do not place tightly fitting diapers or plastic pants on the baby. They can increase the chance that betamethasone will be absorbed through the skin. Such absorption can result in side effects and affect the child's growth. Whenever this medicine is used on a child, keep in touch with your doctor.

Use betamethasone exactly as prescribed by your doctor. Do not use it more often or longer than your doctor has ordered. If this medicine is applied too often, the chances of absorption through the skin and of side effects are increased. Using too much on thin skin areas such as the face, armpits and groin can result in thinning of the skin and stretch marks.

Unless directed by your doctor, do not bandage or otherwise wrap the area of skin being treated. Betamethasone is absorbed more quickly and in greater amounts when the treated area is covered. Check with your doctor or pharmacist if you have any questions.

Your doctor has prescribed this medicine for a specific skin problem. Do not apply it to other parts of your body or use it for other problems without your doctor's permission. Using betamethasone other than as directed by your doctor can create problems. This medicine should not be used against many bacterial, viral and fungal skin infections. Do not apply cosmetics, lotions or any other skin preparation to the area being treated unless you first check with your doctor.

To select the best treatment for you and your baby, tell your doctor if you are pregnant, plan to become pregnant or are breast-feeding.

DOSAGE

Your doctor will determine how often you should use betamethasone and how much you should use for each application. Carefully follow the instructions on your prescription label, and ask your doctor or pharmacist to explain any part of the instructions you do not understand.

Betamethasone comes in ointment, cream, gel, lotion and aerosol forms. Before applying it, clean your skin. Then apply a small amount and rub it in gently. If you are using the aerosol form, avoid breathing in the vapors from the spray. Do not use the aerosol near heat or an open flame or while smoking.

If you forget a dose, apply it as soon as you remember. Then apply the other applications at evenly spaced intervals. *Do not use twice as much to make up for the missed application.*

STORAGE

When your doctor tells you to stop using betamethasone, throw away any unused portion of the medication.

Keep betamethasone in the container it came in. Store the aerosol form away from heat and direct sunlight. Keep this medicine out of the reach of children. Do not allow anyone else to use your betamethasone; another person's skin problem may be very different from yours.

Fluocinolone and Fluocinonide
(floo oh sin′ oh lone) (floo oh sin′ oh nide)

PRODUCT INFORMATION
Brand names for fluocinolone: Fluonid, Flurosyn, Synalar, Synemol
Brand names for fluocinonide: Lidex, Lidex-E, Topsyn

USES
Fluocinolone and fluocinonide are closely related steroids or cortisone-like drugs that are applied to the skin to relieve the redness, itching and discomfort of many skin problems. The drugs control symptoms of a disease but do not cure it.

UNDESIRED EFFECTS
When you apply any form of these medicines (ointment, cream, gel or solution), you can expect a mild temporary stinging.

The drug can cause burning, itching, blistering or peeling of the skin not present before its use. Check with your doctor if you develop any skin reactions or signs of irritation or infection.

PRECAUTIONS
Before you start to use fluocinolone or fluocinonide, tell your doctor if you have an infection. These medicines can hide the symptoms of infection or make it worse.

If you are using either of these medicines on a baby's diaper area, do not place tightly fitting diapers or plastic pants on the baby. They can increase the chance that the medicine will be absorbed through the baby's skin. Such absorption can cause side effects and affect the baby's growth. Have your doctor check the baby frequently while you are using this medicine.

Do not use fluocinolone or fluocinonide more often or for a longer time than ordered by your doctor. If these medicines are applied too often, the chances of absorption through the skin and of side effects are increased. Thinning of the skin and stretch marks can occur if you use too much of these medicines on thin skin areas such as the face, armpits and groin.

Do not bandage or wrap the area of skin being treated unless your doctor has told you to do so. These medicines are absorbed more quickly and in larger amounts when the treated area is covered. If you have any questions, check with your doctor or pharmacist.

Do not use these medicines for any problem except the one for which they were prescribed; do not apply them to other parts of your body unless you have your doctor's permission. These medicines should not be used on many bacterial, viral and fungal skin infections, and only your doctor can determine the kind of skin problem you have. Do not apply cosmetics, lotions or any other skin preparation to the area being treated unless you first check with your doctor.

Be sure to tell your doctor if you are pregnant or plan to become pregnant while you are using these medicines in order to select the best treatment for both you and your baby.

DOSAGE

Your doctor will determine how often you should use these medicines and how much you should apply at each dose. Carefully follow the instructions on your prescription label, and ask your doctor or pharmacist to explain any part of the instructions you do not understand.

Fluocinolone and fluocinonide come in ointment, cream, gel or solution forms. Apply small amounts to clean skin and rub in gently. If your doctor has directed you to use a bandage or plastic film over the medicine, be sure you understand how to do this properly. Carefully follow your doctor's directions.

If you forget a dose, apply it as soon as you remember. Then apply the other doses at evenly spaced intervals. *Do not apply a double dose to make up for a missed one.*

If the skin problem for which either of these medicines was prescribed continues or gets worse, contact your doctor.

STORAGE

When your doctor tells you to stop using these medicines, throw away any unused portions.

Keep fluocinolone and fluocinonide in the containers they came in. Keep them out of the reach of children. Do not allow anyone else to use your medicine; another person's skin problem may be very different from yours.

Flurandrenolide

(flure an dren' oh lide)

PRODUCT INFORMATION

Brand names: Cordran, Cordran-N, Cordran SP

USES

Flurandrenolide is a steroid or cortisone-like medicine that is applied to the skin to relieve the redness, itching and discomfort of many skin problems. It controls symptoms of a skin disease but does not cure it.

UNDESIRED EFFECTS

When you apply the cream, lotion or ointment forms of this medicine, you probably will experience a mild temporary stinging.

Flurandrenolide can cause burning, itching, blistering or peeling of the skin not present before its use. Contact your doctor if you have any skin reactions or signs of infection or irritation that were not present before you started to apply flurandrenolide.

PRECAUTIONS

Before you start using flurandrenolide, tell your doctor if you have an infection. This medicine hides the symptoms of infection and can make an infection worse.

If you are using this medicine on a baby's diaper area, do not place tightly fitting diapers or plastic pants on the baby. They can increase the chance that flurandrenolide will be absorbed through the baby's skin. Such absorption can cause side effects and affect your baby's growth. The baby should be checked regularly by the doctor to determine the effect of the medicine.

Do not use flurandrenolide more often or longer than prescribed by your doctor. If applied too often, this medicine is likely to be absorbed into the skin and cause side effects. If you use too much of this medicine on thin skin areas such as the face, armpits and groin, thinning of the skin and stretch marks may result.

Unless your doctor has told you to do so, do not bandage or wrap the area of skin being treated. When the treated area is covered, flurandrenolide is absorbed more quickly and in larger amounts. If you have any questions, check with your doctor or pharmacist.

Do not apply this medicine to areas of the body other than those for which it was prescribed without your doctor's permission. Flurandrenolide should not be used on many bacterial, viral and fungal infections. If you develop a problem on another part of your body, see your doctor. Check with your doctor before you apply cosmetics, lotions or any other skin preparation to the area being treated.

Before you start to use flurandrenolide, tell your doctor if you are pregnant or plan to become pregnant while using this medicine. The safe use of this medicine for pregnant women has not been established.

DOSAGE

Your doctor will determine how often you should use this medicine and how much you should apply at each dose. Carefully follow the instructions on your prescription label, and ask your doctor or pharmacist to explain any part of the instructions you do not understand.

Flurandrenolide comes in cream, lotion and ointment forms and as a dressing tape. If you are using the cream, lotion or ointment, apply it to clean skin in small amounts and rub it in gently. The tape should be applied according to the directions. Do not use the tape under your arms, between your toes or in the groin area.

If you forget a dose, apply it as soon as you remember. Then apply the other doses at evenly spaced intervals. *Do not apply a double dose to make up for the missed one.*

STORAGE

When your doctor tells you to stop using flurandrenolide, throw away any unused portion. If your condition does not improve or if it gets worse, contact your doctor.

Keep flurandrenolide in the container it came in, and keep it out of the reach of children. Do not allow anyone else to use your flurandrenolide; another person's skin problem may be very different from yours and may require medical attention.

Hydrocortisone
(hye dro cor′ ti sone)

PRODUCT INFORMATION
Brand names: Acticort, Aeroseb-HC, Alphaderm, Anusol HC, Bactin, Carmol-HC, Cetacort, Cortaid, Cort-Dome, Cortef, Cortenema, Cortifoam, Cortiprel, Cortril, Cotacort, Cremesone, Delacort, Dermacort, Dermolate, Econsone, Eldecort, Epicort, Epifoam-HC, HC, Heb-Cort, Hexaderm, Hycort, Hytone, Kort, Lexocort, Microcort, My-Cort, Nutracort, Orabase HCA, Proctocort, Proctofoam-HC, Rectoid, Relecort, Texacort, Ulcort, Westcort and others

USES
Hydrocortisone is a steroid or cortisone-like medicine that is applied to the skin to relieve the redness, itching and discomfort of many skin problems. The drug controls a skin disease but does not cure it.

The paste form of hydrocortisone is applied to inflamed areas of ulcers in the mouth to provide temporary relief. Hydrocortisone enema and hydrocortisone foam are used with other types of therapy to relieve the inflammation of mild to moderate ulcerative colitis. Hydrocortisone rectal suppositories help relieve the redness and swelling of hemorrhoids.

UNDESIRED EFFECTS
When applied to the skin, the cream, gel, lotion, solution or aerosol forms of hydrocortisone will cause a mild temporary stinging.

Hydrocortisone can cause burning, itching, blistering or peeling of the skin not present before its use. With all forms of this medicine, if you have any skin reaction or signs of irritation or infection, contact your doctor.

PRECAUTIONS
Before you start to use any form of hydrocortisone, tell your doctor if you have an infection. This medicine may make the infection worse or hide its symptoms until it becomes a serious problem.

If you are using this medicine for a problem in your mouth, contact your doctor if your condition does not improve in one week, if it gets worse or if you notice signs of a throat or mouth infection.

When you use this medicine on a baby's diaper area, do not place tightly fitting diapers or plastic pants on the baby; they can increase the chance of absorption through the baby's skin. Absorption of hydrocortisone can result in side effects and affect your baby's growth. The baby should be checked regularly by a doctor to determine the effect of the medicine.

Use hydrocortisone exactly as directed by your doctor. Do not use it more often or longer than your doctor has ordered. If this medicine is used too often, there is a greater chance that it will be absorbed through the skin and cause side effects. If too much of this medicine is used on areas with thin skin such as the face, armpits and groin, it can cause thinning of the skin and stretch marks.

Do not bandage or wrap the area of skin being treated unless your doctor has told you to do so. Covering the treated area can cause the medicine to be absorbed more quickly and in larger amounts. Contact your doctor or pharmacist if you have any questions.

Your doctor has prescribed hydrocortisone for a particular skin problem. Do not use it on other parts of your body. See your doctor if you develop a problem on another part of your body. This medicine should not be used against many bacterial, viral and fungal infections. Do not apply cosmetics, lotions or any other skin preparation to the skin area being treated without your doctor's permission.

Before you start to use hydrocortisone, tell your doctor if you are pregnant, plan to become pregnant or are breast-feeding.

DOSAGE

Your doctor will determine how often you should use this medicine and how much you should apply at each dose. Carefully follow the instructions on your prescription label, and ask your doctor or pharmacist to explain any part of the instructions you do not understand.

Hydrocortisone comes in cream, gel, lotion, solution and aerosol forms to be applied to the skin and in enema, foam and suppository forms to be placed in the rectum. It is also available in an oral paste form. Your doctor will select the best form for your particular problem.

The cream, gel, lotion or solution should be applied to clean skin in small amounts and rubbed in gently. If your doctor has directed you to use a bandage or plastic film over the medicine, be sure you understand how to do this properly. Carefully follow your doctor's instructions.

The aerosol spray should be used according to the directions that come with it. Do not breathe in the vapors from the spray. Do not use the spray near heat, close to an open flame or while smoking.

The enema form comes with instructions that you should follow carefully. Lie on your left side while taking the enema and for 30 minutes afterward. Try to hold the enema for at least an hour or, better still, overnight. Keep in touch with your doctor while you are using the hydrocortisone enema so your progress can be checked and you can be told when to start using it less frequently.

Hydrocortisone rectal foam also comes with directions. Carefully read them before you use this form. A special applicator is provided and always should be used to apply the foam. *Do not insert any part of the aerosol container into the rectum.* After using the applicator, pull it apart and clean it thoroughly with warm water.

To use a rectal suppository, remove the foil wrapper and dip the tip of the suppository into water. Lie on your side, draw your top knee up to your chest and insert the suppository. Push it well up into the rectum with your finger and hold it there for a few moments. If the suppository is too soft to insert because it has been stored in a warm place, chill it in the refrigerator for 30 minutes or run cold water over it before removing the foil wrapper.

If you are using the oral paste form, press—but do not rub—a small amount of paste onto the area to be treated until the paste sticks and forms a smooth, slippery film. Apply hydrocortisone film at bedtime (so the medicine can work overnight) and after meals.

If you forget to apply a dose of hydrocortisone, do so as soon as you remember and then apply the other doses at evenly spaced intervals. *Do not apply a double dose to make up for a missed dose.*

STORAGE

When your doctor tells you to stop using hydrocortisone, throw away any unused portions.

Keep hydrocortisone in the container it came in. Store the aerosol container away from heat and direct sunlight. Keep this medicine out of the reach of children.

Do not allow anyone else to use your hydrocortisone; another person's skin problem may be very different from yours and may require medical attention.

MISCELLANEOUS

Isotretinoin
(eye soe tret' i noyn)

PRODUCT INFORMATION
Brand name: Accutane

USES

Isotretinoin is used to treat severe acne that has not responded to treatment with oral or topical anti-infectives. It also has been used investigationally for other skin disorders including psoriasis.

UNDESIRED EFFECTS

The most common side effects of isotretinoin are dry nose and mouth; red, cracked and sore lips; and red, itching and inflamed eyes. Contact your doctor if these side effects are severe. You should also contact your doctor if you experience pain or stiffness in the bones, muscles or joints; a rash; skin peeling; or infections.

PRECAUTIONS

Tell your doctor if you ever had a bad reaction to vitamin A or tretinoin (retinoic acid). Because taking isotretinoin can make some medical conditions worse, tell your doctor if you have diabetes, a high amount of triglycerides (fats) in your blood or a family history of high triglycerides in the blood.

Although it is not common, isotretinoin can make some people more sensitive to sunlight and sunlamps so limit your exposure to them while taking isotretinoin. Use a sunscreen preparation or wear protective clothing if you will be exposed to direct sunlight.

Limit your intake of alcoholic beverages while taking isotretinoin because they may increase the amount of triglycerides (fats) in your blood. Ask your doctor for advice on how much alcohol you should drink.

Because isotretinoin is similar to vitamin A, discontinue taking any vitamin supplements that contain vitamin A to avoid possible toxic reactions while taking isotretinoin.

Women who are pregnant, intend to become pregnant or are breast-feeding infants should tell their doctors before taking isotretinoin. Isotretinoin has been reported to cause serious harm to the unborn baby when taken during pregnancy. An effective method of birth control should be used while taking this drug and for one month after stopping it. If you think you may be pregnant, stop taking isotretinoin.

DOSAGE

Isotretinoin comes in capsules to be taken by mouth. Your prescription label tells you how much and how often to take the drug. Follow carefully the instructions on the label, and ask your doctor or pharmacist to explain any part you do not understand.

It may take four to six weeks before improvement is seen, and your skin may actually look worse during the first few weeks of taking isotretinoin. Ask your doctor if you have questions about how long to take this drug.

If you forget to take a dose, take the missed dose as soon as you remember it. However, if you remember a missed dose near the time you are scheduled to take the next dose, take only the regularly scheduled dose. *Do not take a double dose to make up for a missed dose.*

STORAGE

Keep isotretinoin in the container it came in, tightly closed and away from light. Keep this medication out of the reach of children, and do not let anyone else take it without a doctor's supervision.

Tretinoin
(tret' i noyn)

PRODUCT INFORMATION
Brand name: Retin-A
Other names: Retinoic Acid, Vitamin A Acid

USES

Tretinoin is used to treat acne. It promotes the peeling of affected skin areas and unclogs pores. Tretinoin therapy will control acne but not cure it.

Tretinoin also has been used investigationally for the treatment of flat warts and some skin conditions such as psoriasis.

UNDESIRED EFFECTS

Tretinoin may cause redness, warmth and stinging of the skin. If these problems are severe, use less than a full dose each time you apply this medication; gradually increase the amount you use until you are able to use a full dose without experiencing discomfort. If you have any questions regarding how much medication to use, ask your doctor or pharmacist.

Tretinoin may also cause temporary lightening or darkening of the skin.

PRECAUTIONS
Try to stay out of direct sunlight, wind and cold weather as much as you can. Do not use a sunlamp while using tretinoin. Use a sunscreen preparation or wear protective clothing if you will be exposed to direct sunlight. Do not use this medication while you have a sunburn. Do not use medicated or abrasive soaps or cleansers, soaps and cosmetics that dry the skin a lot, or soaps, cleansers or other cosmetic products containing a lot of alcohol, astringents, spices or lime. If you have any questions about what kinds of soaps or cleansers you may use, ask your pharmacist.

Do not wash your face more than two or three times a day while using this medication.

DOSAGE
Your doctor has determined how often you should use this medication and how much you should use each time. It is usually applied once a day at bedtime. Follow carefully the instructions on your prescription label, and ask your doctor or pharmacist to explain any part you do not understand.

Tretinoin comes in cream, gel, and liquid forms for use on the skin. To use tretinoin, follow these steps:
1. Wash your hands and the affected area with soap and water and let them dry thoroughly.
2. Use your fingertips, a gauze pad, cotton swab or a prepared swab to apply the medication.

Your acne may seem to get worse during the first few weeks you use this medication. Nevertheless, continue to use it. Do not expect to see results until about three weeks after you begin using the medication, and do not expect maximum results until about six weeks after you begin. Ask your doctor if you may use cosmetics. If you can, always be sure to clean the skin thoroughly with soap and water to remove the cosmetics before applying the medication.

Do not let the medication touch your eyes, nose, mouth or open wounds.

Do not use this medication more often than once a day.

STORAGE
Keep the container of this medication closed tightly. Store it at room temperature, away from excess heat and moisture.

Keep this medication out of the reach of children.

Asthma and Other Breathing Problems

DRUGS USED TO TREAT ASTHMA AND OTHER BREATHING PROBLEMS

Asthma

Asthma is a condition characterized by repeated attacks of wheezing, shortness of breath, difficulty in breathing and, occasionally, pain in the chest. During an asthma attack, the air passages—primarily the bronchi in the lungs—narrow and go into spasm. The spasms occur in response to stimulation or irritation by, for example, pollen from trees or flowers or from emotional stress, excitement or numerous other causes. When the air passages are in spasm, air flow is partially obstructed, causing wheezing, shortness of breath and difficult breathing.

Narrowing of the air passages also occurs in bronchial infection, pulmonary emphysema and some kinds of congestive heart failure. It is often difficult even for a doctor to diagnose asthma and to distinguish it from other conditions that cause breathing problems.

Drugs used to treat asthma are called bronchodilators. They relax the muscle spasm in the air passages and relieve shortness of breath. Relief usually is quick— within an hour for tablets taken orally and within 20 minutes for products used by inhalation. If a bronchodilator does not provide excellent and rapid relief from an asthma attack, the patient should seek medical attention immediately.

Some drugs are useful only in *preventing* attacks of asthma and will not help to stop an attack once it has started. Other drugs can be used to stop an attack once it is underway.

Drugs described here, with the exception of cromolyn (page 218), are used in the treatment and prevention of asthma, chronic bronchitis, emphysema and other lung diseases. Cromolyn is not a bronchodilator and is used only to prevent asthma.

Steroids, in the form of an inhalation or tablets taken orally, may be used to treat bronchial asthma. By injection, steroids also can be used to treat acute episodes of asthma. Prolonged treatment of asthma with steroids should be reserved for patients with disabling asthma that is not responsive to other drugs.

BRONCHODILATORS

Albuterol
(al byoo′ ter ole)

PRODUCT INFORMATION
Brand names: Proventil, Ventolin

USES
Albuterol is a bronchodilator used to relieve wheezing, shortness of breath and

troubled breathing caused by asthma, bronchitis and emphysema. It relaxes and increases the size of the air passages to the lungs, making it easier to breathe.

It is longer acting (up to six hours) and may cause less of an increase in heart rate than isoproterenol.

UNDESIRED EFFECTS

The most common side effects of albuterol are dryness of the mouth and throat, nervousness, restlessness and trouble sleeping. You can experience dryness of the mouth and throat after using the inhalation form of this medicine. The dryness can be relieved by rinsing your mouth with water after each inhalation. The other effects, which can result after you take any form of albuterol, tend to decrease as you continue to take it and as your body adjusts to it. If they continue or bother you, contact your doctor.

Less often, albuterol will cause dizziness or lightheadedness, flushing or redness of the face or skin, headache, nausea or vomiting, trembling, increase in sweating, fast or pounding heartbeat or weakness. Contact your doctor if these effects are severe. It may be necessary to adjust your dosage or change your medication.

More serious side effects, which require medical attention if they occur, are chest pain and irregular heartbeat. Stop using albuterol and contact your doctor if you experience either of these effects.

Contact your doctor if your sputum (the matter you cough up during an asthma attack) becomes thickened or changes color from clear white to yellow, green or gray. These changes may be signs of an infection that requires immediate treatment.

PRECAUTIONS

Before you start to take albuterol, tell your doctor if you ever had an unusual reaction to this drug or to similar drugs, including amphetamines, ephedrine, epinephrine, isoproterenol, metaproterenol, norepinephrine, phenylephrine, phenylpropanolamine, pseudoephedrine or terbutaline.

Albuterol can make certain medical conditions worse. Be sure to tell your doctor if you have diabetes, heart or blood vessel disease, high blood pressure or an overactive thyroid.

Tell your doctor what prescription or nonprescription drugs you are taking, including amphetamines, any of the albuterol-like drugs, other medicines for your heart or for asthma or other breathing problems, beta blockers such as propranolol (medicine for high blood pressure), MAO inhibitors (isocarboxazid, pargyline, phenelzine and tranylcypromine) or antidepressant medications. If you do not know the names of the drugs or what they were prescribed for, bring them in their labeled containers to your doctor or pharmacist.

Use this medicine only as you have been directed by your doctor. Do not use more of it and do not use it more often than instructed. *Keep all appointments for checkups.*

If you are pregnant or are nursing a baby, tell your doctor so that you receive the albuterol treatment that is best for both you and your baby.

DOSAGE

Your doctor will determine how often you should take albuterol and how much you should take at each dose. Carefully follow the instructions on your prescription label, and ask your doctor or pharmacist to explain any part of the instructions you do not understand.

Albuterol comes as an aerosol inhalation and as tablets to be swallowed.

If you use the aerosol form, turn the inhaler upside down to use it. Place the mouthpiece in your mouth, and close your lips and teeth around it. Breathe out as much air through your nose as you possibly can. Then take a deep breath through the mouthpiece and, at the same time, press down on the container. Be sure the mist goes into your throat and is not blocked by your teeth or tongue.

Hold your breath for five seconds, remove the inhaler and exhale through your nose. Wait one to five minutes to see whether you need another inhalation. Do not take more than two inhalations at one time.

If you give a treatment to a young child, it may be best to hold the child's nose closed to be sure the medication goes into the throat.

After each use, wash the mouthpiece of the inhaler with warm water. Be sure to follow your doctor's instructions on the use of this medication. Do not take it more often than prescribed, and do not take more inhalation treatments than indicated without checking with your doctor. Drink a lot of fluids each day.

If you are taking this drug on a regular schedule and forget a dose, take the missed dose as soon as you remember. If you remember a missed dose near the time you are to take the next one, take only your regularly scheduled dose. *Do not take a double dose.*

STORAGE
Keep this medication away from excessive heat and in the container it came in. Keep this medication out of the reach of children.

Ephedrine
(e fed' rin)

PRODUCT INFORMATION
Brand names: Ectasule Minus, Ephedsol and others

Brand names of some of the many products containing ephedrine in combination with other bronchodilators and other drugs: Amesec, Bronkolixir, Bronkotabs, Marax, Mudrane, Quadrinal, Quibron, Tedral and others

USES
Ephedrine is used as a bronchodilator to relax the nerves of the lungs and enlarge the air passages to relieve wheezing, shortness of breath and difficult breathing. It is used in the prevention and treatment of asthma, chronic bronchitis, emphysema and other lung diseases. It also will relieve nasal congestion caused by hay fever and other allergies and is found in some cold products.

The injectable form of ephedrine is used to treat severe asthma attacks and, along with other measures, to treat shock. The oral forms often are used with other drugs to relieve the symptoms of myasthenia gravis.

UNDESIRED EFFECTS

The most common side effects of ephedrine are nervousness, restlessness and trouble sleeping. If you take the last dose for the day a few hours before bedtime, you should be able to sleep. Nervousness and restlessness may go away as you continue to take this medication and as your body adjusts to it. If these problems are persistent or severe, contact your doctor. Your doctor may want to adjust the dosage or change your medication.

Less often, ephedrine may cause difficult or painful urination, dizziness or lightheadedness, a feeling of warmth, headache, loss of appetite, nausea or vomiting, trembling, troubled breathing, increase in sweating, paleness, fast or pounding heartbeat or weakness. If you experience these effects, contact your doctor.

More serious effects of ephedrine are chest pain and irregular heartbeat. Stop taking the medicine and contact your doctor if you experience either of these effects.

High doses of ephedrine may give you hallucinations (seeing, hearing or feeling things that are not there) and mood or mental changes. If you have any of these problems, stop taking the medicine and contact your doctor.

PRECAUTIONS

Before you start to take a product containing ephedrine, tell your doctor or pharmacist if you have diabetes, an enlarged prostate, glaucoma, heart or blood vessel disease or an overactive thyroid. Ephedrine can make these conditions worse and should be taken only under a doctor's supervision.

Tell your doctor or pharmacist what prescription or nonprescription drugs you are taking. Ephedrine can increase or decrease the effects of amphetamines, digitalis drugs (heart medicine), medicine for high blood pressure such as propranolol, guanethidine or reserpine, other medicine for asthma, other medicine for hay fever or allergies, medicine to decrease bleeding after delivery of a baby (ergonovine or methylergonovine) and medicine for depression. If you do not know the names of the drugs you are taking or what they were prescribed for, bring them in their labeled containers to your doctor or pharmacist.

Because many products containing ephedrine are available without a prescription, be sure to use them only as directed on the package label or as instructed by your doctor. Do not take ephedrine more often than recommended on the label. If you have any questions, check with your doctor or pharmacist.

No one who ever had an unusual reaction to medicines chemically similar to ephedrine (amphetamines, epinephrine, isoproterenol, metaproterenol, norepinephrine, phenylephrine, phenylpropanolamine, pseudoephedrine or terbutaline) should take ephedrine or products containing ephedrine.

Do not use ephedrine or products containing ephedrine if you are breast-feeding a baby. It will be passed to the baby through your milk. If you are pregnant, do not use any products containing ephedrine unless your doctor tells you to.

DOSAGE

If your doctor has prescribed ephedrine, he or she has determined how often you should take this medicine and how much you should take at each dose. Carefully follow the instructions on your prescription label, and ask your doctor or pharmacist to explain any part of the instructions you do not understand. If you have obtained ephedrine or a product containing it without a prescription, follow the instructions on the label or in the package.

Ephedrine comes in capsules, extended-release capsules, tablets and liquid form (all to be taken orally) and as a nasal solution and spray. If you are taking the extended-release capsules, be sure to swallow them whole. Do not crush, break or chew them before swallowing. If the capsule is too large to swallow, empty the contents into applesauce, jelly, honey or syrup. Stir to mix and then swallow without chewing.

Measure doses of the liquid with a specially marked measuring spoon to make sure you have an accurate dose.

If you forget to take a dose of ephedrine, take it as soon as you remember and then take the remaining doses for that day at evenly spaced intervals. If it is almost time for another dose, omit the missed dose and take only the regularly scheduled dose. *Do not take a double dose to make up for the missed dose.*

STORAGE

Keep ephedrine in the container it came in, and keep it out of the reach of children. Do not allow anyone else to take your ephedrine.

Epinephrine
(ep i nef′ rin)

PRODUCT INFORMATION

Brand names: Adrenalin, Bronkaid, Medihaler-Epi, microNEFRIN, Primatene, Sus-Phrine, S-2, Vaponefrin and others

USES

Epinephrine is used as a bronchodilator to treat asthma, chronic bronchitis, emphysema and other lung diseases. It acts on the muscles and blood vessels of the lungs to open air passages by relieving muscle spasm, swelling and congestion. As a result, wheezing, shortness of breath and difficult breathing are relieved.

Epinephrine injection is used frequently in the *emergency* treatment of allergic reactions to insect stings, medicines, food and other substances. Some inhalation preparations of epinephrine are available without a prescription.

UNDESIRED EFFECTS

Use of inhaled epinephrine can cause dryness of the mouth and throat. If you rinse your mouth with water after using this medicine, you may be able to prevent this dryness. Coughing and other signs of bronchial irritation can occur after inhaling epinephrine. If these effects are severe, contact your doctor. Your doctor may want to change the strength of the solution you are using.

With the injectable form of epinephrine and sometimes with the inhalation form (because this medicine can be absorbed into the body through the tissues of the air passages), other effects may occur. The following effects usually decrease as you continue to use epinephrine and as your body adjusts to it: dizziness or lightheadedness; flushing or redness of the face or skin; headache; nausea or vomiting; nervousness, restlessness or trouble sleeping; trembling; troubled breathing; increase in sweating; paleness or weakness; and fast or pounding heartbeat. Contact your doctor if any of these effects are persistent or severe.

More serious side effects of epinephrine, which may require medical attention, are chest pain and irregular heartbeat. If you experience either of these effects, stop using the medicine and contact your doctor.

PRECAUTIONS

Do not take epinephrine if you ever had an unusual reaction to epinephrine or any of the medicines similar to it, such as amphetamines, ephedrine, isoproterenol, metaproterenol, norepinephrine, phenylephrine, phenylpropanolamine, pseudoephedrine or terbutaline.

Before you start to use epinephrine, tell your doctor or pharmacist if you have diabetes, glaucoma, brain damage, heart or blood vessel disease, high blood pressure or an overactive thyroid. This medicine can make these conditions worse.

Tell your doctor or pharmacist what prescription or nonprescription drugs you are taking, including any of the epinephrine-like drugs (see above), oral medicine for diabetes, insulin, medicine for high blood pressure (such as guanethidine, propranolol or reserpine), medicine for pheochromocytoma or blood vessel disease (such as phenoxybenzamine, phentolamine or tolazoline), medicine for angina attacks (such as nitroglycerin), other medicine for asthma or breathing problems, sedatives or tranquilizers, medicine for depression, medicine to decrease bleeding after delivery of a baby (ergonovine or methylergonovine) and antihistamines. If you do not know the names of the drugs you are taking or what they were prescribed for, bring them in their labeled containers to your doctor or pharmacist.

Do not use the solution for inhalation or injection if it has turned pinkish to brownish in color or if it is cloudy. This means the epinephrine has deteriorated and may no longer be effective.

Do not use the inhalation form of epinephrine without a doctor's prescription unless a doctor has diagnosed your problem as asthma. If you still have trouble breathing 20 minutes after using the inhalation form or if your condition gets worse, stop using the medicine and check with your doctor.

Use epinephrine exactly as directed. Do not use any more of it and do not use it any more often than recommended on the label. *Keep all appointments for checkups.*

If you have diabetes, epinephrine may cause your blood sugar levels to rise. Contact your doctor if you notice a change in the results of your urine sugar test.

Tell your doctor if you are pregnant or are nursing a baby. Epinephrine should not be used by women who are pregnant or think they may be or by women who are breast-feeding babies.

DOSAGE

Your doctor will determine how often you should use epinephrine and how much you should use at each dose. Carefully follow the instructions on your prescription label, and ask your doctor or pharmacist to explain any part of the instructions you do not understand.

Epinephrine comes in three forms—inhalation, aerosol inhalation and injection. If you use the inhalation form in a nebulizer or a combination nebulizer and respirator, be sure you understand exactly how to use it. If you have any questions, check with your doctor or pharmacist.

If you use the aerosol form, keep the spray away from your eyes. Do not take more than two inhalations at one time, unless directed otherwise by your doctor. Wait one or two minutes after the first inhalation to determine if you need a second one. Save your applicator because refill units of this medicine may be available.

If you use the injection form and plan to give yourself injections, be sure you know how to do this properly. If you have any questions, check with your doctor or pharmacist.

STORAGE

Keep all forms of epinephrine in the containers they came in, and store them away from heat and direct sunlight. Keep epinephrine out of the reach of children. Do not allow anyone else to use it.

Isoetharine
(eye soe eth' a reen)

PRODUCT INFORMATION
Brand names: Bronkometer, Bronkosol

USES

Isoetharine is a bronchodilator that opens the air passages to the lungs, permitting air to move in and out more easily. It is used to treat asthma, bronchitis and emphysema.

Isoetharine is slightly longer acting and causes less of an increase in heart rate than isoproterenol.

UNDESIRED EFFECTS

The most common side effects of isoetharine are fast heartbeat, palpitation of the heart, weakness, tremors or shaking, feeling of excitement, difficulty in sleeping and nausea and vomiting. Contact your doctor if these side effects persist or are bothersome. It may be necessary to reduce the dosage or frequency with which you are taking it. If fast heartbeat or palpitations occur, stop taking this medication and contact your doctor.

PRECAUTIONS
Before you start to take isoetharine, tell your doctor if you ever had an unusual reaction to this drug or to similar drugs, including albuterol, amphetamines, ephedrine, epinephrine, isoproterenol, metaproterenol, norepinephrine, phenylephrine, phenylpropanolamine, pseudoephedrine or terbutaline.

Before you begin to use this medication, tell your doctor about all prescription and nonprescription medications you are taking, including Primatene, beta blockers such as propranolol (for high blood pressure), isoetharine-like drugs, amphetamines, and other medicines for your heart, asthma or other breathing problems. Isoetharine may make certain medical conditions worse. Be sure to tell your doctor if you have diabetes, high blood pressure, heart or blood vessel disease or an overactive thyroid.

Use this medication only as directed by your doctor. Do not use it more often than every four hours.

If you are pregnant or are nursing a baby, tell your doctor. Your doctor can then select the isoetharine treatment that is best for you and your baby.

DOSAGE
Isoetharine is used after acute asthma attacks or on a regular basis in treating chronic airway spasms in asthma, bronchitis or emphysema.

Your doctor will determine how often you should take this drug. Carefully follow the instructions on your prescription label, and ask your doctor or pharmacist to explain any part of the instructions you do not understand.

Isoetharine comes in a liquid that is to be inhaled with the use of a special inhaler. To use the inhaler, place the mouthpiece in your mouth. Take a deep breath and squeeze the bulb of the inhaler at the same time. Hold your breath for four or five seconds. Breathe out.

STORAGE
Keep this medication in the container it came in, and keep the container away from excess heat or light. Keep this medication out of the reach of children.

Isoproterenol
(eye soe proe ter' e nole)

PRODUCT INFORMATION
Brand names: Aerolone, Iprenol, Isuprel, Medihaler-Iso, Norisodrine, Proterenol, Vapo-N-Iso

USES
Isoproterenol is used as a bronchodilator to relieve wheezing, shortness of breath and troubled breathing caused by asthma, chronic bronchitis, emphysema or other lung diseases. It does this by relaxing the muscles in the air passages in the lungs

and by counteracting histamine, one of the body's natural substances that can cause spasm of the airways.

Isoproterenol is also used to treat certain heart disorders.

UNDESIRED EFFECTS

The most common effects of isoproterenol are dryness of the mouth and throat, nervousness, restlessness and trouble sleeping. You can experience dryness of the mouth and throat after using an inhalation form of this medicine. The dryness can be relieved by rinsing your mouth with water after each inhalation. The other effects, which can result after you take any form of isoproterenol, tend to decrease as you continue to take it and as your body adjusts to it. If they continue or bother you, contact your doctor.

Less often, isoproterenol will cause dizziness or lightheadedness, flushing or redness of the face or skin, headache, nausea or vomiting, trembling, increase in sweating, fast or pounding heartbeat or weakness. Contact your doctor if these effects are severe. Your doctor may want to adjust your dosage or change your medication.

More serious side effects, which require medical attention if they occur, are chest pain and irregular heartbeat. Stop using isoproterenol and contact your doctor if you experience either of these effects.

Isoproterenol may cause your saliva to turn pink or red. This effect is harmless and happens only because isoproterenol turns red when it is exposed to air.

Contact your doctor if your sputum (the matter you cough up during an asthma attack) becomes thickened or changes color from clear white to yellow, green or gray. These changes may be signs of an infection that requires immediate treatment.

PRECAUTIONS

Before you start to take isoproterenol, tell your doctor if you ever had an unusual reaction to this drug or to similar drugs, including albuterol, amphetamines, ephedrine, epinephrine, metaproterenol, norepinephrine, phenylephrine, phenylpropanolamine, pseudoephedrine or terbutaline.

Isoproterenol can make certain medical conditions worse. Be sure to tell your doctor if you have diabetes, heart or blood vessel disease, high blood pressure or an overactive thyroid.

Tell your doctor what prescription or nonprescription drugs you are taking, including amphetamines, any of the isoproterenol-like drugs, other medicines for your heart or for asthma or other breathing problems or beta blockers such as propranolol (medicine for high blood pressure). If you do not know the names of the drugs or what they were prescribed for, bring them in their labeled containers to your doctor or pharmacist.

Do not use more than two inhalations of isoproterenol at one time. If, after you have used the inhalation form as instructed, you still have trouble breathing or your condition gets worse, contact your doctor at once.

Use this medicine only as you have been directed by your doctor. Do not use more of it and do not use it more often than instructed. *Keep all of your appointments for checkups.*

If you are using the inhalation form of isoproterenol, do not use the solution if it has turned pinkish or brownish or if it has become cloudy.

If you are pregnant or are nursing a baby, tell your doctor. Your doctor can then select the isoproterenol treatment that is best for both you and your baby.

DOSAGE

Your doctor will determine how often you should take isoproterenol and how much you should take at each dose. Carefully follow the instructions on your prescription label, and ask your doctor or pharmacist to explain any part of the instructions you do not understand.

Isoproterenol comes in a solution for inhalation, aerosol inhalation, tablets to be swallowed and tablets to be dissolved under the tongue. If you use the inhalation solution in a nebulizer, be sure you know exactly how to use it. With the dropper provided, place in the nebulizer only that amount of solution needed for a single day's treatment. If you have any questions, ask your doctor or pharmacist.

If you use the aerosol form, turn the inhaler upside down to use it. Place the mouthpiece in your mouth, and close your lips and teeth around it. Breathe out as much air through your nose as you possibly can. Then take a deep breath through the mouthpiece and, at the same time, press down on the container. Be sure the mist goes into your throat and is not blocked by your teeth or tongue.

Hold your breath for five seconds, remove the inhaler and exhale through your nose. Wait one to five minutes to see whether you need another inhalation. Do not take more than two inhalations at one time.

If you give a treatment to a young child, it may be best to hold the child's nose closed to be sure the medication goes into the throat.

If you take the under-the-tongue tablets, do not chew or swallow them. This medicine is absorbed through the lining of the mouth as it dissolves slowly under your tongue. Do not swallow until the tablets have dissolved completely.

If you take isoproterenol extended-release tablets, be sure to swallow the tablets whole. Do not break, crush or chew these tablets before swallowing them.

STORAGE

Keep isoproterenol in the container it came in and away from heat and sunlight. Save the aerosol container; refill units of this medicine may be available. Keep this medicine out of the reach of children. Do not allow anyone else to take it.

Metaproterenol
(met a proe ter' e nole)

PRODUCT INFORMATION
Brand names: Alupent, Metaprel

USES
Metaproterenol is used as a bronchodilator to relax and increase the size of the

air passages in the lungs and make it easier to breathe. It is used to relieve the wheezing, shortness of breath and difficult breathing associated with asthma, bronchitis, emphysema and other lung diseases.

Although metaproterenol is similar to isoproterenol, metaproterenol works for a longer time and is more effective when taken as a tablet.

UNDESIRED EFFECTS

The most common side effects of metaproterenol are nervousness and restlessness. Generally, these effects tend to decrease as you continue to take metaproterenol and as your body adjusts to it. If they continue or are severe, contact your doctor. Using the inhalation form of metaproterenol may make your mouth and throat dry. To relieve this problem, rinse your mouth with water after each treatment.

You also may notice a bad taste in your mouth. This effect is harmless and will go away when you stop taking metaproterenol.

Less often, metaproterenol will cause dizziness or lightheadedness; headache; muscle cramps in the arms, hands or legs; nausea or vomiting; trembling; increase in sweating; fast or pounding heartbeat; or weakness. If you experience these effects and they are severe, contact your doctor.

More serious side effects are chest pain and irregular heartbeat. If either of these occurs, it requires medical attention. Stop taking the medicine and contact your doctor.

If your sputum (the matter you cough up during an asthma attack) becomes thick or changes color from clear white to yellow, gray or green, contact your doctor. These changes may be signs of an infection that requires immediate treatment.

PRECAUTIONS

People who have had an unusual reaction to metaproterenol in the past or to any of the drugs like metaproterenol should not take this medicine. Tell your doctor if you ever had a reaction to albuterol, amphetamines, ephedrine, epinephrine, isoproterenol, norepinephrine, phenylephrine, phenylpropanolamine, pseudoephedrine or terbutaline.

Before you start to take metaproterenol, tell your doctor if you have diabetes, heart or blood vessel disease, high blood pressure or an overactive thyroid. Metaproterenol may make these conditions worse.

Tell your doctor what prescription or nonprescription drugs you are taking, including amphetamines, other medicine for your heart or for asthma or other breathing problems or beta blockers such as propranolol (medicine for high blood pressure). If you do not know the names of the drugs or what they were prescribed for, take them in their labeled containers to your doctor or pharmacist.

Take this medicine exactly as directed. Do not take more of it and do not take it more often than your doctor has ordered. If you still have trouble breathing after you have used metaproterenol as directed or if your condition gets worse, contact your doctor. *Keep all appointments for checkups.*

Metaproterenol should not be taken by children under the age of six years. It should not be taken by pregnant women or nursing mothers. Be sure to tell your doctor if you are pregnant or think you may be or if you are breast-feeding a baby. This will help your doctor select the best treatment for you and your baby.

DOSAGE
Your doctor will determine how often you should take metaproterenol and how much you should take at each dose. Carefully follow the directions on your prescription label, and ask your doctor or pharmacist to explain any part you do not understand.

Metaproterenol comes in a metered-dose inhaler and in tablets and liquid to be taken by mouth. If you are using the inhaler, turn it upside down and place the mouthpiece in your mouth. Close your lips and teeth around the mouthpiece, and breathe out as much as possible through your nose. Then take a deep breath through the mouthpiece and, at the same time, press down on the container to spray the medication into your mouth. Hold your breath for five seconds. Remove the inhaler from your mouth, and exhale through your nose or mouth. Wait one full minute to decide whether you need another treatment. Do not take more than two inhalations at one time.

If you take tablets or liquid on a regular basis and forget to take a dose, take it as soon as you remember. Take any remaining doses for that day at evenly spaced intervals. If you remember a missed dose at the time you are to take another, take only the regularly scheduled dose. Omit the missed dose entirely. *Do not take a double dose to make up for the missed one.*

STORAGE
Keep metaproterenol in the container it came in. Store it away from heat and direct sunlight. Keep it out of the reach of children. Do not allow anyone else to take your metaproterenol.

Terbutaline
(ter byoo' ta leen)

PRODUCT INFORMATION
Brand names: Brethine, Bricanyl

USES
Terbutaline is used as a bronchodilator to relax the muscles of the air passages in the lungs, making it easier to breathe. It is used to relieve the wheezing, shortness of breath and other breathing problems caused by asthma, bronchitis and emphysema. Terbutaline begins to work in 30 minutes and continues to work for four to eight hours.

UNDESIRED EFFECTS
Nervousness, restlessness and trembling are the most common effects of terbutaline. These effects tend to decrease or disappear as you continue to take terbutaline

and as your body adjusts to it. If they persist or are severe, contact your doctor. Your doctor may want to adjust the dose or change your medication.

Other effects, which do not require medical treatment unless they are severe, are dizziness or lightheadedness, drowsiness, headache, muscle cramps or twitching, nausea or vomiting, increase in sweating, fast or pounding heartbeat and weakness.

PRECAUTIONS

If you ever had an unusual reaction to terbutaline or to drugs like it, you should not take terbutaline. Before you start to take terbutaline, tell your doctor if you ever had a reaction to albuterol, amphetamines, ephedrine, epinephrine, isoproterenol, metaproterenol, norepinephrine, phenylephrine, phenylpropanolamine or pseudo-ephedrine.

If you have diabetes, heart disease, high blood pressure, an overactive thyroid or a history of seizures, tell your doctor before your start to take terbutaline.

Tell your doctor what prescription or nonprescription drugs you are taking, including amphetamines, other medicine for your heart or for asthma or other breathing problems and beta blockers such as propranolol (medicine for high blood pressure). If you do not know the names of the drugs you are taking or what they were prescribed for, bring them in their labeled containers to your doctor or pharmacist.

Take terbutaline exactly as your doctor has directed. Do not take more of it and do not take it more often than your doctor has told you. If you still have trouble breathing after using terbutaline or if your condition becomes worse, contact your doctor at once. *Keep all appointments for checkups.*

If you are breast-feeding a baby or are pregnant or think you may become pregnant while taking terbutaline, tell your doctor. While problems have not been reported, your doctor will want to consider the benefit of this treatment to you against the possible risk to your baby.

DOSAGE

Your doctor will determine how often you should take terbutaline tablets and how much you should take at each dose. Carefully follow the instructions on your prescription label, and ask your doctor or pharmacist to explain any part of the instructions you do not understand.

If you forget to take a dose of terbutaline, take it as soon as you remember and take any remaining doses for that day at evenly spaced intervals. If you remember a missed dose when it is close to the time for you to take another, omit the missed dose and take only the regularly scheduled dose. *Do not take a double dose to make up for the missed dose.*

STORAGE

Keep terbutaline in the container it came in, and keep it out of the reach of children. Do not allow anyone else to take your terbutaline.

Theophyllines
(thee off' i lin)

PRODUCT INFORMATION
Brand names of products containing aminophylline: Aminodur, Lixaminol, Panamin, Somophyllin and others
Brand names of products containing dyphylline: Airet, Dilor, Lufyllin, Neothylline
Brand name of a product containing oxtriphylline: Choledyl
Brand names of products containing theophylline: Bronkodyl, Elixophyllin, Slo-Phyllin, Somophyllin, Sustaire, Synophylate, Theo-Dur, Theolair
Brand names of combination products containing theophylline or one of these related drugs with other drugs: Brondecon, Mudrane, Quibron, Theokin

USES
Aminophylline, dyphylline and oxtriphylline are chemically related to theophylline. These drugs have similar uses, undesired effects and precautions.

Theophylline (and theophylline-related drugs) act as bronchodilators, which means that they open air passages in the lungs to make it easier to breathe. They are particularly effective when wheezing, shortness of breath and other breathing problems are caused by spasm of the air passages. They are used primarily to treat bronchial asthma, chronic bronchitis, emphysema and other lung problems.

UNDESIRED EFFECTS
One common side effect of theophylline (and similar drugs) is irritation of the stomach and bowels. When you start to take this medicine, you may experience nausea, vomiting, stomach pain, abdominal cramps, loss of appetite and, rarely, diarrhea. These effects can be relieved by taking the medicine with meals or a light snack. If you continue to have these problems, contact your doctor.

Theophylline and related drugs also stimulate the central nervous system and can cause headache, irritability, nervousness, restlessness, trouble sleeping and dizziness or lightheadedness. These effects usually are more severe in children than in adults. If you experience these effects and they do not lessen or disappear as you continue to take this medication and as your body adjusts to it, contact your doctor. It may be necessary to adjust the dose or change your medication.

Other effects, which are usually temporary, are flushing or redness of the face and fast breathing.

If you get a skin rash or hives from this medication, it means you are allergic to it. Stop taking it and contact your doctor.

Overdose can be a problem with theophylline and theophylline-related drugs, particularly with the rectal suppository form. Some signs of overdose are cloudy urine, increased urination, mental confusion, muscle twitching, unusual thirst, unusual tiredness or weakness, unusually fast or irregular heartbeat, bloody or black stools and vomiting up blood or material that looks like coffee grounds. Contact your doctor at once if you have any of these effects.

PRECAUTIONS

If you ever had an unusual reaction to aminophylline, caffeine, dyphylline, oxtriphylline or theophylline, tell your doctor before you start to take this medicine.

This medication can make certain medical problems worse. Be sure to tell your doctor if you have an enlarged prostate, heart or blood vessel disease, high blood pressure, kidney or liver disease, overactive thyroid, porphyria or stomach ulcer.

Certain medication should not be taken while you are taking theophylline or similar drugs. Tell your doctor what other prescription or nonprescription drugs you are taking, including erythromycins, lithium, other medicine for your heart or for asthma or other breathing problems, propranolol (medicine for high blood pressure), clindamycin and lincomycin. If you do not know the names of the drugs or what they were prescribed for, bring them in their labeled containers to your doctor or pharmacist.

Many nonprescription medicines for relief of asthma or breathing problems contain theophylline. Taking prescription theophylline with these over-the-counter medications can cause upset stomach, nausea and vomiting or overdose (see Undesired Effects). To avoid taking these drugs together without realizing it, *carefully check the labels of all nonprescription medicines you are taking to make sure that they do not contain theophylline.* If you have any questions, ask your doctor or pharmacist.

Beverages that also stimulate the central nervous system, such as tea, coffee, cocoa and colas, should not be consumed in large amounts while you are taking this medication.

Take your medication exactly as your doctor has directed. It can be harmful if you take more of it, take it more often or take it for a longer time than ordered by your doctor.

Your doctor will want to check your response to this drug, especially for the first few weeks after you begin to take it. *Be sure to keep all your appointments with your doctor.*

This medication may be used by pregnant women without harm to the unborn child. However, it should not be used by women who are breast-feeding babies. Be sure to tell your doctor if you are nursing a baby.

DOSAGE

Theophylline comes in tablets, extended-release tablets, capsules, liquid and sprinkles. Aminophylline also comes in rectal suppositories, solution for enema and an injectable form.

Your doctor will determine which form is best for you and will instruct you how often to take this medicine and how much to take at each dose. Carefully follow the instructions on your prescription label, and ask your doctor or pharmacist to explain any part of the instructions you do not understand.

The tablets should be swallowed whole. Do not break, crush or chew them before swallowing them. They are best taken with a full glass of water 30 minutes to one hour before meals. However, if the tablets upset your stomach, take them with meals or a snack.

Measure the oral liquid with a specially marked measuring spoon to ensure an accurate dose.

Rectal suppositories should be stored in the refrigerator. Take special care to keep them in a part of the refrigerator where they cannot be reached by small children, and be sure the suppositories will not be mistaken for food by either adults or children. Aminophylline suppositories can be harmful if they are chewed or swallowed, especially by small children.

The suppositories come with directions for their use. Carefully follow these directions. Take the suppositories out of the refrigerator a few minutes before using them, and let them warm at room temperature. If you are to use only part of a suppository, cut it lengthwise to the right size before inserting it. Remove the wrapper, and dip the tip of the suppository in water. Lie on your side, draw your top knee up to your chest and insert the suppository well into the rectum with your finger. Hold it there for a few moments, then get up and resume your usual activities. Try not to have a bowel movement for at least an hour after inserting the suppository. If burning or other irritation of the rectal area occurs after you use the suppository and if it continues or becomes worse, contact your doctor.

Theo-Dur Sprinkle capsules may be swallowed whole or opened so that the contents may be sprinkled on soft food.

The solution for enema comes with directions. Follow these directions carefully; if you have any questions about the use of this form, ask your pharmacist. If crystals form in the solution, dissolve them by placing the closed container of solution in warm water.

If you forget to take a dose, take it as soon as you remember and take any remaining doses for that day at evenly spaced intervals. *Do not take a double dose to make up for a missed dose.*

STORAGE

Keep all forms of theophylline in the containers they came in. Store aminophylline suppositories in the refrigerator out of the reach of children. Keep all forms of this medicine out of the reach of children in a place away from excessive heat and moisture. Do not allow anyone else to take this medicine.

OTHER DRUGS FOR ASTHMA

Corticosteroids
(kore ti kos′ ter oids)

The body produces a number of hormones that are essential to good health. When too little of these hormones (cortisones) is produced, corticosteroids may be prescribed to help make up the difference.

In addition, corticosteroids are used to reduce inflammation, redness and swelling in various parts of the body and to relieve allergic reactions.

The oral forms (capsules, tablets and liquid) are used to relieve the symptoms of arthritis, asthma, severe allergies and skin problems. There is also a form that is injected directly into the joint for the treatment of arthritis as well as a form that is taken by inhalation (beclomethasone) for the treatment of asthma.

Included in this group of medicines are both the natural hormone (hydrocortisone) and substances made in the laboratory (dexamethasone, prednisone and triamcinolone) that act in the body like the natural hormone. For complete descriptions of these drugs, see the section on Corticosteroids (pages 321–327) under Drugs Used to Treat Arthritis.

Beclomethasone
(be kloe meth' a sone)

PRODUCT INFORMATION
Brand names: Beclovent Inhaler, Beconase Nasal Inhaler, Vancenase Nasal Inhaler, Vanceril Inhaler

USES
Beclomethasone is a corticosteroid that is used by inhalation to treat asthma. It is used for its local effect in the lungs. When inhaled, it has little effect on the rest of the body, in contrast to the other corticosteroids. Beclomethasone is not used for asthma attacks and does not act as a bronchodilator. It is sometimes used with a bronchodilator or cromolyn.

UNDESIRED EFFECTS
Side effects from inhalation of beclomethasone are very rare when used as directed. Dry mouth and hoarseness have been reported in a few instances.

PRECAUTIONS
Tell your doctor if you are pregnant or are breast-feeding a baby. Corticosteroids taken orally are known to have harmful effects on unborn babies. Although beclomethasone acts primarily in the lungs and may not have adverse effects on unborn or breast-fed babies, its safety has not been determined. You should discuss this problem with your doctor to decide on the best treatment for you and your baby.

If your sputum (the matter you cough up during an asthma attack) becomes thick or changes color from clear white to yellow, gray or green, contact your doctor. These changes may be signs of an infection that requires immediate treatment.

If you are taking an oral corticosteroid along with beclomethasone, you should not suddenly stop taking the oral medication. The dose of the oral medication should be gradually decreased to prevent side effects such as joint and muscle pain, weariness and depression.

Do not use beclomethasone more often or in larger quantities than directed. It may take several months before you feel the full effect of this drug.

Do not use beclomethasone for asthma attacks. Your doctor should have given you a different medication such as a bronchodilator for asthma attacks. If not, contact your doctor.

DOSAGE
Your doctor will tell you how often to use beclomethasone. Carefully follow the instructions on your prescription label and any accompanying instructions, and ask your doctor or pharmacist to explain any part that you do not understand.

To use the inhaler, shake the metal canister well. Put the mouthpiece in your mouth, and close your lips and teeth around it. Breathe out as much air through your nose as you possibly can. Take a deep breath through the mouthpiece and, at the same, press down on the container to spray the medication into your mouth. Be sure that the mist goes into your throat and is not blocked by your teeth or tongue. Parents giving the treatment to young children may hold the child's nose closed to be sure the medication goes into the child's throat. Hold your breath as long as possible. Remove the inhaler from your mouth. Exhale through your nose or mouth. Wait one full minute. If you are still having difficulty breathing, repeat the same process one more time.

To use the nasal inhaler, follow the instructions that accompany it or ask your doctor or pharmacist to instruct you. If you are taking this drug on a regular schedule and forget a dose, take the missed dose as soon as you remember. If you remember a missed dose near the time you are to take the next one, take only your regularly scheduled dose. *Do not take a double dose.* Take the rest of the doses for that day at evenly spaced intervals.

If you are using a bronchodilator by inhalation in addition to beclomethasone, use the bronchodilator first and wait several minutes before using the beclomethasone. This allows the beclomethasone to penetrate deeper into the lungs.

STORAGE
Keep this medication away from excessive heat and out of the reach of children.

Cromolyn
(kroe′ moe lin)

PRODUCT INFORMATION
Brand names: Aarane, Intal

USES
Cromolyn is used to prevent asthma attacks that occur when small cells in the body, known as mast cells, release materials that irritate the airways and make it difficult for persons with asthma to breathe. Cromolyn coats the mast cells so they cannot release these materials.

This medicine is used only to *prevent* asthma attacks. It will not help against an asthma attack that has already started.

UNDESIRED EFFECTS

The most common side effects of cromolyn are cough, hoarseness, dryness of the mouth and throat irritation. Gargling or rinsing your mouth after inhaling this medicine may help to prevent these effects. If these effects continue or are bothersome, contact your doctor.

More serious effects, which may require medical attention, are tightness in the chest, wheezing, troubled breathing or swallowing, difficult or painful urination, frequent urge to urinate, dizziness, joint pain or swelling, muscle pain or weakness, nausea or vomiting, headache, skin rash or itching and swelling of the lips and eyes. If you experience any of these effects, stop using cromolyn and contact your doctor.

PRECAUTIONS

Because cromolyn is available only mixed with lactose powder, tell your doctor if you ever had an unusual reaction to lactose, milk or milk products. You should not take cromolyn if you are allergic to it or to milk.

Before you start taking cromolyn, tell your doctor if you have kidney disease or liver disease. Cromolyn may make these conditions worse.

Do not use cromolyn during an asthma attack because it may make the attack worse. If you have any questions, check with your doctor.

If you are also using a bronchodilator inhaler to help your breathing, use the bronchodilator first, wait several minutes and then use the cromolyn inhaler. If you also are taking a steroid such as cortisone or prednisone for your asthma along with cromolyn, do not stop taking the steroid even if your asthma seems better.

It may take up to four weeks for you to feel the benefits of cromolyn. However, if your symptoms do not improve or if your condition gets worse, contact your doctor. *Keep all appointments for checkups.*

Children under five years of age and pregnant women should not use cromolyn. Safe use of this drug during pregnancy has not been established, although problems have not been reported.

DOSAGE

Cromolyn usually is used four times a day. Your doctor will determine how often you should use it. Carefully follow the instructions on your prescription label, and ask your doctor or pharmacist to explain any part of the instructions you do not understand.

Cromolyn comes in a capsule and is used with a special inhaler. Directions are included with the inhaler. Carefully read the directions before using this medicine. Proper use will lessen the possibility of throat and mouth irritation from the powder.

Do not swallow the capsules. To be effective, this medicine must be inhaled every day in regularly spaced doses as prescribed by your doctor.

Clean your inhaler at least once a week. Take the inhaler apart and rinse it in clean, warm water. *Do not use soap.* Allow the inhaler to dry in the air before you use it again. If properly cared for, the inhaler should last about six months.

If you forget to take a dose of cromolyn, take the missed dose as soon as you remember it. Take any remaining doses for that day at regularly spaced intervals. *Do not take a double dose.*

STORAGE

Keep cromolyn capsules in the container they came in, and store them away from moisture and temperatures of more than 100°F. Keep cromolyn out of the reach of children, and do not allow anyone else to take it.

Stomach and Intestinal Problems

DRUGS USED TO TREAT
STOMACH AND INTESTINAL PROBLEMS

Indigestion and Heartburn

"Indigestion" is a term used to describe a variety of complaints, including nausea, upper abdominal or stomach pain, gas and a sense of fullness in the abdomen that occurs during or after eating. Indigestion can be caused by disease in the gastrointestinal tract (stomach and intestines) or by diseases originating someplace else in the body. Indigestion also can be caused by overeating, eating too fast or eating foods that are highly seasoned, "rich" or unfamiliar to you. Eating during emotional upsets or severe mental stress also can cause indigestion.

"Heartburn" is a popular term for a burning sensation in the stomach or esophagus, the tube connecting the mouth and the stomach. It can occur when partially digested food is retained in the lower esophagus. Heartburn is common with ulcers and gallbladder disease and during pregnancy.

Although indigestion and heartburn can be caused by improper diet, overeating or tension, you should request a physical examination by a doctor if you have these problems persistently.

Antacids are widely used to relieve the symptoms of indigestion and heartburn. Antacids also are commonly prescribed to treat gastric and duodenal ulcers.

Antacids work by neutralizing the acid produced by the stomach. Neutralization of this acid helps to relieve the pain and promotes healing of damaged tissue. Although all antacids work in the same way, their strengths vary because of their different capacities to neutralize acid.

When antacids are part of your treatment for an ulcer, it is extremely important that you take them on a regular schedule as prescribed. It is also important that you carefully follow your doctor's instructions on diet limitations. Some drugs aggravate ulcers, so you should check with your doctor or pharmacist before using other drugs, including nonprescription drugs, while under treatment for an ulcer.

ANTACIDS

Aluminum Hydroxide and Magnesium Hydroxide
(a loo′ min um hye drox′ ide) (mag nee′ zhum hye drox′ ide)

PRODUCT INFORMATION
Brand names: Algemol, Alka-Med, Aludrox, Alumid, Creamalin, Delcid, Kolantyl, Maalox, Maalox TC, Magmalin, Neosorb Plus, Neutralox, Rolox, Rulox, WinGel

Brand names of products containing simethicone: Almacone, Alumia Plus, Di-Gel, Gelusil, Maalox Plus, Mygel, Mylanta, Silain-Gel, Simaal, Simeco

USES
Aluminum hydroxide and magnesium hydroxide are antacids that are used together to treat ulcers and to relieve heartburn, stomach gas and upset stomach.

UNDESIRED EFFECTS
This combination medicine can cause nausea, vomiting, diarrhea or constipation. If you experience any of these effects, contact your doctor.

Taking this medicine in large doses or over a long time may remove too much phosphorus from the body. Signs of this problem are loss of appetite, muscle weakness and unusual tiredness. Contact your doctor if you experience these symptoms.

PRECAUTIONS
Before you start to take aluminum hydroxide and magnesium hydroxide, tell your doctor or pharmacist if you have kidney disease. Some antacids may make this condition worse.

This medicine may affect the way your body responds to certain other drugs. Tell your doctor or pharmacist what prescription or nonprescription drugs you are now taking, including digoxin, arthritis medicine, ferrous sulfate, isoniazid, buffered aspirin, anticoagulants (blood thinners), pseudoephedrine (decongestant), tetracycline and tranquilizers.

If you are taking aluminum hydroxide and magnesium hydroxide for an ulcer, carefully follow the diet prescribed by your doctor.

Contact your doctor if you have taken aluminum hydroxide and magnesium hydroxide for one week and the pain has not improved or has become worse. You should not take the maximum dose for more than two weeks unless your doctor tells you to do so.

DOSAGE
If this medicine was prescribed for you, your doctor has determined how often you should take it and how much you should take at each dose. Carefully follow the instructions on your prescription label. If you buy this medicine without a

prescription, carefully follow the directions on the label. Ask your doctor or pharmacist to explain any part of the directions you do not understand.

This medicine comes in tablets and in liquid form. The tablets should be chewed thoroughly before they are swallowed. Shake the liquid well before taking it.

If you forget to take a dose of this medicine, take it as soon as you remember. Take the remaining doses for that day at the regularly scheduled times.

STORAGE

Keep this medicine in the container it came in. Keep it tightly closed, and store the container at room temperature. Keep this medicine out of the reach of children.

Calcium Carbonate

(kal' see um kar' bone ate)

PRODUCT INFORMATION

Brand names: Alka-2, Amitone, Calcilac, Calglycine, Chooz, Dicarbosil, Equilet, Mallamint, Pama No. 1, Titracid, Titralac, Trialka, Tums

USES

Calcium carbonate is an antacid that neutralizes stomach acid. Calcium carbonate is used as a part of total therapy for certain types of stomach ulcers and to relieve indigestion, heartburn and sour stomach.

UNDESIRED EFFECTS

Calcium carbonate can cause constipation, belching and gas. You also can expect a chalky taste with this medicine.

If you take calcium carbonate in large doses or for a long time, or if you drink large amounts of milk while taking this medicine regularly, too much calcium can build up in your body. This build-up could upset your body chemistry and lead to kidney stones. Signs of this problem are nausea, vomiting, loss of appetite, weakness, headache and dizziness. Contact your doctor if you experience these effects.

Contact your doctor if you have severe stomach pain or heartburn a few hours after taking this medicine.

PRECAUTIONS

You should not take calcium carbonate if you have a history of kidney stones; ask your doctor or pharmacist to recommend a different antacid for you.

Before you start to take calcium carbonate, tell your doctor or pharmacist what prescription or nonprescription drugs you are taking, including tetracyclines, digoxin (heart medicine), indomethacin (arthritis medicine), ferrous sulfate, buffered aspirin and anticoagulants (blood thinners). If you do not know the names of the drugs or why they were prescribed, bring them in their labeled containers to your doctor or pharmacist.

You should not take the maximum dose of calcium carbonate for more than two weeks unless your doctor tells you to do so. If you are taking calcium carbonate over a long period, your doctor will want to check your response to this medicine at regular visits. *Be sure to keep all appointments with your doctor.*

DOSAGE
If calcium carbonate has been prescribed for you, your doctor will have determined how often you should take it and how much you should take at each dose. Carefully follow the instructions on your prescription label, and ask your doctor or pharmacist to explain any part of the instructions you do not understand. If you obtain calcium carbonate without a prescription, carefully follow the instructions on the label.

Calcium carbonate comes in tablets and in liquid form. The tablets should be chewed completely.

If you forget to take a dose of this medicine, take it as soon as you remember. Then take the remaining doses for that day on your regular dosage schedule.

STORAGE
Keep calcium carbonate in the container it came in, and keep it out of the reach of children.

Sodium Bicarbonate
(so' dee um bye car' bone ate)

PRODUCT INFORMATION
Brand names of some products containing sodium bicarbonate: Alka-Seltzer, Bell Ans, Bisodol Powder, Citrocarbonate, Soda Mint and others
Other name: Baking Soda

USES
Sodium bicarbonate is an antacid used to relieve occasional acid indigestion, heartburn and sour stomach.

UNDESIRED EFFECTS
The most common side effects of sodium bicarbonate are passing of gas and swelling of the abdomen.

Sodium bicarbonate, taken in large amounts or regularly over a long period, can cause high blood pressure and can seriously upset your body chemistry. If you drink large amounts of milk while taking this medicine regularly, too much calcium may build up in your body. Contact your doctor if you have nausea, vomiting, headache, mental confusion or loss of appetite.

PRECAUTIONS
If you have high blood pressure, heart disease, kidney disease, swelling of the legs and feet or cirrhosis of the liver, you should not take sodium bicarbonate. It

can make these conditions worse. Do not use sodium bicarbonate if you are on a salt-free or sodium-free diet. If you have any questions, check with your doctor or pharmacist.

Sodium bicarbonate can affect the way certain medications act in your body. You should not take sodium bicarbonate if you are taking anticoagulants (blood thinners), digoxin, indomethacin, naproxen or other medicines for arthritis, ferrous sulfate, amphetamines, buffered aspirin or quinidine (medicine for irregular heartbeat). If you do not know the names of the drugs you are taking or why they were prescribed, bring them in their labeled containers to your doctor or pharmacist.

Do not take large doses or use sodium bicarbonate over a long period (regularly for more than two weeks). Too much sodium in your body can cause problems. If you have questions, check with your doctor or pharmacist.

If you are allergic to aspirin, be sure to check the package label of combination products to avoid those that contain aspirin (for example, some types of Alka-Seltzer contain aspirin).

DOSAGE
If sodium bicarbonate has been prescribed for you, carefully follow your doctor's instructions on how often to take it and how much to take at each dose. If you obtain sodium bicarbonate without a prescription, follow the directions on the container; ask your pharmacist to explain any part of the directions you do not understand.

Sodium bicarbonate comes in a powder form. It should be dissolved in a full eight-ounce glass of water. Stir well before you drink it.

STORAGE
Keep this medicine in the container it came in, and keep it out of the reach of children.

ANTIGAS DRUG

Simethicone
(sye meth' eye cone)

PRODUCT INFORMATION
Brand names: Gas-X, Mylicon, Silain
Brand names of some products containing simethicone: Di-Gel, Gelusil, Maalox Plus, Mylanta, Phazyme, Riopan Plus, Silain-Gel and others

USES
Simethicone is an antiflatulent that acts on gas bubbles in the intestinal tract to make it possible for gas to be released by belching or by passing gas. Simethicone is used for gas pain after surgery and for many conditions where gas in the intestines may be a problem.

UNDESIRED EFFECTS
There are no known side effects after taking simethicone. However, if you do experience undesired effects after taking simethicone, contact your doctor.

PRECAUTIONS
Do not use simethicone for infant colic. Safe use of simethicone for infants and children has not been established.

DOSAGE
If this medicine has been prescribed for you, your doctor has determined how often you should take it and how much you should take at each dose. Carefully follow the instructions on your prescription label, and ask your doctor or pharmacist to explain any part of the instructions you do not understand. If you obtain simethicone without a prescription, carefully follow the label instructions on how often to take this medicine and how much to take at each dose.

Simethicone comes in tablets and in liquid form. The tablets should be thoroughly chewed before they are swallowed. Shake the liquid well before each use. Measure the proper dose with the dropper included with the container. Be sure you know how to use the dropper. Ask your pharmacist to explain the use of the dropper if you have any questions.

STORAGE
Keep simethicone in the container it came in, and keep it out of the reach of children.

Constipation

Laxatives may be the most widely misused class of drugs. Excessive use of laxatives stems from the popular belief that "regularity" (one bowel movement per day) is absolutely essential for good health. This idea is heavily promoted through advertisements by manufacturers of laxative products.

In fact, normal frequency of bowel movements can vary from three times per day to three times per week, depending on the individual. The normal frequency for each person is determined by physiology, diet and lifestyle. Laxatives are needed only when you become constipated compared to your regular bowel-movement habits.

Laxatives frequently are used to prepare a person for X-rays or other diagnostic tests. When used for this purpose, your doctor will give you specific instructions.

Several different types of laxatives are available. The bulk-producing laxatives increase the size of the stool, and this increase in size stimulates bowel contractions to produce a bowel movement. The lubricant laxatives coat the stool with oil to prevent them from becoming hard and difficult to pass. Castor oil and glycerin suppositories stimulate the bowel directly to produce a bowel movement.

Before using any laxative, it is important to tell your doctor or pharmacist what drugs you are taking and whether you have any other medical condition, particularly if you have had recent surgery. You should not use any laxative product for more than one week unless directed to by your doctor. Prolonged use of laxatives can be habit-forming and may lead to loss of important nutrients and damage to the bowel.

LAXATIVES
Bulk-forming Laxatives

PRODUCT INFORMATION
Brand names for methylcellulose (meth ill sell' yoo lows): Cellothyl, Cologel
Brand name for malt soup extract: Maltsupex
Brand name for malt soup extract combined with psyllium: Syllamalt
Brand names for psyllium (sil' ee yum): Effersyllium, Konsyl, L.A. Formula, Laxamead, Metamucil, Modane, Mucillium, Mucilose, Reguloid, Serutan, Siblin, Syllact, V-Lax

USES
Bulk-forming laxatives act in a way similar to that of high-fiber-content foods. They absorb water in the intestines and add bulk to the bowel contents. The bulk stimulates muscular contractions in the bowel and helps the bowel to empty. Bulk-forming laxatives begin to work in 12 to 24 hours, but you may not notice their full

laxative effect until a day or two after you start taking them. Although there are several different bulk laxatives, they all work in the same basic way.

These medicines are the preferred drugs for constipation during pregnancy or after childbirth. They are also used after surgery and for patients with conditions (such as heart attack, high blood pressure, blood vessel disease, anal or rectal disease and hernia) in which straining to move the bowels might cause a problem.

UNDESIRED EFFECTS

Side effects with bulk-forming laxatives are rare.

Bulk-forming laxatives can cause blockage of the esophagus or the bowel if they are taken without enough liquid. To prevent this problem, always take these medicines with a full eight-ounce glass of water and be sure to prepare them according to instructions.

PRECAUTIONS

Do not take a bulk-forming laxative if you have abdominal pain, bloating, nausea or vomiting. These symptoms may be of appendicitis or other abdominal problems. Contact your doctor if you have these symptoms.

Do not take bulk-forming laxatives if you have intestinal ulceration, blockage of the bowel or difficulty swallowing. If you need a laxative, check with your doctor or pharmacist about what you may use without problems. Tell your doctor if you have high blood pressure, diabetes or kidney or heart problems.

If you are taking antacids, antibiotics, anticoagulants (blood thinners), aspirin, birth-control pills, heart medicine, nitrofurantoin (antibacterial medicine for urinary tract infections), pain medicine or other laxatives, do not start using bulk-forming laxatives before first checking with your doctor or pharmacist.

Take only as much bulk-forming laxative as directed by your doctor or by the instructions on the package. Do not take it for a longer time than directed. If you take a bulk-forming laxative regularly for a week and still are constipated, contact your doctor.

DOSAGE

If a bulk-forming laxative has been prescribed for you, your doctor has determined how often you should take it and how much to take at each dose. Carefully follow the instructions on your prescription label, and ask your doctor or pharmacist to explain any part of the instructions you do not understand.

If you obtain a bulk-forming laxative without a prescription, be sure to follow the directions on the package carefully. Check with your pharmacist if you have any questions about how often to take this medicine or how much to take.

Bulk-forming laxatives come in powders, flakes, granules, tablets and liquid form. They should be dissolved or diluted according to the directions on the package. All forms should be taken with a full eight-ounce glass of water. *Be sure to drink plenty of fluids while taking any laxative.*

If you forget to take a dose of this medicine, take it as soon as you remember and take any remaining doses for that day at evenly spaced intervals. If you remember a missed dose when it is almost time for you to take another, omit the missed dose entirely and take only the regularly scheduled dose. *Do not take a double dose to make up for the missed dose.*

STORAGE
Keep bulk-forming laxatives in the containers they came in. Keep them out of the reach of children.

Castor Oil
(kas′ tore)

PRODUCT INFORMATION
Brand names: Alphamul, Emulsoil, Neoloid

USES
Castor oil acts on the intestines to speed up the emptying action of the bowel. The result usually is a violent emptying of bowel contents. Although once a commonly used laxative for simple constipation, castor oil now is used almost exclusively to clean the bowel before surgery or before X-ray or scope examination of the bowel.

UNDESIRED EFFECTS
Following a dose of castor oil, you may experience intestinal discomfort, nausea, mild cramps, bowel pain or fainting.

Long-term use of castor oil may make it impossible for you to have a bowel movement without using this laxative. You may lose weight because your food is not nourishing your body as it should. Minerals needed by the body may be removed if you take castor oil too often, and vomiting and muscle weakness can result. Contact your doctor if you have any of these problems.

If you or a child accidentally takes too much castor oil, contact your doctor or a poison control center immediately. Signs of overdose are unusually rapid breathing, abdominal pain, diarrhea, nausea and vomiting.

PRECAUTIONS
Do not take castor oil if you have abdominal pain, bloating, nausea or vomiting. These symptoms may be signs of appendicitis, and you should contact your doctor. Pregnant women, women who are menstruating and people who have bowel obstruction should not use castor oil. If you have any questions, check with your doctor or pharmacist. Tell your doctor if you are breast-feeding or have high blood pressure, diabetes or kidney, heart or intestinal problems.

Tell your doctor what prescription or nonprescription drugs you are taking, especially antacids, antibiotics, anticoagulants (blood thinners), birth-control pills, medicine for your heart or other laxatives. If you do not know the names of the drugs you are taking or why they were prescribed, bring them in their labeled containers to your doctor or pharmacist.

Castor oil should be used only for infrequent bouts of constipation. Frequent or continued use can cause laxative dependence, because castor oil is habit-forming. If you have used castor oil regularly for a week and still are constipated, contact your doctor.

DOSAGE

Castor oil is available as an emulsion; it is usually flavored to mask its disagreeable taste. Shake the emulsion well before using. Carefully follow the instructions on the package for the proper dose, and check with your pharmacist if you have any questions about how much to take.

Mix castor oil with one-half glass (four ounces) or a full eight-ounce glass of water, milk, fruit juice or a soft drink. *Be sure to drink plenty of fluids while taking any laxative.*

STORAGE

Keep castor oil in the container it came in, and keep it out of the reach of children.

Glycerin Suppositories

(gliss' ehr in supp pos' i tor eez)

USES

Glycerin draws water from the bowel itself into the bowel contents, with the result that the bowel is emptied. It is given as a rectal suppository and is particularly useful for constipation in infants and children.

UNDESIRED EFFECTS

Glycerin suppositories have few side effects when used infrequently and for a short time. This medicine may cause rectal discomfort, irritation, burning, bowel pain, cramps or straining without producing a bowel movement. If these effects are bothersome, contact your doctor.

If glycerin suppositories cause a bloody discharge from the rectum, contact your doctor.

Overuse of this medicine may cause continuing diarrhea, which leads to a loss of vitamins and minerals and potentially dangerous decrease in body water. Stop using glycerin suppositories and contact your doctor if continuing diarrhea is a problem.

PRECAUTIONS

Do not use glycerin suppositories if you have abdominal pain, bloating, nausea or vomiting. These symptoms may be signs of appendicitis or some other problem. Contact your doctor.

Do not use more of this medicine than directed by your doctor or than indicated on the package label. Do not use it for a long time. If you have used glycerin suppositories regularly for a week and still are constipated, contact your doctor.

DOSAGE
If glycerin suppositories have been prescribed for you, your doctor has determined how often you should use them. Carefully follow the instructions on your prescription label, and ask your doctor or pharmacist to explain any part of the instructions you do not understand.

If you obtain these suppositories without a prescription, carefully follow the instructions for use on the package. Check with your pharmacist if you have questions.

To use the suppositories, remove the foil wrapper and moisten the tip of the suppository with water. Then lie on your side, bring your top knee to your chest and insert the suppository well into the rectum with your finger. A bowel movement usually will occur within 15 to 30 minutes.

Be sure to drink plenty of fluids while taking any laxative.

STORAGE
Keep glycerin suppositories in the container they came in, and store them away from heat and direct sunlight. Keep them out of the reach of children. Do not allow anyone else to use your glycerin suppositories.

Mineral Oil

PRODUCT INFORMATION
Brand names: Agoral Plain, Fleet Mineral Oil Enema, Kondremul Plain Emulsion, Neo-Cultol, Nujol, Petrogalar Plain, Saf-Tip Oil Retention Enema, Zymenol

Brand names of some products containing mineral oil: Agoral Marshmallow (with phenolphthalein), Agoral Raspberry (with phenolphthalein), Haley's M-O (with milk of magnesia), Kondremul with Cascara, Kondremul with Phenolphthalein, Milkinol, Petrogalar and Cascara, Petrogalar with Phenolphthalein, Petro-Syllium No. 1 Plain (with psyllium)

USES
Mineral oil puts an oily film over the lining of the bowel to prevent water from leaving the stool. This action keeps the stool soft and aids in emptying the bowel.

Mineral oil often is prescribed after surgery and for people with conditions (such as heart attack, high blood pressure, blood vessel disease, anal or rectal disease and hernia) in which straining to move the bowels might cause problems.

UNDESIRED EFFECTS
When properly used (infrequently and for short periods), mineral oil has few side effects. Seepage from the rectum is a common problem. This seepage can stain clothing, cause irritation and anal itching and increase infection in bleeding hemor-

rhoids or rectal fissures and prevent their healing. Usually leakage can be avoided by taking a smaller dose or by dividing the daily dose into several small doses and taking them at intervals.

Taking mineral oil over a long time can result in your body being unable to absorb and use vitamins A, D, E and K. It also can cause loss of essential minerals and other important nutrients, continuing diarrhea and a potentially dangerous loss of water from the body.

When mineral oil is taken in large doses over an extended period, it can be absorbed into the body and cause tumors in the lymph nodes, liver and spleen.

PRECAUTIONS

Do not take mineral oil if you have abdominal pain, bloating, nausea or vomiting. These symptoms may be signs of appendicitis or other abdominal problems, and you should contact your doctor. Do not take mineral oil if you have stomach or esophagus disease, difficulty in swallowing or hiatal hernia. If you have any questions, check with your doctor or pharmacist. Tell your doctor if you have high blood pressure, diabetes or kidney or heart problems.

Mineral oil may make certain medicines less effective. Tell your doctor what prescription or nonprescription drugs you are taking, especially antacids, antibiotics, anticoagulants (blood thinners), birth-control pills, heart medicine, other laxatives and vitamins A, D, E and K. If you do not know the names of the drugs you are taking or why they were prescribed, bring them in their labeled containers to your doctor or pharmacist.

Check with your doctor before giving oral mineral oil to children under six years of age or to very elderly or very sick persons. They might inhale some of the oil, which can cause inflammation of the lungs.

Do not take mineral oil any longer than directed by your doctor or the instructions on the package. If you take oral mineral oil for a week and still are constipated, contact your doctor.

If you are pregnant, do not use mineral oil. Regular use of this medicine can cause blood problems in the baby. If you have questions, check with your doctor.

DOSAGE

If mineral oil has been prescribed for you, your doctor has determined how often you should take it and how much you should take at each dose. Carefully follow the instructions on your prescription label, and ask your doctor or pharmacist to explain any part of the instructions you do not understand.

If you obtain mineral oil without a prescription, carefully follow the instructions on the package as to the proper use of this medicine. Check with your pharmacist if you have questions.

Mineral oil comes as plain oil and as an oil emulsion to be taken by mouth and as an enema to be given rectally.

The oral forms should be taken on an empty stomach to prevent interference with absorption of vitamins from your food. The laxative will begin to work in six to eight hours. Be sure you know how to use the enema form. If you do not understand the directions on the package, ask your pharmacist to explain them.

Be sure to drink plenty of fluids while taking any laxative.

STORAGE
Keep mineral oil in the container it came in, and keep it out of the reach of children.

STOOL SOFTENER
Docusate
(dock′ you sate)

PRODUCT INFORMATION
Brand names: Bu-Lax, Colace, Comfolax, Dialose, Dialose-Plus, Dilax, Dioeze, Diosuccin, Diosul, Diothron, Di-Sosul, Dosanate, Doss, Doxidan, Doxinate, D.S.S., Duosol, Kasof, Laxinate, Modane, Peri-Colace, Pro-Cal Sof, Regul-Aid, Regutol, Surfak

USES
Docusate softens stools and makes them easier to pass. It often is given to women during pregnancy and after childbirth and to patients after surgery. It also is used to ease bowel movements for people who should avoid straining (people with heart conditions, hernia or hemorrhoids).

UNDESIRED EFFECTS
Side effects with docusate are rare. Occasionally this medicine will cause mild stomach cramps, diarrhea, loose stools or throat irritation. Contact your doctor if these effects bother you.

PRECAUTIONS
Stool softeners may affect the absorption of many oral drugs. *Do not take mineral oil while you are taking this medicine.* Docusate increases the absorption of mineral oil into the body, which can cause liver or spleen problems. Tell your doctor what prescription or nonprescription drugs you are taking, including aspirin and other laxatives.

Tell your doctor if you have abdominal pain, bloating, nausea or vomiting (signs of appendicitis or intestinal disease), high blood pressure, diabetes or kidney or heart problems. Do not take docusate for a longer period than your doctor has directed. If your stools still are hard after this time, ask your doctor or pharmacist whether you should change your diet or do some exercise to relieve your problem.

DOSAGE
If docusate has been prescribed for you, your doctor has determined how often you should take it and how much you should take at each dose. If you obtain this medication without a prescription, carefully follow the directions for use on the package. If you have any questions about the proper use of this medicine or do not

understand the directions on your prescription label, ask your doctor or pharmacist for an explanation.

Docusate comes in capsules, tablets and liquid form. It should be taken with a full eight-ounce glass of water. You may take the liquid by adding it to milk or fruit juice.

If you forget to take a dose, take it as soon as you remember. If you do not remember a missed dose until it is almost time to take another, omit the missed dose completely and take only the regularly scheduled dose. *Do not take two doses at one time. Be sure to drink plenty of fluids while taking any laxative.*

STORAGE

Keep this medicine in the container it came in, and keep it out of the reach of children. Do not allow anyone else to take your docusate.

Diarrhea

Diarrhea is the frequent passage of loose stools. Because individual bowel habits vary widely, diarrhea is defined as an increase of passage of loose stools over an individual's normal pattern.

Diarrhea can be an acute, short-term condition or a chronic problem. In either case, diarrhea is a symptom of some gastrointestinal disorder. The causes of acute diarrhea include infection (bacterial or viral), food poisoning, adverse drug effects and dietary imbalances.

Persistent or recurrent diarrhea may be a signal of more serious disease, particularly if other symptoms are present. Individuals who also experience weight loss, weakness or loss of appetite should contact a physician to determine the underlying cause of their diarrhea.

The biggest dangers associated with diarrhea are dehydration and loss of electrolytes. These problems are particularly dangerous in infants and small children because their supply of water and electrolytes can be depleted very quickly. A child under three years of age experiencing this disorder should always be seen by a doctor so the cause and severity can be evaluated. The doctor may wish to prescribe a special fluid and electrolyte solution.

ANTIDIARRHEALS

Diphenoxylate and Atropine
(dye fen ox' i late) (a' troe peen)

PRODUCT INFORMATION
Brand names: Diphenatol, Elmotil, Enoxa, Lofene, Lomotil, Lonox, Lo-Trol, Low-Quel, SK-Diphenoxylate

USES
Diphenoxylate and atropine relax the intestinal tract. This combination of medications is used to treat certain types of severe diarrhea.

UNDESIRED EFFECTS
This medicine can cause thirst and dry mouth. To relieve these effects, drink a lot of fluids and chew gum or suck hard candies.

Some people get dizzy or drowsy when they take diphenoxylate and atropine. Do not drive a car or operate dangerous machinery until you know how this medicine will affect you.

Other side effects, which may disappear as your body adjusts to the medicine, are blurred vision, depression, fever, flushing, headache, numbness of the hands or feet, rapid heartbeat, skin rash or itching, swelling of the gums and an unusual decrease in urination. Contact your doctor if these effects continue or get worse.

More serious side effects will require medical attention. Contact your doctor if you have bloating, constipation, loss of appetite, nausea and vomiting or stomach pain.

Taking too much diphenoxylate and atropine can be dangerous. Signs of an overdose are fainting, pinpoint pupils, shallow breathing and unusual excitement. If you have these symptoms, contact your doctor or poison control center immediately.

When you stop taking this medicine, your body may need time to adjust. During the adjustment period, contact your doctor if you have muscle cramps, nausea and vomiting, shaking or trembling, stomach cramps or unusual sweating.

PRECAUTIONS

Before you start to take diphenoxylate and atropine, tell your doctor if you have Addison's disease, alcoholism, colitis, difficult urination, emphysema, asthma, bronchitis or other chronic lung disease, enlarged prostate, gallbladder disease or gallstones, glaucoma, heart disease, hiatal hernia, high blood pressure, kidney disease, liver disease, myasthenia gravis or overactive or underactive thyroid. This medicine may make these conditions worse.

Tell your doctor what prescription or nonprescription drugs you are taking, particularly amantadine, haloperidol, medicine for your heart, medicine for ulcers, antihistamines, medicine for allergies or colds, barbiturates, narcotics, prescription medicine for pain, sedatives, tranquilizers, medicine to help you sleep, medicine for seizures, medicine for depression and MAO inhibitors (isocarboxazid, pargyline, phenelzine or tranylcypromine), even if you stopped taking them within the past two weeks.

If you do not know the names of the drugs or what they were prescribed for, bring them in their labeled containers to your doctor or pharmacist.

Do not drink alcoholic beverages while you are taking diphenoxylate and atropine. Do not start taking any of the drugs listed above unless you first check with your doctor or pharmacist. All of them can increase the chance and severity of side effects.

Take diphenoxylate and atropine exactly as prescribed by your doctor. Do not take more of it, do not take it more often and do not take it for a longer period than your doctor has ordered. This medicine can be habit-forming.

If your diarrhea does not stop a few days after you start taking diphenoxylate and atropine or if you develop a fever, contact your doctor.

Check with your doctor if you want to stop taking this medicine. Your doctor may want you to reduce the amount you are taking gradually before you stop completely.

Keep in touch with your doctor while you are taking this medicine. Before you have any surgery, including dental surgery, tell the doctor or dentist in charge that you are taking diphenoxylate and atropine.

To help your doctor choose the best treatment for you and your baby, be sure to say if you are pregnant or are nursing a baby. The effects of these drugs on an unborn child and a breast-fed baby are not known.

DOSAGE

Your doctor will determine how often you should take this medicine and how much you should take at each dose. The effectiveness of diphenoxylate and atropine starts 45 to 60 minutes after it is taken and continues for three to four hours. This medicine often is prescribed to be taken after loose bowel movements occur. Carefully follow the instructions on your prescription label, and ask your doctor or pharmacist to explain any part of the instructions you do not understand.

Diphenoxylate and atropine comes in tablets for adults and in liquid form for children. The liquid comes in a container with a special dropper to measure the exact dose. Be sure you know how to use the dropper properly. If you have any questions, check with your doctor or pharmacist. Be sure to shake the liquid well before each use.

If you are taking this medicine on a schedule and forget to take a dose (and you still have diarrhea), take the dose as soon as you remember it and take any remaining doses for that day at evenly spaced intervals. If you do not have diarrhea, omit the missed dose completely and take only the next regularly scheduled dose. *Do not take a double dose to make up for the missed dose.*

STORAGE

Keep this medicine in the container it came in. Keep it out of the reach of children. An overdose is especially dangerous for children. Do not allow anyone else to take your diphenoxylate and atropine.

Loperamide
(loe per′ a mide)

PRODUCT INFORMATION
Brand name: Imodium

USES

Loperamide is used to control severe or chronic diarrhea. It is a stronger and longer-acting drug than diphenoxylate (another medicine for diarrhea). Loperamide decreases muscular activity in the intestinal tract. It is not habit-forming.

UNDESIRED EFFECTS

Some side effects that may occur are abdominal pain, constipation, fatigue, dry mouth and a rash. To relieve dry mouth, chew gum or suck hard candies. Contact your doctor if these symptoms persist or are bothersome.

Loperamide may cause dizziness or drowsiness. Do not drive a car or operate dangerous machinery until you know how this drug will affect you.

PRECAUTIONS

Loperamide can make certain medical conditions worse. Tell your doctor if you have colitis (a chronic bowel disease).

Do not take loperamide more often than as instructed by your doctor. If your diarrhea does not stop within two days (10 days for chronic diarrhea), contact your doctor.

Tell your doctor if you are pregnant or breast-feeding a baby before beginning to take this drug. It is not known if loperamide can be taken safely during pregnancy or while breast-feeding.

DOSAGE

Loperamide comes in capsules to be taken by mouth. Your doctor will determine how often you should take this medicine and how much you should take at each dose. Follow the instructions on your prescription label, and ask your doctor or pharmacist to explain any part you do not understand. Loperamide is usually taken after loose bowel movements.

Be sure to drink plenty of fluids to replace fluids lost while having diarrhea.

If you are taking loperamide on a schedule and forget to take a dose, take it as soon as you remember and take any remaining doses for that day at evenly spaced intervals. However, if you are not having diarrhea, omit the missed dose completely. *Do not take a double dose to make up for the missed dose.*

STORAGE

Keep this medication in the container it came in, and keep it out of the reach of children.

Paregoric
(par eh gore′ ik)

PRODUCT INFORMATION

Brand names of preparations containing paregoric: Amogel PG, Corrective Mixture with Paregoric, Diabismul, Donnagel-PG, Infantol Pink, Kaodonna-PG, Kenpectin-P, Mul-Sed, Parepectolin, Quiagel

USES

Paregoric is a mixture of opium, anise oil, benzoic acid, camphor, glycerin and alcohol. Paregoric relaxes the intestines to relieve diarrhea. Paregoric is available alone or in combination with kaolin, pectin and bismuth (substances also used to treat diarrhea).

UNDESIRED EFFECTS

Occasionally, paregoric will cause nausea and stomach upset. If these problems occur, you may take paregoric with food or milk. If stomach upsets continue or are severe, contact your doctor. Paregoric makes some people drowsy. Do not drive a car or operate dangerous machinery until you know how it will affect you.

When paregoric is taken in low doses for a short time, it rarely is habit-forming. However, if you take this medicine over a long period (for example, as a treatment for diarrhea resulting from chronic inflammation of the bowel), your body may need time to adjust when you stop taking it. During this adjustment period, contact your doctor if you have convulsions or seizures, hallucinations (seeing, hearing or feeling things that are not there), increased dreaming, muscle twitching, nausea or vomiting, nightmares, trembling, trouble sleeping or unusual nervousness or restlessness.

Taking too much paregoric can be dangerous. If you accidentally take too much, contact your doctor immediately or go to the nearest hospital emergency room. Signs of an overdose are constipation, unusually slow heartbeat, shortness of breath and difficulty breathing.

PRECAUTIONS

Because paregoric can make some medical conditions worse, tell your doctor if you have emphysema, asthma, any other chronic lung disease, enlarged prostate, liver disease or a history of drug abuse or dependence.

Tell your doctor what prescription or nonprescription drugs you are taking, including antihistamines, medicine for allergies or colds, barbiturates, narcotics, sedatives, tranquilizers, medicine to help you sleep, prescription medicine for pain, medicine for seizures, medicine for depression and MAO inhibitors (isocarboxazid, pargyline, phenelzine or tranylcypromine), even if you stopped taking them within the past two weeks. If you do not know the names of the drugs or what they were prescribed for, bring them in their labeled containers to your doctor or pharmacist.

Do not drink alcoholic beverages while taking paregoric. Do not start taking any of the drugs listed above without first checking with your doctor or pharmacist. All of them can increase the chance and severity of side effects.

Take paregoric exactly as your doctor has prescribed it. Do not take more of it, do not take it more often and do not take it for a longer period than your doctor has ordered. If you take this medicine for a long time, do not stop taking it unless you first check with your doctor. Your doctor may want you to reduce the amount you take gradually before you stop completely.

To help your doctor select the best treatment for you and your baby, tell your doctor if you are pregnant or are nursing a baby.

DOSAGE

Your doctor will determine how often you should take paregoric and how much you should take at each dose. Paregoric usually is prescribed to be taken after each loose bowel movement. Carefully follow the instructions on your prescription label, and ask your doctor or pharmacist to explain any part of the instructions you do not understand.

Paregoric comes in liquid form. Use a specially marked measuring spoon to be sure you get an accurate dose.

If you are taking paregoric on a regular dosage schedule and forget to take a dose, do one of the following: (1) If you still have diarrhea, take the missed dose as soon as you remember it and take any remaining doses for that day at evenly spaced intervals. (2) If you do not have diarrhea any longer, omit the missed dose entirely and take only the regularly scheduled dose. *Do not take a double dose to make up for the missed one.*

STORAGE

Keep paregoric in the container it came in, and store it away from heat and direct sunlight. Keep this medicine out of the reach of children. Do not allow anyone else to take your paregoric.

Nausea and Vomiting

Nausea and vomiting are symptoms common to a wide variety of illnesses. Some common causes of vomiting are:

- infections, including the "flu" and gastroenteritis
- food poisoning
- disturbances of the inner ear
- motion sickness
- radiation therapy
- drugs; nausea and vomiting may be side effects or symptoms of an overdose
- serious illness, including appendicitis, migraine headache, and hormonal imbalance

If you experience vomiting for more than two days or have stomach or abdominal pain, contact your doctor. If you notice blood in the vomit (sometimes blood looks like coffee grounds rather than being bright red), contact your doctor.

An infant who is vomiting should be seen by a doctor if simple causes (for example, overfeeding) are not obvious.

ANTIEMETICS

Hydroxyzine

Hydroxyzine is also used to treat nausea and vomiting. See the section on Hydroxyzine (page 446) under Drugs Used to Treat Psychiatric Problems.

Meclizine
(mek′ li zeen)

PRODUCT INFORMATION
Brand names: Antivert, Bonine, Dizmiss, Motion Cure, Wehvert

USES
Meclizine is an antihistamine that is not used to treat allergies. It is particularly useful in preventing the nausea, vomiting and dizziness caused by motion sickness. It also is used to treat the dizziness caused by certain ear conditions such as Meniere's disease.

UNDESIRED EFFECTS

One common effect of meclizine is dry mouth. To relieve this dryness, drink fluids, chew gum or suck hard candy or ice chips.

Like other antihistamines, meclizine may make you drowsy or less alert than normal. Do not operate dangerous machinery or drive a car until you know how this medicine will affect you.

Occasionally, meclizine will cause blurred vision, difficult or painful urination, headache, loss of appetite, nervousness, trouble sleeping, skin rash, unusually fast heartbeat or upset stomach. If you experience these effects, contact your doctor.

PRECAUTIONS

Before you start to take meclizine, tell your doctor if you have an enlarged prostate, a stomach ulcer, urinary tract blockage or glaucoma. This medicine can make these conditions worse.

Tell your doctor what prescription or nonprescription drugs you are taking, including barbiturates, medicine for seizures, narcotics, other antihistamines, medicine for allergies and colds, prescription medicine for pain, sedatives, tranquilizers and medicine to help you sleep. If you do not know the names of the drugs or what they were prescribed for, bring them in their labeled containers to your doctor or pharmacist.

Do not drink alcoholic beverages while you are taking meclizine. Do not start taking any of the drugs listed above without first checking with your doctor or pharmacist. All of them can increase the drowsiness caused by meclizine.

Take meclizine exactly as directed. Do not take more of it and do not take it more often than your doctor has ordered.

If you are taking large amounts of aspirin (for arthritis or other conditions), be sure your doctor knows this before you start taking meclizine on a regular basis. Meclizine may cover up the warning signals of aspirin overdose (e.g., ringing in the ears).

Meclizine should not be taken by children under 12 years because its safe use for this age group has not been established. Meclizine should not be taken by nursing mothers because it may dry up their milk.

Before you start to take meclizine, tell your doctor if you are pregnant or plan to become pregnant while taking this medicine. The effects of this medicine on an unborn child are not known.

DOSAGE

When meclizine is used for motion sickness, you should take it one hour before you start to travel. If you are taking meclizine for the dizziness caused by an ear condition, your doctor has determined how often you should take it and how much to take at each dose. Carefully follow the instructions on your prescription label, and ask your doctor or pharmacist to explain any part of the instructions you do not understand.

Meclizine comes in regular tablets and chewable tablets. The chewable tablets may be chewed or swallowed whole.

If you forget to take a dose of meclizine, take it as soon as you remember. Then take any remaining doses for that day at evenly spaced intervals. *Do not take more than one dose at a time.*

STORAGE
Keep meclizine in the container it came in, and keep it out of the reach of children.

Prochlorperazine

Prochlorperazine is also used to treat nausea and vomiting. See the section on Prochlorperazine (page 479) under Drugs Used to Treat Psychiatric Problems.

Trimethobenzamide
(trye meth oh ben′ za mide)

PRODUCT INFORMATION
Brand names: Tegamide, Ticon, Tigan

USES
Trimethobenzamide acts on the portion of the brain that controls the vomiting center. Trimethobenzamide is used to control nausea and vomiting caused by radiation therapy and certain diseases.

UNDESIRED EFFECTS
Trimethobenzamide may cause some people to become drowsy, dizzy or lightheaded. Do not drive a car or operate dangerous machinery until you know how this medicine will affect you.

Other effects, which may disappear as your body adjusts to this medicine, are blurred vision, diarrhea, headache and muscle cramps. If these effects continue or bother you, contact your doctor.

More serious side effects are Reye's syndrome (a syndrome of severe and continued vomiting, unusual behavior, tiredness, and seizures), blood problems and liver problems, which will need medical attention. Contact your doctor if you have back pain, mental depression, seizures, severe or continued vomiting, shakiness or tremors, sore throat and fever, an unusual feeling of tiredness or yellowing of the eyes and skin.

PRECAUTIONS
If you are allergic to benzocaine or other local anesthetics, you should not use the suppository form of this medicine, which contains benzocaine. If you have any questions, check with your doctor or pharmacist.

Tell your doctor what prescription or nonprescription drugs you are taking, including antihistamines, medicine for allergies or colds, barbiturates, narcotics, phenothiazines (chlorpromazine, fluphenazine, perphenazine, prochlorperazine, promazine, thioridazine or trifluoperazine), prescription medicine for pain, sedatives, tranquilizers, medicine to help you sleep and medicine for seizures. If you do not know the names of the drugs or what they were prescribed for, bring them in their labeled containers to your doctor or pharmacist.

Do not drink alcoholic beverages while you are taking trimethobenzamide. Do not start taking any of the drugs listed above without checking first with your doctor. All of them can increase the chance and severity of side effects.

Because trimethobenzamide is used only to relieve or prevent nausea and vomiting, take it exactly as prescribed by your doctor. Do not take more of it and do not take it more often than your doctor has ordered.

Do not give this medicine to a child unless you have your doctor's permission.

If you are using trimethobenzamide to control a child's nausea and vomiting, be especially careful not to give more than prescribed. Side effects may be especially serious in children.

Before you start to take trimethobenzamide, tell your doctor if you are pregnant or are nursing a baby. Safe use of this drug in pregnant women and breast-feeding mothers has not been established.

DOSAGE

Your doctor will determine when you should take trimethobenzamide and how much to take at each dose. Carefully follow the instructions on your prescription label, and ask your doctor or pharmacist to explain any part of the instructions you do not understand.

Trimethobenzamide comes in capsules to be taken orally and in rectal suppositories. To use the suppositories, first remove the foil wrapper and dip the tip of the suppository into water. Then lie on your side, draw your top knee up to your chest, insert the suppository well into your rectum and hold it in place for a few minutes. Try not to have a bowel movement for at least one hour after inserting the suppository.

If the suppository is too soft to insert, leave on the wrapper and refrigerate the suppository for 30 minutes or run cold water over it.

STORAGE

Keep trimethobenzamide in the container it came in, and keep it out of the reach of children.

Ulcer Pain

An ulcer is an area of the stomach or duodenum (intestine) that has lost its normal lining. As a result, the area is exposed to acid and enzymes that digest food. The breakdown of the stomach lining may be caused by excess formation of acid or enzymes. It also may result from a decreased resistance to acid in the lining.

Factors related to ulcer development include:

- smoking—smokers have a higher rate of stomach and intestinal ulcers than other people do, but the exact reason is not known
- heredity—close relatives of individuals with stomach or intestinal ulcers have an increased risk of developing ulcers
- drugs—some medications can cause ulcers, particularly when used in large doses or over a long time. Aspirin is a well-known cause of ulcers, as are steroids and anti-inflammatory agents used to treat arthritis
- stress—stress caused by emotional states, surgery, extensive burns, infection and other diseases may induce ulcers

Treatment of ulcers almost always includes antacid therapy. Medications that reduce the amount of acid produced also are used. Although bland diets have been recommended, some studies suggest that spicy foods are not harmful for people with ulcers. It may be helpful to eat smaller meals more frequently to keep some food in the stomach at all times. The food prevents stomach acid from coming in direct contact with the stomach lining. The drug sucralfate adheres to damaged ulcer tissue, protecting it from stomach acid and enzymes.

ANTISPASMODICS
Belladonna Alkaloids and Phenobarbital
(bell a don′ a al′ ka loyds) (fee noe bar′ bi tal)

PRODUCT INFORMATION
Brand names: Barbidonna, Belladenal, Belladenal-S, Bellalphen, Donnatal, Hybephen, Hyoscophen, Kinesed

USES
This combination of drugs helps to relieve cramping pain of the stomach, intestines and bladder. This medicine often is prescribed as part of a total treatment of ulcers.

UNDESIRED EFFECTS
One common side effect of this medicine is dryness of the mouth, nose and throat.

To relieve the dryness, chew gum, suck hard candy or ice chips or drink plenty of fluids.

This medicine makes some people drowsy, dizzy or less alert than normal. Do not drive a car or operate dangerous machinery until you know how this medicine will affect you.

Belladonna alkaloids often will make you sweat less and increase the chance of a heatstroke. Use extra care not to become overheated during exercise and hot weather, and avoid hot baths and saunas while you are taking this medicine.

Other effects, which may disappear as your body adjusts to this medication, are constipation, flushing of the skin, headache, mental confusion, rapid heartbeat, blurred vision, clumsiness, decreased sexual ability, difficulty urinating, nausea and vomiting, nervousness and reduced sense of taste. If these effects are persistent or severe, contact your doctor.

This medicine also may make your eyes more sensitive to light. Wear sunglasses to relieve this discomfort.

Rarely, this medicine will cause effects that require medical attention. Contact your doctor if you have eye pain, hallucinations (seeing, hearing or feeling things that are not there), skin rash, slurred speech, sore throat and fever, unusual bleeding or bruising or yellowing of the eyes or skin.

PRECAUTIONS

If you ever had an unusual reaction to atropine, belladonna or any barbiturate, you should not take this medicine. If you have any questions, check with your doctor or pharmacist.

This combination of drugs can make certain medical conditions worse. Before you start to take this medicine, tell your doctor if you have difficulty urinating, glaucoma, kidney disease, liver disease, lung disease, enlarged prostate, rapid heartbeat, spastic paralysis (in children) or brain damage (in children).

Tell your doctor what prescription or nonprescription drugs you are taking, including amantadine, antacids, anticoagulants (blood thinners), corticosteroids, digitalis, digitoxin, griseofulvin, medicine for Parkinson's disease, other medicine for intestinal or stomach cramping, medicine for ulcers, antihistamines, medicine for allergies or colds, medicine for seizures, narcotics, prescription medicine for pain, barbiturates, sedatives, tranquilizers, medicine to help you sleep, medicine for depression and MAO inhibitors (isocarboxazid, pargyline, phenelzine or tranylcypromine), even if you stopped taking them within the past two weeks.

If you do not know the names of the drugs you are taking or what they were prescribed for, bring them in their labeled containers to your doctor or pharmacist.

Do not drink alcoholic beverages while taking this medicine. Do not start taking any of the drugs listed above without first checking with your doctor or pharmacist. All of them can increase the chance and severity of side effects.

Because antacids and medicine for diarrhea can make belladonna less effective, do not take them within one hour of belladonna. If you have questions, check with your doctor or pharmacist.

Take this medicine exactly as directed by your doctor. Do not take more or less of it, do not take it more often and do not take it for a longer period than ordered by your doctor.

Before you start to take this medicine, tell your doctor if you are pregnant or intend to become pregnant while using it. If you do become pregnant while taking this medicine, notify your doctor promptly.

DOSAGE
Your doctor will determine how often you should take this medicine and how much you should take at each dose. Carefully follow the instructions on your prescription label, and ask your doctor or pharmacist to explain any part of the instructions you do not understand.

If you forget to take a dose, take it as soon as you remember. Then take any remaining doses for that day at evenly spaced intervals. *Do not take a double dose.*

STORAGE
Keep this medicine in the container it came in and out of the reach of children.

Dicyclomine
(dye sye' kloe meen)

PRODUCT INFORMATION
Brand name: Bentyl

USES
Dicyclomine acts on the nerves and muscles to relieve spasms in the stomach and intestines. Dicyclomine is used to relieve stomach cramps and cramping or spasms of the intestines caused by ulcers, colitis and other gastrointestinal problems.

UNDESIRED EFFECTS
Dicyclomine may make some people drowsy or dizzy. Do not drive a car or operate dangerous machinery until you know how this medicine will affect you.

Because dicyclomine may make you sweat less, there is an increased chance of heatstroke. Use extra care not to become overheated during exercise and hot weather, and avoid hot baths and saunas while you are taking this medicine.

Other side effects, which may go away as your body adjusts to dicyclomine, include a bloated feeling, headache, decreased sexual ability, mental confusion (especially in the elderly), nausea and vomiting, nervousness and rapid pulse. Contact your doctor if these effects continue or are severe. If you have heart trouble and this medicine changes the rate of your heartbeat, notify your doctor.

Contact your doctor if you experience constipation, difficult urination or skin rash.

PRECAUTIONS
You should not take dicyclomine if you have certain medical problems. Before

starting to take this medicine, tell your doctor if you have difficulty urinating, enlarged prostate, glaucoma, hiatal hernia, intestinal blockage, liver disease, myasthenia gravis or severe ulcerative colitis.

Tell your doctor what prescription or nonprescription drugs you are now taking, including amantadine, antacids, antihistamines, haloperidol, medicine for depression, medicine for diarrhea, medicine to help you sleep, medicine for Parkinson's disease, medicine for ulcers, sedatives or tranquilizers. If you do not know the names of the drugs or what they were prescribed for, bring them in their labeled containers to your doctor or pharmacist.

If you have taken MAO inhibitors (isocarboxazid, pargyline, phenelzine or tranylcypromine) within the past two weeks or are taking them now, tell your doctor.

Do not drink alcoholic beverages while you are taking dicyclomine. Do not start taking any of the drugs listed above unless you first check with your doctor or pharmacist. All of them can increase the chance and severity of side effects.

Take this medicine exactly as prescribed by your doctor. Do not take more or less of it, do not take it more often and do not take it for a longer period than your doctor has ordered.

It is best not to take this medicine within one hour of taking antacids or medicine for diarrhea. If you have any questions, check with your doctor or pharmacist.

Before you start taking dicyclomine, it is wise to tell your doctor if you are pregnant or are nursing a baby, although no harm to the baby has been reported as a result of using dicyclomine.

DOSAGE

Your doctor will determine how often you should take dicyclomine and how much you should take at each dose. Carefully follow the instructions on your prescription label, and ask your doctor or pharmacist to explain any part of the instructions you do not understand.

Dicyclomine comes in capsules, tablets and liquid form. If this medicine upsets your stomach, you may take it with solid food or milk.

If you forget to take a dose of dicyclomine, take it as soon as you remember. Take any remaining doses for that day at evenly spaced intervals. *Do not take a double dose to make up for a missed one.*

STORAGE

Keep dicyclomine in the container it came in, and keep it out of the reach of children.

Isopropamide
(eye so proe′ pa mide)

PRODUCT INFORMATION
Brand name: Darbid

Brand names of combination products containing prochlorperazine maleate: Combid, Isopro T.D., Prochlor-Iso, Pro-Iso

USES
Isopropamide is sometimes used in the treatment of peptic ulcer disease (ulcers) and some stomach and intestinal disorders.

UNDESIRED EFFECTS
Dry mouth is a common side effect of isopropamide. To relieve this effect, chew gum or suck hard candy. Isopropamide can cause blurred vision. This effect tends to decrease or disappear as your body adjusts to the medicine. However, contact your doctor if this effect persists or is severe.

If you experience difficulty or pain on urination, contact your doctor.

Isopropamide may cause drowsiness. Use caution when driving a car or operating dangerous machinery until you know how this drug will affect you.

PRECAUTIONS
Before you start to take any product containing isopropamide, tell your doctor if you have glaucoma, enlarged prostate or obstruction of the stomach, small intestine or neck of the bladder.

Tell your doctor what other prescription or nonprescription drugs you are taking. If you do not know the names of the drugs or what they were prescribed for, bring them in their labeled containers to your doctor or pharmacist.

DOSAGE
Carefully follow the instructions on your prescription label, and ask your doctor or pharmacist to explain any part of the instructions you do not understand. Your doctor has determined when you should take this drug and how much you should take at each dose.

If you miss a dose of isopropamide, take only the next regularly scheduled dose at the time it is due. *Do not take a double dose to make up for the missed one.*

STORAGE
Keep isopropamide in the container it came in, and keep it out of the reach of children. Do not allow anyone else to take your isopropamide.

Propantheline
(proe pan' the leen)

PRODUCT INFORMATION
Brand name: Pro-Banthine

USES
Propantheline relieves cramping pain and spasms in the stomach and intestines.

Because propantheline also reduces the amount of acid formed in the stomach, it is used to treat stomach ulcers.

UNDESIRED EFFECTS

One common side effect of propantheline is dryness of the mouth, nose and throat. To relieve this dryness, chew gum, suck hard candy or ice chips or drink plenty of fluids.

This medicine makes some people drowsy, dizzy or less alert than usual. Do not drive a car or operate dangerous machinery until you know how propantheline will affect you.

Other side effects, which may disappear as your body adjusts to propantheline, include a bloated feeling, headache, rapid pulse, reduced sweating, blurred vision, decreased sexual ability, increased sensitivity of eyes to light, mental confusion (especially in elderly people), nausea and vomiting, nervousness, reduced sense of taste and tiredness. If any of these effects bother you, contact your doctor.

More serious side effects, although they do not occur often, will require medical attention. Contact your doctor if you have constipation, difficulty in urinating, eye pain or skin rash.

PRECAUTIONS

Propantheline can make certain medical conditions worse. Before you start to take this medicine, tell your doctor if you have asthma, bronchitis, difficult urination, emphysema, enlarged prostate, glaucoma, hiatal hernia, high blood pressure, intestinal blockage, kidney disease, liver disease, myasthenia gravis, overactive thyroid or severe ulcerative colitis.

Tell your doctor what prescription or nonprescription drugs you are taking, including amantadine, antacids, antihistamines, medicine for allergies or colds, haloperidol, medicine for your heart, medicine for diarrhea, medicine for Parkinson's disease, medicine to help you sleep, sedatives, tranquilizers and medicine for ulcers. If you do not know the names of the drugs or what they were prescribed for, bring them in their labeled containers to your doctor or pharmacist.

Do not drink alcoholic beverages while you are taking propantheline. Do not start taking any of the drugs listed above unless you first check with your doctor. All of them can increase the chance and severity of side effects.

Propantheline may make your eyes more sensitive to light than normal. Wear sunglasses to help decrease the discomfort caused by bright light.

Because this medicine can make you sweat less, it may increase the chance of heatstroke. While you are taking propantheline, try not to become overheated (for example, avoid strenuous exercise, being out in hot weather, saunas and steam baths).

Do not take propantheline for stomachache due to gas, for sour stomach or for any problem other than the one for which it was prescribed.

To help select the best treatment for you and your baby, tell your doctor if you are pregnant.

DOSAGE
Your doctor will determine how often you should take propantheline and how much to take at each dose. Carefully follow the instructions on your prescription label, and ask your doctor or pharmacist to explain any part of the instructions you do not understand.

Propantheline comes in tablets. It is usually taken four times a day, before or with meals and at bedtime. Do not take propantheline within one hour of taking an antacid or medicine for diarrhea. If these medicines are taken too close together, propantheline may be less effective.

If you forget to take a dose of propantheline, take the missed dose with some food as soon as you remember. Take any remaining doses for that day at evenly spaced intervals. *Do not take more than one dose at a time.*

STORAGE
Keep propantheline in the container it came in, and keep it out of the reach of children.

MISCELLANEOUS
Cimetidine
(sye met' i deen)

PRODUCT INFORMATION
Brand name: Tagamet

USES
Cimetidine is used to treat and prevent the recurrence of gastrointestinal ulcers. It decreases the amount of acid produced by the stomach. Cimetidine is also used to treat other conditions in which the stomach produces too much acid.

UNDESIRED EFFECTS
Cimetidine may cause diarrhea, muscle pain, rash, headache and dizziness or drowsiness. These side effects are usually mild and may decrease or disappear as your body adjusts to the medicine. If they are persistent or severe, contact your doctor. It may be necessary to decrease the dose you are taking.

Other less common side effects include swelling or soreness of the breasts, fever, sore throat and mental confusion (particularly in the elderly or severely ill). If you experience any of these effects, contact your doctor.

PRECAUTIONS
Cimetidine can make certain medical conditions worse. Tell your doctor if you have kidney or liver disease.

Cimetidine can affect the way your body responds to certain medications, including anticoagulants (warfarin-type blood thinners), benzodiazepines (especially chlordiazepoxide and diazepam), beta blockers (atenolol, metoprolol, nadolol, pindolol, propranolol and timolol), phenytoin and theophylline.

Before you begin to take cimetidine, tell your doctor or pharmacist what prescription and nonprescription medications you are taking. If you do not know the names of the drugs or what they were prescribed for, take them in their labeled containers to your doctor or pharmacist.

You may have to take cimetidine for up to eight weeks before your ulcer heals completely. *Keep all appointments with your doctor* so your response to this medication can be monitored.

If you have ulcers, do not smoke cigarettes. Smoking apparently inhibits ulcer healing.

This drug is passed from a mother to her unborn child and to a nursing baby through the milk. It is not known if cimetidine is safe for the baby. If you are pregnant, plan to become pregnant or are breast-feeding, tell your doctor before starting to take cimetidine.

DOSAGE
Cimetidine comes in tablets, in oral liquid form and in an injectable form.

Your doctor will determine how much cimetidine you should take at each dose. Cimetidine may be taken four times a day (with meals and at bedtime), once a day at bedtime (to prevent recurrence of ulcers) or twice a day. Your doctor will decide which dosage schedule you should follow. Follow the instructions on your prescription label carefully, and ask your doctor or pharmacist to explain any part you do not understand.

If you are taking antacids, do not take them within one hour of cimetidine. Antacids may interfere with the absorption of cimetidine.

If you forget to take a dose of cimetidine, take it as soon as you remember. If you do not remember until it is almost time for the next dose, omit the missed dose and take only the scheduled dose. *Do not take a double dose to make up for a missed dose.*

STORAGE
Keep cimetidine in the container it came in, and keep it out of the reach of children. Do not allow anyone else to take your cimetidine.

Ranitidine
(ra nye′ te deen)

PRODUCT INFORMATION
Brand name: Zantac

USES
Ranitidine is used to treat some types of gastrointestinal ulcers. It decreases the amount of acid produced by the stomach. Ranitidine is also used to treat other

conditions in which the stomach produces too much acid. Although its effectiveness is not known, ranitidine has been used investigationally to prevent recurrence of ulcers.

UNDESIRED EFFECTS
Ranitidine may cause headache, constipation, nausea, abdominal pain, dizziness or a rash. If these problems are bothersome, contact your doctor.

Other less common side effects include swelling or soreness of the breasts, fever, sore throat and mental confusion (particularly in the elderly or severely ill). If you experience any of these effects, contact your doctor.

PRECAUTIONS
Ranitidine can make certain medical conditions worse. Tell your doctor if you have kidney or liver disease.

Before you begin to take ranitidine, tell your doctor what prescription and nonprescription medications you are taking, particularly propantheline because it may increase the absorption of ranitidine. If you do not know the names of the drugs or what they were prescribed for, take them in their labeled containers to your doctor or pharmacist.

If you have ulcers, do not smoke cigarettes. Smoking apparently inhibits ulcer healing.

Although most ulcers heal within four weeks, you may have to take ranitidine for up to eight weeks before complete healing occurs. *Keep all appointments with your doctor* so your response to this medication can be monitored.

Ranitidine is passed from a mother to a nursing baby through the milk. Tell your doctor if you are pregnant, plan to become pregnant or are breast-feeding. It is not known if it is safe to take ranitidine during pregnancy or while breast-feeding.

DOSAGE
Ranitidine comes in tablets. Your doctor has determined how much you should take at each dose. Ranitidine is usually taken twice a day (or once a day at bedtime to prevent ulcer recurrence). Follow the instructions on your prescription label carefully, and ask your doctor or pharmacist to explain any part you do not understand.

If you are taking antacids, do not take them within one hour of ranitidine. Antacids may affect the absorption of ranitidine.

If you forget to take a dose, take it as soon as you remember. If you do not remember until it is almost time for the next dose, omit the missed dose and take only the scheduled dose. *Do not take a double dose to make up for a missed dose.*

STORAGE
Keep ranitidine in the container it came in, and keep it out of the reach of children.

Sucralfate
(soo′ kral fate)

PRODUCT INFORMATION
Brand name: Carafate

USES
Sucralfate is used to treat ulcers. It adheres to damaged ulcer tissue and protects against acid and enzymes so healing can occur.

UNDESIRED EFFECTS
Sucralfate usually does not cause problems. The most common side effect of sucralfate is constipation. Other problems that can occur include diarrhea, nausea, indigestion, stomach discomfort, rash, itching, back pain, dizziness and sleepiness. If these side effects are bothersome, contact your doctor.

PRECAUTIONS
It may take up to eight weeks for ulcers to heal. Do not stop taking this medication without your doctor's permission. *Keep all appointments with your doctor and the laboratory.* Contact your doctor immediately if you experience any signs of internal bleeding (passing red or black stools or coughing up or vomiting material that is bright red or looks like coffee grounds).

Before you begin to take sucralfate, tell your doctor what prescription and nonprescription drugs you are taking including antacids, cimetidine, phenytoin and tetracycline. If you do not know the names of the drugs or what they were prescribed for, bring them in their labeled containers to your doctor or pharmacist.

Although problems have not been reported with the use of sucralfate during pregnancy or while breast-feeding, tell your doctor if you are pregnant or nursing a baby.

DOSAGE
Sucralfate comes in tablets. Your doctor will determine how often you should take it and how much you should take at each dose. Follow the instructions on your prescription label, and ask your doctor or pharmacist to explain any part you do not understand. Sucralfate is usually taken four times a day, before meals and at bedtime. It should be taken on an empty stomach one hour before meals. If you are taking antacids, do not take them within 30 minutes of taking sucralfate. If you also are taking cimetidine, phenytoin or tetracycline, do not take any of them within two hours of taking sucralfate.

If you forget to take a dose of this medication, take it as soon as you remember. However, if it is time for the next scheduled dose, omit the missed dose and take only the scheduled dose. *Do not take a double dose to make up for a missed dose.*

STORAGE
Keep this medication in the container it came in, and keep it out of the reach of children.

Sulfasalazine
(sul fa sal′ a zeen)

PRODUCT INFORMATION
Brand names: Azulfidine, Porasul, S.A.S.-500, Sulcolon

USES
Sulfasalazine is a sulfa drug used to treat ulcerative colitis, a chronic inflammatory bowel disease accompanied by attacks of bloody diarrhea. It is usually taken on a long-term basis (up to one year) to decrease the frequency and severity of relapses of the disease.

Sulfasalazine has also been used investigationally to treat other bowel diseases (Crohn's disease and granulomatous colitis) and a skin disease (scleroderma).

UNDESIRED EFFECTS
Sulfasalazine may cause nausea, vomiting, diarrhea and loss of appetite. You may take this medication after food to decrease stomach irritation. If these symptoms appear after you have taken the drug for a few days without problems, your dose may be too high. Check with your doctor about reducing your dose if these side effects persist.

Sulfasalazine may cause an allergic reaction. Stop taking this medicine and contact your doctor if you develop a rash, hives and itching (early signs of allergic reaction). Less frequently, sulfasalazine will cause more serious allergic reactions. If you get fever, aching of the joints or muscles, difficulty in swallowing or skin problems (redness, blistering, peeling or loosening of the skin), stop taking the medicine and contact your doctor immediately.

Sulfasalazine also can cause blood problems and liver problems. Stop taking the medicine and contact your doctor if you experience unusual bleeding or bruising, unusual weakness and tiredness, fever, pale skin or sore throat (symptoms of blood problems) or yellowing of the eyes or skin (symptoms of liver problems).

Sulfasalazine may cause an orange-yellow discoloration of the urine; this effect is harmless. Sulfasalazine rarely will cause kidney or thyroid problems. If you notice blood in your urine, lower back pain, pain or burning while urinating or a swelling of the front part of the neck (goiter), stop taking the medicine and contact your doctor immediately.

Some people who take sulfasalazine become more sensitive to sunlight than they are normally. Limit the amount of time you spend in sunlight or under sunlamps until you know how you react to sulfasalazine, especially if you sunburn easily. This sensitivity to sunlight can continue for many months after you stop taking sulfasalazine. If you become severely sunburned, contact your doctor.

PRECAUTIONS

Before you start taking sulfasalazine, tell your doctor if you ever had a bad reaction to aspirin or other salicylates or an allergic reaction to any sulfa drug, a diuretic (water pill), oral diabetes medicine or oral medicine for glaucoma. Your doctor should also know if you have a history of allergy, hay fever or asthma.

To select the best treatment for you, your doctor needs to know if you have G6PD deficiency (an inherited blood disease), porphyria, intestinal or urinary tract obstruction, kidney disease or liver disease or if you ever had anemia produced by a drug.

Certain other medicines, when taken with sulfasalazine, will affect the way your body responds to this drug. Tell your doctor what other prescription or nonprescription drugs you are taking, including antibiotics (especially penicillins), oral anticoagulants (blood thinners), oral diabetes medicines, digoxin, folic acid, iron, methenamine (a urinary antiseptic), methotrexate (a psoriasis or antitumor medicine), phenylbutazone or oxyphenbutazone (for arthritis), phenytoin (a medicine for seizures), probenecid or sulfinpyrazone (gout medicines) or any medicine to make your urine more alkaline, such as sodium bicarbonate or sodium citrate. If you do not know the names of the drugs you are taking or what they were prescribed for, bring them in their labeled containers to your doctor or pharmacist.

Sulfasalazine should not be taken by children under two years of age, pregnant women who are at term (ninth month) or nursing mothers. Tell your doctor if you are nursing a baby, are pregnant or intend to become pregnant while taking this medicine.

Keep all appointments with your doctor and the laboratory so your response to this medication can be monitored with regular blood counts, urine tests and tests for thyroid, liver and kidney function.

Before having any surgery with a general anesthetic, including dental surgery, be sure to tell the doctor or dentist that you are taking sulfasalazine.

DOSAGE

Your doctor has determined how much sulfasalazine you should take and how often you should take it. Carefully follow the instructions on your prescription label, and ask your doctor or pharmacist to explain any part of the instructions you do not understand.

Sulfasalazine comes in regular tablets, enteric-coated tablets and liquid form. It may be taken after food to decrease stomach irritation. While you are taking this medicine, drink at least eight full eight-ounce glasses of water or other liquids (coffee, tea, soft drinks, milk and fruit juice) every day. This practice will help protect your kidneys from problems sulfasalazine can cause.

Both the tablets and the liquid should be taken with a full eight-ounce glass of water. Shake the container of liquid before each use to distribute the medication evenly. Measure doses of liquid with a specially marked measuring spoon to ensure an accurate dose.

If you forget to take a dose of sulfasalazine, take it as soon as you remember. However, if you remember a missed dose when it is close to the time for another, omit the missed dose and take only the scheduled dose. *Do not take a double dose.*

STORAGE

Store sulfasalazine in the container it came in, and keep it out of the reach of children.

Allergies, Colds and Coughs

DRUGS USED TO TREAT
ALLERGIES, COLDS AND COUGHS

Allergies, Colds and Coughs

The common cold is caused by a number of different viruses that are spread only by contact with persons who are already infected. Although chill and dampness do not cause colds, they may make a person more susceptible to catching one.

Symptoms of a cold usually begin one to four days after contact with the virus. They include nasal congestion and discharge, sneezing, sore throat, headache, chills and cough. In some cases, a mild fever may occur.

In healthy persons, the symptoms last five to seven days and complications are rare. Children and the elderly are more likely to develop complications such as sinus infection, ear infections and pneumonia. It is for this reason that antibiotics sometimes are prescribed for individuals with the common cold. Antibiotics are ineffective against the cold itself but they do prevent bacterial infections.

Cough results from irritation of the throat by postnasal drip. Cough is one of the body's natural reflexes that serves to keep the airways clear. Two types of medications are used to treat coughs—cough suppressants and expectorants. The cough suppressants are best used for dry coughs. Expectorants are used to thin phlegm and make it easier to cough up. In either case, it is very helpful to drink a lot of fluids. In severe cases, a humidifier may be used to keep the throat moist.

The symptoms of allergies are similar to those of the common cold. Nasal congestion, running nose, sneezing and itching, watery eyes usually are present. Pollens are the most common causes of allergic reactions and the seasonal appearance of symptoms is directly related to the amount of pollen in the air. Although pollens are the most common causes of allergic reactions, dust, animal dander, feathers and many other things can cause allergic reactions.

Several types of medications are used to treat allergies, including antihistamines and decongestants. Both types help relieve nasal congestion. Antihistamines act to prevent part of the allergic reaction itself, while the decongestants relieve symptoms after they occur. Many combination products are available that contain both types of medication.

ANTIHISTAMINES

USES
Histamine is a natural substance that is present throughout the body. It remains stored in cells until something that produces an allergic reaction (for example, pollen) comes in contact with the body. When this happens, histamine is released to produce allergy symptoms such as itching, watery eyes, rashes and runny nose.

Antihistamines are drugs that relieve allergy symptoms by counteracting the effects of histamine. These ingredients are present in many nonprescription cough medicines and cold products. Because drowsiness is a common side effect of some antihistamines, they are used in some nonprescription sleep aids.

UNDESIRED EFFECTS
When used correctly at recommended dosages, antihistamines rarely cause serious side effects. They may cause drowsiness, dryness of the mouth and stomach upset. These effects usually are minor, but if they are severe or persistent, you should contact your doctor or pharmacist.

PRECAUTIONS
Use of alcohol, tranquilizers, sleeping pills, narcotics and medications for seizures may increase the drowsiness caused by antihistamines. Check with your doctor or pharmacist before taking antihistamines with these other medications.

Because antihistamines can cause drowsiness, you should not drive or operate dangerous machinery until you know how antihistamines will affect you.

If you have an enlarged prostate, heart disease, high blood pressure, glaucoma, thyroid problems or ulcers, check with your doctor or pharmacist before taking antihistamines.

Women who are pregnant or breast-feeding should check with their doctor before using antihistamines.

Brompheniramine
(brome fen eer' a meen)

PRODUCT INFORMATION
Brand names: B.P.E., Bromphen, Dimetane, Puretane, Rolabromophen, Spentane, Steraphenate, Veltane and others

Brand names of some products containing brompheniramine: Brocon, Dimetapp, Dynohist, Histapp, Phenatapp, Poly-Histine, Puretapp and others

USES
See the general statement titled Antihistamines.

Brompheniramine is one of a group of drugs called antihistamines. These drugs are used to counteract the effects of histamine, one of the body's natural substances.

Antihistamines relieve the symptoms of allergy such as itching, watery eyes and runny nose by counteracting histamine. Antihistamines also are used for allergic reactions to bee stings, poison ivy and poison oak. Brompheniramine is available alone or in combination with decongestants, cough medicine, expectorants and pain medicine.

UNDESIRED EFFECTS
See the general statement titled Antihistamines.
One common effect of brompheniramine is dryness of the mouth. This can be relieved by chewing gum, sucking hard candies or drinking fluids.

Brompheniramine also can upset your stomach. If it does, take it with meals or a snack. Contact your doctor if this does not help or if the upsets are severe.

Brompheniramine causes some people to become dizzy or drowsy. Do not drive a car or operate dangerous machinery until you know how this medicine will affect you. With children, the effect can be just the opposite and they may become nervous or restless or have trouble sleeping.

Other side effects include blurred vision, difficult or painful urination, headache, loss of appetite, skin rash, unusual increase in sweating and unusually fast heartbeat. If you experience any of these effects, contact your doctor or pharmacist.

PRECAUTIONS
See the general statement titled Antihistamines.
Before you start taking brompheniramine, tell your doctor if you have an enlarged prostate, heart disease, high blood pressure, glaucoma, overactive thyroid, stomach ulcer or urinary tract blockage. People with these conditions should not take antihistamines such as brompheniramine. If you are considering using one of the products that can be obtained without a prescription, discuss this with your pharmacist.

Tell your doctor or pharmacist what prescription or nonprescription drugs you are taking, including barbiturates, medicine for seizures, narcotics, other medicine for hay fever or allergies, prescription medicine for pain, sedatives, tranquilizers, medicine to help you sleep and medicine for depression. If you do not know the names of the drugs you are taking or what they were prescribed for, bring them in their labeled containers to your doctor or pharmacist.

Do not start to take any of the drugs listed above while you are taking brompheniramine unless you first check with your doctor or pharmacist.

Do not drink alcoholic beverages while you are taking brompheniramine. Alcohol can increase the chance or severity of drowsiness and dizziness.

Antihistamines are used to relieve or prevent the symptoms of allergy and should be used only as directed. Do not take more of this medicine than your doctor or label instructions prescribe.

If you are pregnant or are breast-feeding a baby, do not take brompheniramine unless your doctor prescribes it for you and is aware of your pregnancy or the fact that you are breast-feeding.

DOSAGE
If your doctor prescribes brompheniramine or a product containing this drug, he

or she will tell you how often to take it and how much to take at each dose. Carefully follow the instructions on your prescription label and ask your doctor or pharmacist to explain any part of the instructions you do not understand. If you obtain brompheniramine without a prescription, follow the instructions on the label or in the carton carefully. If you have any questions about this, check with your pharmacist. Do not give brompheniramine to infants without your doctor's approval.

Brompheniramine is available in liquid, tablets and extended-release tablets. If you are taking the extended-release tablets, be sure to swallow them whole. Do not break, crush or chew them before swallowing.

STORAGE
Keep brompheniramine in the container it came in, and keep it out of the reach of children.

Chlorpheniramine
(klor fen eer' a meen)

PRODUCT INFORMATION
Brand names: Allerbid, AL-R, Chloramate, Chlor-Span, Chlortab, Chlor-Trimeton, Ciramine, Histaspan, Histex, Panahist, Phenetron, T.D. Alermine, Teldrin and others

Brand names of some of the many products containing chlorpheniramine: Anamine, Anatuss, Chlorfed, Codimal, Colrex, Comhist, Comtrex, Contac, Coricidin, Corilin, Coryban-D, CoTylenol, Decon-Aid, Deconamine, Decon-Tuss, Demazin, Extendryl, 4-Way Cold Tablets, Fedahist, Guistrey, Histabid, Hista-Clopine, Histadyl, Histalet, Historal, Isoclor, Korigesic, Kronohist, Naldecon, Napril, Nasalspan, Neotep, Nilcol, Nolamine, Norel Plus, Novafed, Novahistine, Ornade, P-V-Tussin, Pediacof, Probacon, Pseudo-Hist, Quelidrine, Rhinex, Romex, Ru-Tuss, Ryna, Rynatan, Rynatuss, Singlet, Sinovan, Sinulin, Sudafed-Plus, Triaminic, Tusquelin, Tussar, Tussi-Organidin, Tuss-Ornade and others

USES
See the general statement titled Antihistamines.

Chlorpheniramine is an antihistamine that causes less drowsiness and more central nervous system stimulation than some antihistamines. It is particularly suited for daytime relief of the symptoms of colds and allergies. In addition to being used alone, chlorpheniramine is combined with pain medicine, other antihistamines, cough suppressants, decongestants, expectorants and bronchodilators.

UNDESIRED EFFECTS
See the general statement titled Antihistamines.

One of the most common effects of chlorpheniramine is dryness of the mouth. This can be relieved by sucking hard candies, chewing gum or drinking fluids.

Chlorpheniramine may upset your stomach or give you stomach pains. If you take the medicine with a glass of milk, a snack or at mealtime, these problems may be helped. If they continue or are severe, contact your doctor.

Chlorpheniramine makes some people drowsy or dizzy. Do not drive a car or operate dangerous machinery until you know how this medicine will affect you. This effect is more common with older people. Children, on the other hand, may become restless and nervous and have trouble sleeping after they have been taking chlorpheniramine. If these effects continue for a period of time or are bothersome, contact your doctor.

Other side effects of chlorpheniramine include blurred vision, difficult or painful urination, headache, loss of appetite, skin rash, unusual increase in sweating and unusually fast heartbeat. If you experience these effects, contact your doctor.

PRECAUTIONS
See the general statement titled Antihistamines.

If you have certain medical conditions, you probably should not take chlorpheniramine or other antihistamines because these medicines can make the conditions worse. Since several of the products containing chlorpheniramine are available without a prescription, you should have medical advice concerning their use if you have an enlarged prostate, heart disease, high blood pressure, glaucoma, overactive thyroid, stomach ulcer or urinary tract blockage. Check with your doctor or pharmacist if you have any of these conditions.

Tell your doctor or pharmacist what prescription or nonprescription drugs you are taking, particularly barbiturates, medicine for seizures, narcotics, other medicines for allergy, medicine for pain, sedatives, tranquilizers, medicine to help you sleep, medicine for depression and MAO inhibitors (isocarboxazid, pargyline, phenelzine and tranylcypromine). If you do not know the names of the drugs or what they were prescribed for, bring them in their labeled containers to your doctor or pharmacist.

While you are taking chlorpheniramine, do not drink alcoholic beverages or start to take any of the drugs listed above unless you first check with your doctor or pharmacist. All of these drugs can increase the chance or severity of drowsiness or dizziness.

Because chlorpheniramine is intended only to relieve the symptoms of your medical problem, it should be used with care. Do not take more than recommended and do not take it more often than prescribed by your doctor or directed on the package label.

Before having surgery (including dental surgery) with a general anesthetic, tell the doctor or dentist that you are taking chlorpheniramine.

To help your doctor select the best treatment for you and your baby, tell your doctor if you are pregnant or are breast-feeding. This drug can be passed to your unborn baby or breast-fed baby and also may decrease the quantity of your milk.

DOSAGE
Carefully follow the instructions of your doctor or pharmacist or those on the package of chlorpheniramine products that you purchase without a prescription. If you have any questions about the instructions, check with your pharmacist.

Do not give chlorpheniramine to infants without your doctor's approval. Chlorpheniramine is available in liquid, tablets, extended-release tablets and extended-release capsules. If you are taking the extended release tablets or capsules, be sure to swallow them whole. Do not crack, crush or chew them. Take all tablets and capsules with a full glass of water, or with food if they upset your stomach. To ensure an accurate dose of liquid, use a specially marked measuring spoon.

STORAGE
Keep chlorpheniramine in the container it came in, and keep it out of the reach of children.

Cyproheptadine
(si proe hep' ta deen)

PRODUCT INFORMATION
Brand name: Periactin

USES
See the general statement titled Antihistamines.
Cyproheptadine, an antihistamine, is used to relieve the symptoms of hay fever, bee stings, poison ivy, poison oak and colds. It also is used to treat some types of migraine headaches and, in some cases, to help gain weight.

UNDESIRED EFFECTS
See the general statement titled Antihistamines.
One of the most common side effects of cyproheptadine, dryness of the mouth and throat, can be relieved by sucking on hard candy, chewing gum or drinking fluids.

Cyproheptadine may upset your stomach when you first begin to take it. To lessen this problem, take the medicine with milk or solid food.

Cyproheptadine makes some people drowsy or dizzy. Do not drive a car or operate dangerous machinery until you know how this medicine will affect you.

These effects may go away as your body adjusts to the medicine. If they continue or are severe, contact your doctor.

Other side effects of cyproheptadine include blurred vision, difficult or painful urination, headache, increased appetite or weight gain, nervousness, restlessness or trouble sleeping (especially in children), skin rash, unusual increase in sweating and unusually fast heartbeat. If you experience these effects and they are troublesome, contact your doctor.

PRECAUTIONS
See the general statement titled Antihistamines.
Before you start to take cyproheptadine, tell your doctor if you have an enlarged prostate, heart disease, high blood pressure, glaucoma, an overactive thyroid, a

stomach ulcer or urinary tract blockage. Cyproheptadine can make these conditions worse.

Tell your doctor what prescription or nonprescription drugs you are taking. Certain other drugs should not be taken with cyproheptadine, including medicine for seizures, narcotics, other medicines for allergy, prescription medicine for pain, sedatives, tranquilizers, medicine to help you sleep and medicine for depression. If you do not know the names of the drugs you are taking or what they were prescribed for, bring them in their labeled containers to your doctor or pharmacist.

Do not start to take any of the drugs listed above while you are taking cyproheptadine unless you first check with your doctor. Before you have surgery with a general anesthetic, including dental surgery, tell the doctor or dentist in charge that you are taking cyproheptadine.

Take this medicine exactly as directed. Do not take more of it and do not take it more often than your doctor has indicated.

Do not drink alcoholic beverages while you are taking cyproheptadine, because alcohol can increase the chance and severity of drowsiness.

To help your doctor select the best treatment for you and your baby, tell the doctor if you are pregnant or are breast-feeding. Cyproheptadine can be passed to your unborn child or your breast-fed baby. It also can decrease the amount of your milk.

DOSAGE

Your doctor will determine how often you should take cyproheptadine and how much you should take at each dose. Carefully follow the instructions on your prescription label and ask your doctor or pharmacist to explain any part of the instructions you do not understand.

Cyproheptadine comes in liquid and tablets. Take the tablets with a full eight-ounce glass of water or, if this medicine upsets your stomach, with a glass of milk or solid food. Use a specially marked measuring spoon to ensure a liquid dose that is accurate.

If you forget to take a dose, take it as soon as you remember it and take the remaining doses for the day at evenly spaced intervals. *Do not take a double dose to make up for the missed dose.*

STORAGE

Keep cyproheptadine in the container it came in, and keep it out of the reach of children. Do not allow anyone else to take your cyproheptadine.

Dexbrompheniramine

(dex brome fen eer′ a meen)

PRODUCT INFORMATION

Brand names: Disophrol, Drixoral

USES
See the general statement titled Antihistamines.

Dexbrompheniramine is an antihistamine very closely related to brompheniramine in chemical structure and in action. However, dexbrompheniramine is almost twice as effective as brompheniramine. Dexbrompheniramine is available only in combination with the decongestant pseudoephedrine. This combination is used to relieve the symptoms of respiratory allergies.

UNDESIRED EFFECTS
See the general statement titled Antihistamines.

Two common effects of dexbrompheniramine are dryness of the mouth and throat and upset stomach. Dryness can be relieved by chewing gum, sucking on hard candy or drinking fluids. Stomach upset is less likely if you take this medicine with a glass of milk or with food. If these effects are severe or continue in spite of what you do, check with your doctor.

Although dexbrompheniramine causes less drowsiness than some other antihistamines, it can make some people drowsy or dizzy, particularly older people. Do not drive a car or operate dangerous machinery until you know how this medicine will affect you. Drowsiness or dizziness may decrease or disappear as your body adjusts to dexbrompheniramine. If it does not or is severe, contact your doctor.

Dexbrompheniramine can have just the opposite effect on children, making them nervous or restless and making it difficult for them to sleep. If these effects occur, contact your doctor. The doctor may want to adjust the dose or change the medication.

Other effects of dexbrompheniramine include blurred vision, difficult or painful urination, headache, loss of appetite, skin rash, unusual sweating or unusually fast heartbeat. Contact your doctor if these effects are severe.

PRECAUTIONS
See the general statement titled Antihistamines.

Before you start to take one of the products containing dexbrompheniramine, tell your doctor if you have an enlarged prostate, heart disease, high blood pressure, glaucoma, an overactive thyroid, a stomach ulcer or urinary tract blockage. Dexbrompheniramine can make these conditions worse.

Tell your doctor what prescription or nonprescription drugs you are taking, especially barbiturates, medicine for seizures, narcotics, other medicines for allergy, prescription medicine for pain, sedatives, tranquilizers, medicine to help you sleep and medicine for depression. If you do not know the names of the drugs you are taking or what they were prescribed for, bring them in their labeled containers to your doctor or pharmacist.

Do not drink alcoholic beverages while you are taking dexbrompheniramine. They can increase the chance of or the severity of drowsiness. Do not start to take any of the drugs listed above until you first check with your doctor.

Before you have surgery with a general anesthetic, including dental surgery, tell the doctor or dentist that you are taking dexbrompheniramine.

Take dexbrompheniramine exactly as prescribed by your doctor. Do not take more of it and do not take it more often than instructed.

If you are pregnant or breast-feeding, check with your doctor before using dexbrompheniramine.

Products containing dexbrompheniramine should not be given to children under the age of 12.

DOSAGE

Your doctor will determine how often you should take a product containing dexbrompheniramine and how much you should take at each dose. Carefully follow the instructions on your prescription label and ask your doctor or pharmacist to explain any part of the instructions you do not understand.

Dexbrompheniramine and pseudoephedrine are combined in tablets and extended-release tablets. If you are taking the extended-release tablets, be sure to swallow them whole. They should not be broken, crushed or chewed before being swallowed.

If you forget to take a dose of the medicine, take it as soon as you remember and then take the remaining doses for that day at evenly space intervals. *Do not take a double dose to make up for a missed dose.*

STORAGE

Keep dexbrompheniramine in the container it came in, and keep it out of the reach of children. Do not allow anyone else to take your dexbrompheniramine.

Diphenhydramine
(dye fen hye′ dra meen)

PRODUCT INFORMATION
Brand names: Allerben, Benadryl, Bendylate, Benylin, Fenylhist, SK-Diphenhydramine, Tussat, Valdrene

USES
See the general statement titled Antihistamines.

Diphenhydramine is an antihistamine with many more uses than other drugs of this type. In addition to being used to treat the symptoms of allergy (itchy, watery eyes and runny nose), it is also used to prevent motion sickness, to induce sleep and to decrease the stiffness and tremors of Parkinson's disease.

UNDESIRED EFFECTS
See the general statement titled Antihistamines.

Drowsiness, dizziness and lack of coordination are the most common side effects of diphenhydramine. While they are desired effects when this medicine is used to induce sleep, they can be problems when your activities require mental alertness. Do not drive a car or operate dangerous machinery until you know how this medicine will affect you.

Older people are more likely to experience drowsiness after they take diphenhydramine and may require a smaller dose. Young children, however, may have the opposite effect with restlessness, nervousness and difficulty sleeping. Contact your doctor if these effects are severe. The doctor may want to adjust the dose or change the medication.

Diphenhydramine causes less upset stomach than other antihistamines and may even be used to stop vomiting. However, if you should experience stomach upset or pain, take this medicine with a glass of milk or food. If stomach upsets continue or are severe, contact your doctor.

Other effects of diphenhydramine include blurred vision, difficult or painful urination, dryness of the mouth and throat, headache, loss of appetite, skin rash, unusual increase in sweating and unusually fast heartbeat. Contact your doctor if these effects continue beyond the first few days you take this medicine.

PRECAUTIONS
See the general statement titled Antihistamines.

Because diphenhydramine can make some medical problems worse, tell your doctor if you have an enlarged prostate, heart disease, high blood pressure, glaucoma, an overactive thyroid, a stomach ulcer or urinary tract blockage.

Certain medications, when you take them with diphenhydramine, can increase the chance of or severity of side effects. These include medicine for seizures, narcotics, other medicines for allergy, prescription medicines for pain, sedatives, tranquilizers, medicine to help you sleep and medicine for depression. Tell your doctor what prescription or nonprescription drugs you are taking. If you do not know the names of the drugs or what they were prescribed for, bring them in their labeled containers to your doctor or pharmacist.

Do not drink alcoholic beverages while you are taking diphenhydramine. They will increase the drowsiness and dizziness. Do not start to take any of the drugs listed above unless you have permission from your doctor.

Take diphenhydramine exactly as directed by your doctor. Do not take more of it and do not take it more often than instructed.

Before having surgery with a general anesthetic, including dental surgery, tell the doctor or dentist in charge that you are taking diphenhydramine.

Diphenhydramine should not be taken by pregnant women or by nursing mothers. Be sure to tell your doctor if you are pregnant or if you are breast-feeding.

DOSAGE
Your doctor will determine how often you should take diphenhydramine and how much you should take at each dose. Carefully follow the instructions on your prescription label and ask your doctor or pharmacist to explain any part of the instructions you do not understand.

Diphenhydramine comes in capsules, tablets and liquid. Use a specially marked measuring spoon to measure a dose of liquid so that your dose will be accurate.

If you forget to take a dose of this medicine, take it as soon as you remember. Then take the remaining doses for that day at evenly spaced intervals. *Do not take a double dose to make up for a missed dose.*

STORAGE
Keep diphenhydramine in the container it came in, and keep it out of the reach of children. Do not allow anyone else to take your diphenhydramine.

Phenyltoloxamine
(fen ill toe lox' a meen)

PRODUCT INFORMATION
Brand names of products containing phenyltoloxamine: Naldecon, Norel Plus, Poly-Histine-D, Sinubid

USES
See the general statement titled Antihistamines.

Phenyltoloxamine is an antihistamine that is combined with other antihistamines, decongestants or pain medicines to relieve sinus congestion resulting from allergy, colds or infection.

UNDESIRED EFFECTS
See the general statement titled Antihistamines.

Phenyltoloxamine can cause upset stomach, diarrhea or stomach pain. If you have any of these effects, take phenyltoloxamine with solid food or with a glass of milk.

Phenyltoloxamine causes some people to become drowsy, dizzy or less alert than usual. This is especially true for older people. Do not drive a car or operate dangerous machinery until you know how this medicine will affect you.

Children often have effects that are just the opposite—trouble sleeping, nervousness, unusually fast heartbeat, weakness and even convulsions.

Dryness of the mouth, nose or throat occurs frequently after taking phenyltoloxamine. Chewing gum or sucking on hard candies can relieve this.

Other side effects of phenyltoloxamine are blurred vision, difficult or painful urination and hives. Such effects, if they occur, often will disappear as your body adjusts to the medication. If they are persistent or severe, contact your doctor.

PRECAUTIONS
Before you start to take any product containing phenyltoloxamine, tell your doctor if you have heart disease, high blood pressure, an enlarged prostate, glaucoma, an overactive thyroid, a stomach ulcer or urinary tract blockage.

There are several drugs that you should not take with phenyltoloxamine because they increase the possibility of side effects. These include barbiturates; medicine for seizures; narcotics; other antihistamines or medicine for hay fever, other allergies or colds; prescription pain medicine; sedatives; tranquilizers; medicine to help you sleep and medicine for depression. Tell your doctor what other prescription or nonprescription drugs you are taking. If you do not know the names of the drugs or what they were prescribed for, bring them in their labeled containers to your doctor or pharmacist. Be sure not to start to take any of the drugs mentioned above while you are taking a product with phenyltoloxamine in it unless you first check with your doctor.

Alcohol will increase the drowsiness caused by phenyltoloxamine and should be used sparingly or not at all while you are taking this medicine. If you have any questions about this, check with your doctor or pharmacist.

Tell your doctor if you are pregnant or think you might be or if you are breast-feeding. This will help your doctor select the best treatment for you and your baby.

DOSAGE
Your doctor will determine how often you should take a product containing phenyltoloxamine and how much to take at each dose. Carefully follow the instructions on your prescription label. Do not take more than prescribed nor take it more often than recommended. If you have questions about your prescription instructions, ask your doctor or pharmacist.

STORAGE
Keep a product containing phenyltoloxamine in the container it came in. Keep it out of the reach of children.

Promethazine
(proe meth′ a zeen)

PRODUCT INFORMATION
Brand names: Phenergan, Quadnite, Remsed, ZiPAN
Brand name of a combination product containing aspirin and caffeine: Synalgos

USES
See the general statement titled Antihistamines.
Promethazine is a very versatile antihistamine. In addition to relieving symptoms of allergy, it is used as a sedative or tranquilizer before surgery and may be combined with medicine for pain for greater relief of pain. In addition, promethazine can be used to prevent and treat nausea from anesthesia and motion sickness.

UNDESIRED EFFECTS
See the general statement titled Antihistamines.
The most common effects of promethazine are drowsiness and mental confusion. Do not drive a car, operate dangerous machinery or perform other tasks that require mental alertness until you know how this medicine will affect you.

If promethazine makes your mouth and throat dry, suck hard candies, chew gum or drink fluids.

Promethazine also can cause blurred vision, difficult or painful urination, headache, loss of appetite, nervousness, restlessness or difficulty sleeping (especially in children), skin rash, unusual sweating or unusually fast heartbeat. If you experience these effects, they should decrease as you continue to take promethazine and as your body adjusts to it. However, if they are persistent or severe, contact your doctor.

Rarely, a person who takes promethazine will be unusually sensitive to sunlight. Restrict the amount of time you spend in sunlight until you know whether this will happen to you. If you experience a severe sunburn, contact your doctor.

Occasionally promethazine may affect the facial muscles or make swallowing difficult. If either of these effects occurs, contact your doctor.

PRECAUTIONS
See the general statement titled Antihistamines.

Promethazine can make certain medical problems worse. To help your doctor select the treatment best for you, tell your doctor if you have seizures, blood disorders, an enlarged prostate, heart disease, high blood pressure, glaucoma, an overactive thyroid, a stomach ulcer or urinary tract blockage.

When taken with promethazine, certain medications can increase the chance of or the severity of side effects. Tell your doctor what prescription or nonprescription drugs you are taking, including barbiturates, medicine for seizures, narcotics, other medicine for allergy, prescription medicine for pain, sedatives, tranquilizers, medicine to help you sleep and medicine for depression. If you do not know the names of the drugs or what they were prescribed for, bring them in their labeled containers to your doctor or pharmacist.

Do not drink alcoholic beverages while you are taking promethazine; this will increase your drowsiness. Do not start to take any of the drugs listed above until you first check with your doctor.

Take promethazine exactly as your doctor prescribes. Do not take more of it and do not take it more often than instructed.

It is not known whether promethazine can be passed from a mother to her unborn baby or whether it is passed through the milk to a nursing baby. However, it would be wise to tell your doctor if you are pregnant or are breast-feeding a baby before you start to take this medicine.

DOSAGE
Your doctor will determine how often you should take promethazine and how much you should take at each dose. Carefully follow the instructions on your prescription label and ask your doctor or pharmacist to explain any part of the instructions you do not understand.

Promethazine comes in capsules, tablets, liquid and suppositories. It is best to take capsules and tablets with a full eight-ounce glass of water. Liquid doses, to be accurate, should be measured with a specially marked spoon.

Suppositories should be used in the following way. Remove the wrapper or covering from the suppository and dip the tip of the suppository in water. Lie on your left side and raise your right knee to your chest. Insert the suppository into the rectum and hold it there for a few moments. You may then get up and resume your normal activities. Try to avoid having a bowel movement for about one hour after inserting the suppository. If you have any questions about this, check with your doctor or pharmacist.

If you forget to take a dose, take it as soon as you remember. Take any remaining doses for that day at evenly spaced intervals. If you remember a missed dose when it is time for you to take another, omit the missed dose entirely and take only the regularly scheduled dose. *Do not take a double dose to make up for the missed dose.*

STORAGE
Keep promethazine in the container it came in, and keep it out of the reach of children. Do not allow anyone else to take your promethazine.

Trimeprazine
(trye mep' ra zeen)

PRODUCT INFORMATION
Brand name: Temaril

USES
See the general statement titled Antihistamines.

Trimeprazine relieves the itching caused by allergic skin rashes such as poison ivy and poison oak. It is one of a class of drugs called antihistamines. These work by counteracting the effects of histamine, a substance found naturally in the human body. Histamine causes some of the effects of allergies, such as itching, watery eyes and runny nose.

UNDESIRED EFFECTS
See the general statement titled Antihistamines.

One common effect of trimeprazine is dryness of the mouth. This can be relieved by chewing gum, sucking hard candies or drinking fluids. Trimeprazine can also upset your stomach. If it does, take it with meals or a snack. Contact your doctor or pharmacist if this does not help or if the upsets are severe.

Other side effects include blurred vision, weakness and drowsiness.

PRECAUTIONS
See the general statement titled Antihistamines.

Before you start taking trimeprazine, tell your doctor or pharmacist if you have asthma, glaucoma, ulcers or difficulty in urinating.

Do not start taking sleeping pills, tranquilizers or muscle relaxants while taking trimeprazine unless you first check with your doctor or pharmacist.

Because trimeprazine causes drowsiness, do not drive a car or operate dangerous machinery until you know how this drug will affect you.

Alcohol can increase the chance or severity of dizziness or drowsiness.

Be sure to take only the exact amount of medication prescribed by your doctor at each dose. Do not take more.

Trimeprazine should not be taken during pregnancy. Harmful effects have been reported in babies born to women who have taken this drug.

DOSAGE

Trimeprazine comes in regular tablets, long-acting capsules and liquid. Follow the instructions on the package or labeling and ask your doctor or pharmacist to explain any part that you do not understand.

If you forget to take a dose, take it as soon as you remember it. Take any remaining doses for that day at evenly spaced intervals.

STORAGE

Keep this medication in the container it came in and out of the reach of children.

Tripelennamine
(tri pel enn' a meen)

PRODUCT INFORMATION
Brand name: PBZ

USES
See the general statement titled Antihistamines.

Tripelennamine is an antihistamine used to prevent or relieve the symptoms of hay fever, bee stings, poison oak and poison ivy. Tripelennamine counteracts the effects of histamine, one of the body's natural substances, which causes some of the symptoms of allergy such as itchy, watery eyes and runny nose.

UNDESIRED EFFECTS
See the general statement titled Antihistamines.

Upset stomach and stomach pain are two common side effects of tripelennamine. If this medicine upsets your stomach, take it with a glass of milk or with solid food. Contact your doctor if upsets continue or are severe. Tripelennamine also can make your mouth and throat dry. To relieve this, suck on hard candies, chew gum or drink fluids.

Tripelennamine makes some people drowsy or dizzy. Do not drive a car or operate dangerous machinery until you know how this medicine will affect you. As your body adjusts to tripelennamine, the drowsiness and dizziness should decrease. Contact your doctor if they are troublesome.

Other, less common effects of tripelennamine are blurred vision, difficult or painful urination, headache, loss of appetite, nervousness, restlessness or trouble sleeping (especially in children), skin rash, unusual increase in sweating and unusually fast heartbeat. These effects usually decrease as your body adjusts to the medication. However, if they are persistent or severe, contact your doctor. Your doctor may want to adjust your dose or change your medication.

PRECAUTIONS
See the general statement titled Antihistamines.

Tripelennamine can make certain medical conditions worse. Be sure to tell your doctor if you have an enlarged prostate, heart disease, high blood pressure, glaucoma, an overactive thyroid, a stomach ulcer or urinary tract blockage.

Tell your doctor what prescription or nonprescription drugs you are taking, including barbiturates, medicine for seizures, narcotics, other medicine for allergy, prescription medicine for pain, sedatives, tranquilizers, medicine to help you sleep and medicine for depression. These drugs when taken with tripelennamine can increase the chance of or the severity of side effects.

If you do not know the names of the drugs you are taking or what they were prescribed for, bring them in their labeled containers to your doctor or pharmacist.

Do not drink alcoholic beverages while you are taking tripelennamine because alcohol can increase the severity of drowsiness and dizziness. Do not start to take any of the drugs listed above until you first check with your doctor.

Tripelennamine should be taken exactly as directed by your doctor. Do not take more of it and do not take it more often than instructed.

Before having surgery with a general anesthetic, including dental surgery, tell the doctor or dentist in charge that you are taking tripelennamine.

Tripelennamine should not be taken by women who are pregnant or breast-feeding. Tell your doctor if you are breast-feeding or if you are pregnant. This information will help your doctor select the treatment best for you and your baby.

DOSAGE
Your doctor will determine how often you should take tripelennamine and how much you should take at each dose. Carefully follow the instructions on your prescription label and ask your doctor or pharmacist to explain any part of the instructions you do not understand.

Tripelennamine comes in liquid, regular tablets and extended-release tablets. If you are taking the extended-release tablets, be sure to swallow them whole. Do not break, crush or chew them before swallowing. To get an accurate dose of the liquid, use a specially marked measuring spoon. Take this medicine with milk or solid food if it upsets your stomach.

If you forget to take a dose, take it as soon as you remember. Then take the remaining doses for that day at evenly spaced intervals. If you remember a dose when it is almost time for another, omit the missed dose entirely and take only the regularly scheduled dose. *Do not take a double dose to make up for the missed one.*

STORAGE
Keep this medicine in the container it came in, and keep it out of the reach of children. Do not allow anyone else to take your tripelennamine.

Triprolidine
(trye proe' li deen)

PRODUCT INFORMATION
Brand name: Actidil
Brand names of products containing triprolidine: Actifed, Acti-Prem

USES
See the general statement titled Antihistamines.

Triprolidine is an antihistamine used to prevent or relieve the symptoms of hay fever, bee stings, poison ivy and poison oak. Triprolidine causes less drowsiness than some other antihistamines and therefore is particularly good for daytime use.

UNDESIRED EFFECTS
See the general statement titled Antihistamines.

Triprolidine often causes dry mouth and throat, which can be relieved by chewing gum, sucking hard candies or drinking fluids. Triprolidine also can upset your stomach or give you stomach pain. To prevent this, take triprolidine with milk or solid food. If stomach upsets continue or are severe, contact your doctor.

Although it causes less drowsiness than some other antihistamines, triprolidine can make some people drowsy or dizzy. Do not drive a car or operate dangerous machinery until you know how this drug will affect you.

Other effects of triprolidine that are less common are blurred vision, difficult or painful urination, headache, loss of appetite, nervousness, restlessness or difficulty sleeping (especially in children), skin rash, unusual sweating and unusually fast heartbeat. When these effects occur, they tend to disappear after you take the medicine for a few days. Contact your doctor if these effects are persistent or severe. Your doctor may want to adjust your dose or change your medication.

PRECAUTIONS
See the general statement titled Antihistamines.

Before you start to take triprolidine, tell your doctor if you have heart trouble, high blood pressure, an enlarged prostate, glaucoma, an overactive thyroid, a stomach ulcer or urinary tract blockage. This drug may make these medical conditions worse.

Tell your doctor what prescription or nonprescription drugs you are taking, particularly barbiturates, medicine for seizures, narcotics, other medicine for allergy, prescription medicine for pain, sedatives, tranquilizers, medicine to help you sleep and medicine for depression. If you do not know the names of the drugs or what they were prescribed for, bring them in their labeled containers to your doctor or pharmacist.

Do not drink alcoholic beverages while you are taking triprolidine, and do not start to take any of the drugs listed above until you first check with your doctor. All these drugs can increase the chance of and the severity of drowsiness.

Triprolidine should be taken exactly as prescribed by your doctor. Do not take more of it and do not take it more often than directed.

Before having surgery with a general anesthetic, including dental surgery, tell the doctor or dentist that you are taking triprolidine.

Triprolidine should not be taken by women who are breast-feeding and probably should not be used by pregnant women, since it is not known whether triprolidine is safe for the unborn child.

DOSAGE

Your doctor will determine how often you should take triprolidine and how much you should take at each dose. Carefully follow the instructions on your prescription label and ask your doctor or pharmacist to explain any part of the instructions you do not understand.

Triprolidine comes in liquid and tablets. Measure a dose of liquid medicine with a specially marked spoon to assure an accurate dose. Take this medicine with milk or solid food if it upsets your stomach.

If you forget to take a dose, take it as soon as you remember and take the remaining doses for that day at evenly spaced intervals. If you remember a missed dose when it is time to take another, omit the missed dose entirely and take only the regularly scheduled dose. *Do not take a double dose to make up for the missed dose.*

STORAGE

Keep triprolidine in the container it came in. Keep this medicine out of the reach of children, and do not allow anyone else to take your triprolidine.

DECONGESTANTS

Decongestant medications are used to relieve stuffy or runny nose caused by colds. Decongestants are available as oral tablets, as capsules, in liquid form and as nasal sprays and drops.

Oxymetazoline
(ox i met az' oh leen)

PRODUCT INFORMATION

Brand names: Afrin, Afrin Pediatric Nose Drops, Bayfrin, Dristan Long Lasting, Duramist Plus, Duration, Neo-Synephrine 12 Hour, Neo-Synephrine 12 Hour Children's Drops, Nōstrilla Long Acting, Sinex Long Acting

USES

Oxymetazoline shrinks swollen blood vessels in the nose, reducing congestion and making it easier to breathe. Oxymetazoline is sprayed or dropped into the nose for temporary relief of congestion caused by colds or allergies.

UNDESIRED EFFECTS

When oxymetazoline is used for short periods of time in recommended doses, side effects are rare.

When sprayed or dropped into the nose, oxymetazoline may cause sneezing or temporary burning, dryness or stinging of the inside of the nose.

If oxymetazoline is used for too long a period or is used too often, it may be absorbed into the body and cause more serious side effects. If you develop headache or lightheadedness, an increase in runny or stuffy nose, pounding heartbeat or trouble in sleeping, stop using this medicine and contact your doctor.

PRECAUTIONS

Before you start taking oxymetazoline, tell your doctor or pharmacist if you have ever had an unusual reaction to nasal decongestants. You are more likely to have a reaction to oxymetazoline if you have ever had one after use of another nasal decongestant.

You should use oxymetazoline with caution if you have blood vessel disease, diabetes, high blood pressure or an overactive thyroid. Before you use this medicine tell your doctor or pharmacist if you have any of these medical problems. Do not exceed the dosage or use this medication more often than specified on the label if you have any of these medical problems.

Tell your doctor or pharmacist what other prescription or nonprescription drugs you are taking, particularly whether you are now taking or have taken in the past two weeks any MAO inhibitors (isocarboxazid, pargyline, phenelzine and tranylcypromine). If you do not know the names of the drugs you are taking or what they were prescribed for, bring them in their labeled containers to your doctor or pharmacist.

Use oxymetazoline only as directed. Do not use more of it, do not use it more often and do not use it longer than three days without first checking with your doctor; otherwise, your runny or stuffy nose may get worse and you may increase the chance of side effects.

DOSAGE

Carefully follow the instructions on the package label and ask your doctor or pharmacist to explain any part of the instructions you do not understand.

Oxymetazoline comes in nose drops or spray.

If you are using nose drops, follow these instructions:

1. Blow your nose gently.
2. Wash your hands thoroughly with soap and water.
3. Check the dropper tip for chips or cracks.
4. The nose drops must be kept clean. Avoid touching the dropper against the nose or anything else.
5. Draw the medicine into the dropper.

6. Lie on a flat surface, such as a bed, hang your head over the edge and tilt your head back as far as is comfortable.
7. Place the prescribed number of drops into the nose.
8. To allow the medication to spread in the nose, remain in this position for a few minutes.
9. Replace the dropper in the bottle right away.
10. Wash your hands to remove any medicine.

If you are using nose spray, follow these instructions:

1. Blow your nose gently.
2. Wash your hands thoroughly with soap and water.
3. Hold your head erect and spray once or twice into each nostril. Sniff the medicine into your nose as you spray.
4. Wait three to five minutes for the medicine to work.
5. Blow your nose again and repeat the spraying, if needed.
6. Rinse the tip of the spray bottle with hot water.
7. Wipe the tip dry with a clean tissue and replace the cap.
8. Wash your hands to remove any medicine.

If you miss a dose of oxymetazoline, take only the next regularly scheduled dose at the time it is due. Do not take the missed dose and *do not take a double dose*. If you have any questions about this, check with your doctor or pharmacist.

STORAGE

Keep oxymetazoline in the container it came in, and keep it out of the reach of children. Do not allow anyone else to use your oxymetazoline so your infection will not spread.

Phenylephrine

(fen ill ef' rin)

PRODUCT INFORMATION

Brand names: Alconefrin, Allerest, Coricidin, Doktors Nose Drops, Duration Mild 4 Hour, Neo-Synephrine, Nōstril, Rhinall, Sinarest Nasal, Sinex, Sinophen, Vacon

Brand name of a nasal solution containing pheniramine maleate and phenylephrine hydrochloride: Dristan

Brand name of a nasal solution containing phenylephrine hydrochloride, pyrilamine maleate and naphazoline hydrochloride: 4-Way Nasal Spray

USES

Phenylephrine applied to the inside of the nose relieves nasal congestion caused by hay fever, other allergies, colds and sinus problems. Application of this medicine inside the nose also may help open inflamed ears.

Although there are oral products (tablets, capsules and liquids) combining phenylephrine with antihistamines and other decongestants, these combinations do not appear to be more effective than phenylephrine alone. This medicine is available without a prescription, but your doctor may recommend the proper use or dose of this drug for your particular condition.

UNDESIRED EFFECTS

When phenylephrine is applied, it can cause a temporary burning, stinging or dryness in the nose.

If large amounts of this medicine are used or if an excess amount of the drops is swallowed, they can be absorbed into the body and cause more serious side effects. Stop using phenylephrine and contact your doctor if you experience headache or dizziness, an increase in runny or stuffy nose, pounding or unusually fast heartbeat, trembling, trouble in sleeping or unusual nervousness.

PRECAUTIONS

Do not use phenylephrine if you have ever had any unusual reaction to nasal decongestants; if you have, you are much more likely to have a reaction to this medicine. If you have any questions about this, check with your doctor or pharmacist.

People with blood vessel disease, diabetes, heart disease, high blood pressure or an overactive thyroid should not use phenylephrine. Before you start to use this medicine, tell your doctor or pharmacist if you have any of these medical problems.

Tell your doctor or pharmacist what other prescription or nonprescription drugs you are taking, particularly medicine for depression and MAO inhibitors (isocarboxazid, pargyline, phenelzine and tranylcypromine). If you do not know the names of the drugs or what they were prescribed for, bring them in their labeled containers to your doctor or pharmacist.

This medicine should be used only as directed. Do not use more of it, do not use it more often and do not use it for more than three days without first checking with your doctor. If you do, your nasal stuffiness may get worse and you will increase the chance of side effects.

DOSAGE

Carefully follow the instructions on the prescription label or container and ask your doctor or pharmacist to explain any part of the instructions you do not understand.

Phenylephrine comes in drops, spray and jelly, all of which are applied to the inside of the nose.

If you are using nose drops, follow these instructions:
1. Blow your nose gently.
2. Wash your hands thoroughly with soap and water.
3. Check the dropper tip for chips or cracks.
4. The nose drops must be kept clean. Avoid touching the dropper against the nose or anything else.
5. Draw the medicine into the dropper.

6. Lie on a flat surface, such as a bed, hang your head over the edge and tilt your head back as far as is comfortable.
7. Place the prescribed number of drops into the nose.
8. To allow the medication to spread in the nose, remain in this position for a few minutes.
9. Replace the dropper in the bottle right away.
10. Wash your hands to remove any medicine.

If you are using nose spray, follow these instructions:

1. Blow your nose gently.
2. Wash your hands thoroughly with soap and water.
3. Hold your head erect and spray once or twice into each nostril. Sniff the medicine into your nose as you spray.
4. Wait three to five minutes for the medicine to work.
5. Blow your nose again and repeat the spraying, if needed.
6. Rinse the tip of the spray bottle with hot water.
7. Wipe the tip dry with a clean tissue and replace the cap.
8. Wash your hands to remove any medicine.

To use the nasal jelly, first blow your nose. Then place a dab of jelly about the size of a pea in your nose with your finger. Sniff the jelly well back into your nose. Wipe the tip of the tube with a clean, damp tissue and replace the cap immediately.

If you forget to use a dose, use only the regularly scheduled dose at the next regular time. Do not use the missed dose and *do not use a double dose.*

STORAGE

Keep phenylephrine in the container it came in, and keep it out of the reach of children. Do not spread infection by allowing another person to use your phenylephrine.

Phenylpropanolamine

(fen ill proe pa nole′ a meen)

PRODUCT INFORMATION

Brand names: Dexatrim Caffeine-Free Extra Strength, Dietac, Propadrine, Rhindecon

Some brand names of products containing phenylpropanolamine: Anatuss, Anorexin, Appedrine, Bayer Cold Tablets, Bayer Cough Syrup, Brocon, Codimal, Comtrex, Congespirin, Contac, Control Capsules, Coricidin, Coryban-D, Daycare, Decon-aid, Decon-tuss, Dexatrim, Dextrotussin, Dimetane, Dimetapp, Dorcol, Entex, 4-Way Cold Tablets, Fiogesic, Histabid, Histalet, Histatapp, Hycomine, Kronohist, Naldecon, Napril, Nilcol, Nolamine, Norel Plus, Novahistine, Ornacol, Ornade, Ornex, Poly-Histine, Probacon, Prolamine, Puretapp, Resolution I, Rhinex, Robitussin, Ru-Tuss, S-T Forte, SineAid, Sinubid, Sinulin, Triaminic, Triaminicol, Tuss-Ornade, Vicks Formula 44D

USES

Phenylpropanolamine shrinks swollen blood vessels to reduce swelling in the nose and air passages. It is taken by mouth to relieve the discomfort caused by colds, hay fever and other allergies. This drug comes alone or in products combining phenylpropanolamine with other drugs. Phenylpropanolamine is available without a prescription but your doctor may recommend the proper dose for your particular condition.

Phenylpropanolamine is also used orally as a diet aid.

UNDESIRED EFFECTS

Phenylpropanolamine can cause nervousness, restlessness, trouble in sleeping and dizziness. These effects tend to decrease as your body adjusts to the medicine. If they are severe or persistent, contact your doctor.

Less frequently this medicine will cause more serious reactions. Stop taking phenylpropanolamine and contact your doctor if you experience headache, tightness in the chest, irregular heartbeats or unusually fast heartbeats.

Phenylpropanolamine makes some people drowsy. Do not drive a car or operate dangerous machinery until you know how this drug will affect you.

PRECAUTIONS

Before you start taking phenylpropanolamine, tell your doctor or pharmacist if you have ever had an unusual reaction to medicines similar to phenylpropanolamine such as amphetamines, ephedrine, epinephrine, isoproterenol, metaproterenol, norepinephrine, phenylephrine, pseudoephedrine and terbutaline.

Certain medical problems may become worse if you take phenylpropanolamine. People with diabetes, an enlarged prostate, glaucoma, heart or blood vessel disease, high blood pressure or an overactive thyroid should use phenylpropanolamine with caution and should not take more of it or take it more often than specified on the label.

Phenylpropanolamine can affect the way your body responds to certain other medications, including other drugs similar to phenylpropanolamine (see the list above), amphetamines, many medicines for high blood pressure, digitalis (heart medicine) and medicine for depression. Tell your doctor what other prescription or nonprescription drugs you are taking. Your doctor also will need to know if you are taking MAO inhibitors (isocarboxazid, pargyline, phenelzine and tranylcypromine) or if you have taken them within the past two weeks. If you do not know the names of the drugs you are taking or what they were prescribed for, bring them in their labeled containers to your doctor or pharmacist.

Avoid using alcohol, pills to help you sleep and narcotics while you are taking phenylpropanolamine. These will increase the drowsiness caused by phenyl-propanolamine.

Be sure to take this medication exactly as your doctor has prescribed it. Do not take more. If you think you need more to relieve your symptoms, check with your doctor.

If you are pregnant or think you may be, tell your doctor before you start to take phenylpropanolamine.

DOSAGE
Carefully follow the instructions on the package label and ask your doctor or pharmacist to explain any part of the instructions you do not understand.

Phenylpropanolamine comes in capsules, tablets and liquid. If you are taking the extended-release capsules, be sure to swallow them whole. Do not crack, break or chew them.

To ensure an accurate dose of liquid, measure your dose with a specially marked spoon.

If you forget to take a dose, take it as soon as you remember. However, if you remember a missed dose at the time you are scheduled to take another, take only one dose. *Do not take a double dose to make up for the missed one.*

STORAGE
Keep phenylpropanolamine in the container it came in, and keep it out of the reach of children. Do not allow anyone else to take your phenylpropanolamine which was prescribed for your particular condition.

Pseudoephedrine
(soo doe a fed′ rin)

PRODUCT INFORMATION
Brand names: Cenafed, Neofed, Neo-Synephrinol, Novafed, Sinufed, Sudafed, Sudrin

Brand names of some products containing pseudoephedrine: Actifed, Acti-Prem, Afrinol, Chlorafed, Chlor-Trimeton, Codimal, CoTylenol, Deconamine, Dimacol, Disophrol, Drixoral, Emprazil, Fedahist, Fedrazil, Histalet, Historal, Isoclor, Lo-Tussin, Nasalspan, Novafed, Nucofed, Polaramine, Poly-Histine, Pseudobid, Pseu-do-Hist, Rhinosyn, Robitussin DAC, Rondec, Ryna, Tripodrine, Tussend

USES
Pseudoephedrine shrinks swollen blood vessels in the nose, lungs and ears. It is used to relieve the congestion and discomfort caused by colds, allergies, and certain types of ear problems. Several cold and cough preparations containing pseudoephedrine are available with or without a doctor's prescription.

UNDESIRED EFFECTS
When you start to take pseudoephedrine, it may make you nervous or restless or give you trouble sleeping. These effects tend to decrease or disappear as you continue to take it and as your body adjusts to the medicine. If they are persistent or severe, contact your doctor.

Less frequently, pseudoephedrine can cause difficult or painful urination, dizziness or lightheadedness, headache, nausea or vomiting, trembling, troubled breathing, an unusual increase in sweating, unusual paleness, unusually fast or pounding heartbeat or weakness. Try taking a smaller amount of the medicine each day. If these effects continue, stop taking the medicine and contact your doctor.

Very large doses of pseudoephedrine can result in hallucinations, irregular heartbeat or unusually slow heartbeat and shortness of breath. If you experience any of these effects, stop taking the medicine and contact your doctor.

PRECAUTIONS

Before you start taking pseudoephedrine, tell your doctor if you have ever had any unusual reaction to medicines similar to pseudoephedrine, such as amphetamines, ephedrine, epinephrine, isoproterenol, metaproterenol, norepinephrine, phenylephrine, phenylpropanolamine or terbutaline. If you have had a reaction to any of these medicines, you may have a reaction to pseudoephedrine.

Certain medical problems may become worse if you take pseudoephedrine. Tell your doctor if you have diabetes, an enlarged prostate, glaucoma, heart or blood vessel disease, high blood pressure or an overactive thyroid. Because many nonprescription remedies for coughs, colds and hay fever contain pseudoephedrine, ask your pharmacist about the ingredients of such remedies before you buy them. You should not take pseudoephedrine if you have any of the medical conditions named above unless your doctor specifically says you may.

Pseudoephedrine can affect the way your body responds to certain other medications, including amphetamines, many medicines for high blood pressure, digitalis glycosides (heart medicine) and medicine for depression. Tell your doctor or pharmacist what other prescription or nonprescription medications you are taking. If you do not know the names of the drugs or what they were prescribed for, bring them in their labeled containers to your doctor or pharmacist.

Tell your doctor if you are breast-feeding. Pseudoephedrine is passed through the milk and can have an undesired effect on the baby.

Excessive consumption of coffee or tea may increase the restlessness or insomnia that pseudoephedrine can cause. You may want to reduce the amount of these beverages you drink while you are taking this drug.

Contact your doctor if any new symptoms or health problems develop while you are taking pseudoephedrine or if your symptoms do not improve within five days.

DOSAGE

Your doctor will determine how often you should take pseudoephedrine and how much you should take at each dose. Carefully follow the instructions on your prescription label and ask your doctor or pharmacist to explain any part of the instructions you do not understand.

Pseudoephedrine comes in capsules, syrup and tablets. Usually it begins to work within 15 minutes to a half hour after it is taken and takes full effect in about an hour.

If you are taking the extended-release capsule or the extended-release tablet, swallow it whole. Do not crush, break or chew it before swallowing it. If the capsule is too large to swallow, you may mix its contents with jam or jelly and swallow without chewing.

To help prevent trouble in sleeping, take the last dose of pseudoephedrine several hours before bedtime. If you have any questions about this dosage procedure, ask your doctor or pharmacist.

If you forget to take a dose of pseudoephedrine, take the next dose at the regularly scheduled time. Do not take the missed dose and *do not take a double dose.*

STORAGE
Keep this medicine in the container it came in. Keep pseudoephedrine out of the reach of children, and do not allow anyone else to take your pseudoephedrine.

EXPECTORANTS

Expectorants are used to help thin the mucus in the air passages. This makes it easier to cough up the mucus and clear the air passages. It also will help if you drink a lot of water while you are using expectorants. In severe cases, a vaporizer may be used to help thin the mucus.

Guaifenesin
(gwye fen' i sen)

PRODUCT INFORMATION
Brand names: Guaiatuss, 2G, Robitussin Syrup and others

Brand names of products containing guaifenesin: Actifed-C Expectorant, Adatuss, Anatuss, Asbron G, Brondecon, Bronkolixir, Chlor-Trimeton Expectorant, Conex Expectorant, Coricidin Cough Syrup, Coryban-D Cough Syrup, Co-Xan, Dimacol, Dimetane Expectorant, Donatussin Syrup, Dorcol, Emfaseem, Entex, Entuss, Fedahist Expectorant, Guistrey, Histalet X, Isoclor Expectorant, Lo-Tussin, Lufyllin, Mudrane, Nasalspan, Neothylline-GG, Nilcol, Novahistine Expectorant, P-V-Tussin, Polaramine Expectorant, Pseudo-Hist Expectorant, Quibron Elixir, Rhinex-DM, Rhinspec, Robitussin A-C, Romex, Ryna-Cx, S-T Forte, Slo-Phyllin-GG, Sorbutuss, Synophylate-GG, Tedral Expectorant, Triaminic, Tussend Cough Syrup, Unproco, Verequad, Vicks Cough Syrup and others

USES
Guaifenesin, also known as glyceryl guaiacolate, thins the mucus in air passages and makes it easier to cough it up. Guaifenesin relieves coughs of colds, tuberculosis and whooping cough. Guaifenesin is combined with decongestants, antihistamines, narcotics and bronchodilators to treat coughs.

UNDESIRED EFFECTS
When taken in larger amounts than those required for effective expectorant action, guaifenesin may cause vomiting. However, at usual doses upset stomach as an effect of taking this medicine is rare.

PRECAUTIONS
Many of the combination products containing guaifenesin are available without a prescription. Discuss with your pharmacist the other drugs in these products to be sure you do not take something you should not, such as phenylpropanolamine if you have high blood pressure or isopropamide if you have glaucoma.

DOSAGE
If your doctor has prescribed guaifenesin, carefully follow the instructions on the prescription label. If you purchase this medicine without a prescription, follow the directions included in the package or on the label. Do not take more and do not take it more often than recommended.

If you forget to take a dose of this medicine, take it as soon as you remember and then take the remaining doses for that day at evenly spaced intervals. If you remember a missed dose at the time you are to take another, take only the scheduled dose. Do not take the missed dose and *do not take a double dose*.

STORAGE
Keep guaifenesin in the container it came in, and keep it out of the reach of children.

Terpin Hydrate
(ter′ pin hye′ drate)

PRODUCT INFORMATION
Brand names of products containing terpin hydrate: Terpin Hydrate and Codeine Elixir, Tussaminic Tablets

USES
Terpin hydrate, in the form of an elixir with or without codeine, is used to relieve coughs. However, five milliliters of the elixir (the usual dose) contains only about one-fourth of the effective dose of terpin hydrate. The high alcohol content of the elixir (more than 40 percent) makes it unwise to give doses larger than five milliliters. Therefore, the elixir usually contains codeine, a narcotic that acts on the cough center of the brain to lessen coughing (see the monograph on Codeine for side effects).

UNDESIRED EFFECTS
Although side effects are rare, terpin hydrate can cause nausea, and the alcohol in the product can cause drowsiness.

PRECAUTIONS
Terpin hydrate cough medicines contain more than 40 percent alcohol. Avoid alcoholic beverages while you are taking terpin hydrate.

DOSAGE
Carefully follow the instructions on your prescription label or package label if you are taking a nonprescription product.

If you forget to take a dose, take it as soon as you remember it. However, if it is almost time for you to take the next dose, take only the regularly scheduled dose.

STORAGE
Keep this medication in the container it came in, and keep it out of the reach of children.

COUGH SUPPRESSANTS

Cough suppressants act on a portion of the brain that stimulates the cough reflex. These medications are best used to stop a dry, hacking cough that irritates the throat and may prevent sleep. It is best not to use this type of medication if a lot of mucus is being coughed up.

Codeine
(koe′ deen)

Codeine is a narcotic which acts on the cough center in the brain to decrease coughing. It is used alone or combined with other cough medicines, expectorants, decongestants and antihistamines to relieve cough and cold symptoms. In higher doses, it also is used to relieve pain.

Dextromethorphan
(dex troe meth ore′ fan)

PRODUCT INFORMATION
Brand names of some of the many products containing dextromethorphan: Albatussin, Anatuss, Bayer Cough Syrup, Chloraseptic DM, Codimal DM, Comtrex, Coricidin, Coryban-D, CoTylenol, Daycare, Dextrotussin, Dimacol, Dorcol, Guaifenesin-Dextromethorphan Syrup, Histalet, Nilcol, Nyquil, Ornacol, Phenergan, Quelidrine, Rhinex-DM, Robitussin-DM, Romex, Rondec-DM, Sorbutuss, Triaminic-DM, Triaminicol, Tusquelin, Tussaminic, Tussar DM, Tussi-Organidin, Unproco, Vicks Formula 44 and 44D and others

USES

Dextromethorphan, like codeine, acts on the cough center in the brain to stop coughing. Dextromethorphan's effect on the cough reflex is about equal to that of codeine, but dextromethorphan has fewer side effects than codeine. Dextromethorphan is a common ingredient in cough preparations available without a prescription.

UNDESIRED EFFECTS

Although side effects are rare after you take dextromethorphan, it can cause nausea and drowsiness. These effects tend to decrease or disappear as your body becomes adjusted to the medicine. However, if they continue or are severe, contact your doctor or pharmacist.

PRECAUTIONS

Before you start to take a product containing dextromethorphan, tell your doctor or pharmacist what prescription or nonprescription drugs you are taking.

DOSAGE

If your doctor has prescribed a cough preparation containing dextromethorphan, carefully follow the instructions on how often to take the cough preparation and how much to take at each dose. If you have selected a cough preparation that does not require a prescription, carefully follow the directions on the bottle. Do not take more of this medicine, take it more often or take it longer than instructed.

If you forget to take a dose, take it as soon as you remember. However, if it is almost time for you to take another dose, omit the missed dose entirely and take only the regularly scheduled dose.

STORAGE

Keep this medicine in the container it came in, and keep it out of the reach of children.

Hydrocodone

(high dro co' dohn)

PRODUCT INFORMATION

Brand names: Codone, Dicodid

Brand names of products containing hydrocodone: Adatuss, Citra-Forte, Codimal DH, Duradyne DHC, Entuss, Hycodan, Hycomine, Hycotuss, Norcet, P-V-Tussin, Pseudo-Hist, S-T Forte, Triaminic, Tussend, Tussionex, Vicodin

USES

Hydrocodone is a narcotic that acts on the cough center in the brain to stop coughing. The ability of hydrocodone to stop coughing is slightly greater than that of codeine. Hydrocodone also dries the nose and throat.

This drug is used alone or with other cough suppressants, expectorants, antihistamines, decongestants and pain medicine to relieve the symptoms of colds and allergies.

UNDESIRED EFFECTS
Although side effects are uncommon with usual doses, hydrocodone can cause nausea and constipation. Drink plenty of fluids and contact your doctor if these effects continue over a period of time or are severe.

Rarely, hydrocodone will cause difficulty in breathing. If you have this problem, stop taking the medicine and contact your doctor.

Hydrocodone makes some people drowsy and dizzy. Do not drive a car or operate dangerous machinery until you know how this drug will affect you.

PRECAUTIONS
Before you start to take hydrocodone, tell your doctor if you have ever had any problem with this drug in the past or if you have asthma, emphysema, an underactive thyroid, an enlarged prostate, adrenal disease (Addison's disease) or kidney or liver disease.

Certain other medications should not be taken with hydrocodone. These include other narcotics, barbiturates, sedatives, tranquilizers, medicine to help you sleep and medicine for depression. Tell your doctor what prescription or nonprescription drugs you are taking. If you do not know the names of the drugs or what they were prescribed for, bring them in their labeled containers to your doctor or pharmacist.

Do not start to take any of the drugs listed above without first checking with your doctor.

Do not drink alcoholic beverages while you are taking hydrocodone. Alcohol can increase the chance and severity of side effects.

Before you have surgery with a general anesthetic, including dental surgery, tell the doctor or dentist that you are taking hydrocodone.

Do not take hydrocodone any longer that your doctor has told you to take it. Do not take any more of it nor take it more often than your doctor has instructed. To do so could cause problems because hydrocodone is habit-forming.

To help your doctor select the treatment best for you and your baby, tell your doctor if you are pregnant or are breast-feeding a baby. Safe use of this drug in pregnancy has not been established and hydrocodone is passed to a nursing baby through the milk.

DOSAGE
Your doctor will determine how often you should take hydrocodone and how much you should take at each dose. Carefully follow the instructions on your prescription label and ask your doctor or pharmacist to explain any part you do not understand.

Hydrocodone alone is available in tablets, and the combination products are available in liquid, tablets and capsules.

If you forget to take a dose, take it as soon as you remember. However, if you remember a missed dose when it is almost time for you to take another dose, omit the missed dose entirely and take only the regularly scheduled dose. *Do not take a double dose.*

STORAGE

Keep this medicine in the container it came in, and keep it out of the reach of children. Do not allow anyone else to take your hydrocodone.

Arthritis

DRUGS USED TO TREAT ARTHRITIS

Arthritis

Arthritis is an inflammation of the joints. The joints become painful, red, tender, swollen and stiff. There are many different types of arthritis, but the most common ones are osteoarthritis and rheumatoid arthritis.

Osteoarthritis occurs later in life and usually is characterized by painful and knobby swelling of the fingers. Rheumatoid arthritis starts in middle age, usually involves many joints and causes you to feel stiff all over.

A type of arthritis that involves primarily the back and joints of the lower back is ankylosing spondylitis.

Gout is a type of arthritis that occurs mostly in men and usually is sudden in onset. Pain and swelling occur in the affected joint—frequently the big toe, ankle or knee.

Usually, a salicylate—commonly aspirin—is the first drug you will take for arthritis. If a salicylate does not help, your doctor may prescribe one of the nonsteroidal anti-inflammatory drugs discussed on the following pages. A steroid—a cortisone-like drug—may be injected into a painful arthritic joint. Rarely, use of a steroid by mouth, on a continuing basis, is justified. (See page 392 for the names of additional drugs to treat gout.)

Any of these drugs may relieve the *symptoms* of arthritis and slow down the progression of the disease. However, the basic course of the disease usually is not changed and arthritis is not cured.

Aspirin/Salicylates
(as′ pir in)

PRODUCT INFORMATION
Brand names of products containing aspirin: ASA, Aspergum, Bayer Aspirin, Ecotrin, Empirin, Measurin, St. Joseph's and others

Some common brand names of products containing aspirin and an antacid: Alka-Seltzer, Arthritis Pain Formula, Ascriptin, Bufferin

Brand names of other salicylates besides aspirin that may be taken for arthritis: choline salicylate—Actasal, Arthropan; magnesium salicylate—Durasal, Efficin, Magan, Mobidin; sodium salicylate—Uracel 5

There are also many products containing combinations of salicylates, many of which are available without a prescription.

Some common brand names are: Duragesic, Pabalate, Parbocyl, Persistin, Sal-Eze, Stanback, Trilisate, Zarumin

USES
Aspirin belongs to the group of medicines known as salicylates. Aspirin also is

called acetylsalicylic acid. Salicylates are used to relieve mild to moderate pain, to reduce fever caused by infection and to relieve redness, joint pain and swelling caused by arthritis. Aspirin also helps prevent blood from clotting.

Because aspirin is available without a prescription and is so widely used, it is important to know what problems it can cause and what precautions you should take when using it. Carefully read the label on the container for a nonprescription medicine to determine if the medicine contains aspirin.

UNDESIRED EFFECTS

The most common side effects of aspirin and salicylates are nausea, vomiting and stomach pain. To prevent these effects, take the medicine with meals or with a full eight-ounce glass of water, with a snack or with an antacid. If these measures do not help and stomach upsets continue, contact your doctor.

Less common effects, but ones that require medical attention if they occur, are ringing in the ears, loss of hearing, bloody or black stools, wheezing, tightness in the chest and shortness of breath. If you experience any of these effects, stop taking the drug and contact your doctor.

Taking large doses of aspirin (or salicylates), taking it over a long time or giving it to young children who are dehydrated by fever can cause aspirin poisoning. Some signs of aspirin poisoning are dizziness or mental confusion, rapid breathing, a continuous ringing or buzzing in the ears and severe or continuing headache. Contact your doctor if these effects occur.

Salicylates also can cause allergic reactions. Some symptoms of allergic reaction are itching, hives, runny nose, swelling of the throat, difficulty breathing, chest pains and fainting. If you have any of these symptoms, contact your doctor at once.

PRECAUTIONS

Before you take salicylates or aspirin, tell your doctor or pharmacist if you have ever had a reaction to aspirin, any nonsteroidal anti-inflammatory agents (diflunisal, fenoprofen, ibuprofen, indomethacin, meclofenamate, mefenamic acid, naproxen, oxyphenbutazone, phenylbutazone, piroxicam, sulindac or tolmetin) or other salicylates including methyl salicylate (oil of wintergreen), choline salicylate, magnesium salicylate, sodium salicylate and salsalate.

If you have certain medical conditions, you should not take salicylates or aspirin except on the advice of your doctor. These conditions include anemia, asthma, allergies, history of nasal polyps, glucose-6-phosphate dehydrogenase (G6PD) deficiency, gout, hemophilia or other bleeding problems, Hodgkin's disease, kidney disease, liver disease, heart disease and ulcers or other stomach problems.

Your doctor should supervise your use of aspirin or salicylates if you are taking any of the following medications on a regular basis: acetazolamide, anticoagulants (blood thinners), medicine for gout, medicine for inflammation (such as the inflammation of arthritis), corticosteroids, methotrexate, oral medicine for diabetes and medicine to make your urine more or less acidic. Tell your doctor or pharmacist what prescription or nonprescription drugs you are taking. If you do not know the names of the drugs or what they were prescribed for, bring them in their labeled containers to your doctor or pharmacist.

Children under 12 years of age should not take aspirin for fevers associated with flu or chicken pox because the use of aspirin during these illnesses in children has been associated with a serious illness known as Reye's Syndrome. Discuss this problem with your doctor.

Adults should not take this medicine for more than 10 days in a row unless they are taking it for arthritis.

Do not take more medication than is recommended on the package label unless so directed by your doctor. Contact your doctor if your symptoms do not improve, if they become worse or if your fever lasts for more than three days.

If you are taking aspirin or salicylates on a regular schedule to treat a chronic illness such as arthritis, the medicine will be effective only if you follow your medication schedule carefully. It is also important that your doctor check your response, at regular visits, when you take this medicine over a long time.

If you have diabetes, regular use of eight or more aspirin tablets a day (or large doses of other salicylates) may cause inaccurate results of tests for your urine sugar. If you have any questions, check with your doctor.

If you are taking large doses of salicylates or aspirin or if you are taking it for a long period of time, drinking alcoholic beverages may increase the possibility or severity of stomach problems.

Aspirin is an ingredient in many prescription and nonprescription products. Do not take other medication while you are taking this drug unless you first check the ingredients with your doctor or pharmacist.

If you are pregnant, use aspirin sparingly and avoid taking salicylates. Do not take aspirin or salicylates if you are within two or three months of delivery or if you are breast-feeding. If you have any questions, check with your doctor.

DOSAGE

If you take aspirin for arthritis, you need large doses—probably 12 to 16 tablets of five grains or 300 milligrams each—every day.

Aspirin and salicylates come in chewable tablets, tablets to be swallowed, oral solution and rectal suppositories. Chewable tablets may be chewed, dissolved in liquid, crushed or swallowed whole. Tablets to be swallowed should be taken with meals, with a full glass of water or with antacids.

To use one of the suppositories, remove the foil wrapper and dip the tip of the suppository in water. Then lie on your side, bring your top knee up to your chest and insert the suppository well into your rectum. Hold it there for a few moments; then get up and resume your normal activities. Try not to have a bowel movement for at least an hour after inserting the suppository.

STORAGE

Keep the medication in a tightly closed bottle (preferably one with a childproof cap), and keep it out of the reach of children. Overdose with aspirin is especially dangerous in young children. If you have arthritis, you may ask your pharmacist to put this medication in a bottle without a childproof cap, but keep it out of the reach of children.

Store aspirin and salicylates in a cool, dry place. Do not keep them in the bathroom or in a bathroom medicine cabinet, because the dampness may cause them to lose their effectiveness. Throw away any aspirin that smells like vinegar.

Salsalate
(sal' sa late)

PRODUCT INFORMATION
Brand name: Disalcid

USES
Salsalate is used to treat the pain and inflammation of arthritis. It is not known whether it is effective in reducing fevers.

Salsalate is chemically related to aspirin and other salicylates. It is composed of two aspirin molecules, which are split apart when the drug is metabolized in the body. Since this process does not occur in the stomach, salsalate may cause less stomach irritation than aspirin. Also, salsalate does not have the same effect as aspirin in preventing blood clotting.

UNDESIRED EFFECTS
The most common side effects of salsalate are nausea, vomiting and stomach pain. To prevent these effects, take the medicine with meals or with a full eight-ounce glass of water, with a snack or with an antacid. If these measures do not help and stomach upsets continue, contact your doctor.

Less common effects, but ones that require medical attention if they occur, are ringing in the ears, loss of hearing, bloody or black stools, wheezing, tightness in the chest and shortness of breath. If you experience any of these effects, stop taking the drug and contact your doctor.

Taking large doses of salsalate, aspirin or other salicylates, or taking them over a long time, can cause salicylate poisoning. Some signs of this poisoning are dizziness or mental confusion, rapid breathing, a continuous ringing or buzzing in the ears and severe or continuing headache. Contact your doctor if these effects occur.

Salsalate also can cause allergic reactions. Some symptoms of allergic reaction are itching, hives, runny nose, swelling of the throat, difficulty breathing, chest pains and fainting. If you have any of these symptoms, contact your doctor at once.

PRECAUTIONS
Before you take salsalate, tell your doctor or pharmacist if you have ever had a reaction to aspirin, any nonsteroidal anti-inflammatory agents (diflunisal, fenoprofen, ibuprofen, indomethacin, meclofenamate, mefenamic acid, naproxen, oxyphenbutazone, phenylbutazone, piroxicam, sulindac or tolmetin) or other salicylates

including methyl salicylate (oil of wintergreen), choline salicylate, magnesium salicylate and sodium salicylate.

If you have certain medical conditions, you should not take salsalate except on the advice of your doctor. These conditions include anemia, gout, hemophilia or other bleeding problems, Hodgkin's disease, kidney disease, liver disease, heart disease and ulcers or other stomach problems.

Your doctor should supervise your use of salsalate if you are taking any of the following medications on a regular basis: acetazolamide, anticoagulants (blood thinners), medicine for gout, medicine for inflammation (such as the inflammation of arthritis), corticosteroids, methotrexate, oral medicine for diabetes and medicine to make your urine more or less acidic. Tell your doctor or pharmacist what prescription or nonprescription drugs you are taking. If you do not know the names of the drugs or what they were prescribed for, bring them in their labeled containers to your doctor or pharmacist.

Children under 12 years of age should not take salsalate. Adults should not take this medicine for more than 10 days in a row unless they are taking it for arthritis.

Do not take more medication than is recommended on your prescription label unless so directed by your doctor. Contact your doctor if your symptoms do not improve or if they become worse. The medicine will be effective only if you follow your medication schedule carefully. It is also important that your doctor check your response, at regular visits, when you take this medicine over a long time.

If you have diabetes, regular use of six or more 325-mg tablets (or four or more 500-mg tablets) a day (or large doses of aspirin or other salicylates) may cause inaccurate results of tests for your urine sugar. If you have any questions, check with your doctor.

If you are taking large doses of salsalate and/or aspirin or if you are taking it for a long period of time, drinking alcoholic beverages may increase the possibility or severity of stomach problems.

Aspirin is an ingredient in many prescription and nonprescription products. Do not take other medication while you are taking this drug unless you first check the ingredients with your doctor or pharmacist.

Tell your doctor if you are pregnant or breast-feeding a baby. It is not known if it is safe to take salsalate during pregnancy or while breast-feeding. Do not take aspirin if you are within two or three months of delivery or if you are breast-feeding. If you have any questions, check with your doctor.

DOSAGE

Salsalate is available as tablets. Your doctor will determine how much and how often you should take this drug. Follow the instructions on your prescription label, and ask your doctor or pharmacist to explain any part you do not understand.

This medication may be taken with food, a full glass of water or an antacid to decrease stomach irritation.

If you are taking salsalate on a regular schedule and forget to take a dose, take it as soon as you remember unless it is time for the next dose. Take any remaining doses for that day at evenly spaced intervals. *Do not take a double dose to make up for a missed dose.*

STORAGE
Keep this medication in the container it came in, and keep it tightly closed. If you have arthritis, you may ask your pharmacist to put this medication in a bottle without a childproof cap, but keep it out of the reach of children.

NONSTEROIDAL ANTI-INFLAMMATORY DRUGS
Diflunisal
(dye floo′ ni sal)

PRODUCT INFORMATION
Brand name: Dolobid

USES
Diflunisal is used to relieve mild to moderate pain of many different types, including the pain and swelling caused by arthritis.

UNDESIRED EFFECTS
The most common side effects of diflunisal are headache, nausea, stomach pain and diarrhea. Taking the drug with milk or food may reduce stomach irritation. Contact your doctor if these symptoms persist or are bothersome.

Less common effects, but ones that require medical attention if they occur, are skin rash, swelling of the lower legs, ringing in the ears, bloody or black stools, wheezing and difficulty breathing. If you experience any of these effects, stop taking diflunisal and contact your doctor.

PRECAUTIONS
Before you take diflunisal, tell your doctor or pharmacist if you have ever had a reaction to any nonsteroidal anti-inflammatory agent (fenoprofen, ibuprofen, indomethacin, meclofenamate, mefenamic acid, naproxen, oxyphenbutazone, phenylbutazone, piroxicam, sulindac or tolmetin), salsalate, aspirin or other salicylates (choline salicylate, magnesium salicylate and sodium salicylate). Do not take any of these medications while taking diflunisal unless directed to do so by your doctor.

If you have certain medical conditions, you should not take diflunisal except on the advice of your doctor. These conditions include anemia, hemophilia or other bleeding problems, liver disease, kidney disease, heart disease, high blood pressure and ulcers or other stomach problems.

Your doctor should supervise your use of diflunisal if you are taking anticoagulants (blood thinners), antacids or hydrochlorothiazide on a regular basis. Tell your doctor or pharmacist what prescription and nonprescription drugs you are taking. If you do not know the names of the drugs or what they were prescribed for, bring them in their labeled containers to your doctor or pharmacist.

Avoid taking acetaminophen while taking diflunisal. Be sure to check the label before taking nonprescription medications to see if they contain acetaminophen. Ask your doctor or pharmacist to advise you on which products and how much acetaminophen are safe to take while taking diflunisal.

Do not take more medication than as directed on the prescription label. Contact your doctor if your symptoms do not improve or if they become worse.

If you are taking diflunisal on a regular schedule to treat a chronic illness such as arthritis, the medicine will be effective only if you follow your medication schedule carefully. It is also important that your doctor check your response, at regular visits, when you take this medicine over a long time.

If you are taking large doses of diflunisal for a long period of time, drinking alcoholic beverages may increase the possibility or severity of stomach problems.

Although it is rare, contact your doctor if you have an eye problem while taking this drug.

Tell your doctor if you are pregnant, plan to become pregnant, or are breast-feeding a baby. Diflunisal should not be taken during the last three months of pregnancy. It is not known if it is safe to take diflunisal at any time during pregnancy or while breast-feeding a baby. It is not known if it is safe for children under 12 years of age to take the drug.

DOSAGE
Diflunisal comes in capsule-shaped tablets to be taken by mouth. The tablets should be crushed or chewed. Diflunisal may be taken with water, milk or food to reduce stomach irritation.

If you are taking diflunisal on a regular schedule and forget to take a dose, take it as soon as you remember unless it is time for the next dose. Take any remaining doses for that day at evenly spaced intervals. *Do not take a double dose to make up for a missed dose.*

STORAGE
Keep diflunisal in the container it came in, and keep it tightly closed. Keep all medications out of the reach of children. If you have arthritis, you may ask your pharmacist to put this medication in a container without a childproof cap, but be sure to keep it out of the reach of children.

Fenoprofen
(fen oh proe' fen)

PRODUCT INFORMATION
Brand name: Nalfon

USES

Fenoprofen is used to relieve the pain, redness, tenderness, swelling and stiffness of certain types of arthritis. The drug also is used to relieve mild to moderate pain such as that following surgery or major dental work.

UNDESIRED EFFECTS

The most common side effects of fenoprofen are stomach upsets such as indigestion, nausea, vomiting, stomach pain and diarrhea. To prevent stomach upsets after taking fenoprofen, take it with milk, meals, a snack or an antacid. If these effects continue or are severe, contact your doctor.

Fenoprofen makes some people drowsy, dizzy or less alert. Do not drive a car or operate dangerous machinery until you know how this medicine will affect you.

Other effects, which may go away as you continue to take fenoprofen and as your body adjusts to it, include constipation, headache, loss of appetite, blurred vision, dry mouth, nervousness, trembling, trouble sleeping, increased sweating and fast or pounding heartbeat. Contact your doctor if these effects continue or are bothersome.

More serious side effects can occur, which may require medical attention. Contact your doctor if you have a ringing or buzzing in your ears; skin rash; hives; itching; bloody or tarry stools; partial loss of hearing; vision problems; swelling of the hands, feet, ankles or lower legs; shortness of breath or difficult breathing, wheezing or tightness in the chest; or unusual tiredness or weakness.

PRECAUTIONS

You should not take fenoprofen if you have ever had a bad reaction to it or if you have ever had an unusual reaction to aspirin or other salicylates, diflunisal, ibuprofen, indomethacin, meclofenamate, mefenamic acid, naproxen, oxyphenbutazone, phenylbutazone, piroxicam, sulindac or tolmetin. If you have questions about this, check with your doctor.

Because fenoprofen can make certain medical conditions worse, tell your doctor if you have bleeding problems, heart disease, diverticulitis, kidney disease, a stomach ulcer or other stomach problems.

Tell your doctor what prescription or nonprescription drugs you are taking, including anticoagulants (blood thinners), medicine for diabetes, any other medicine for arthritis, phenytoin and sulfa medicines. If you do not know the names of the drugs or why they were prescribed, bring them in their labeled containers to your doctor or pharmacist.

It may take a few days for you to feel better after you take fenoprofen, and you may have to take it for two to three weeks before you feel the full effects. Take fenoprofen exactly as prescribed. Do not take more of it, take it more often or take it for a longer period than ordered by your doctor. If you think you need more to relieve your symptoms, contact your doctor.

Laboratory tests such as blood tests or kidney and liver function tests may be required while you are taking fenoprofen. If you experience problems with your vision or hearing after you start to take this drug, you should tell your doctor, have your eyes examined and have a test for your hearing. *Be sure to keep all appointments with your doctor and at the laboratory.*

Do not drink alcoholic beverages while you are taking fenoprofen. Do not take aspirin regularly unless you have permission from your doctor. Alcohol or aspirin can increase the chance of stomach upset.

Before you have surgery with a general anesthetic, including dental surgery, tell the doctor or dentist that you are taking fenoprofen.

Because it is not known whether this medicine may be safely used in pregnant women or nursing mothers, tell your doctor if you are pregnant or breast-feeding.

DOSAGE

Your doctor will determine how often you should take fenoprofen and how much you should take at each dose. Carefully follow the instructions on your prescription label, and ask your doctor or pharmacist to explain any part of the instructions you do not understand.

Fenoprofen comes in capsules and tablets. If this medicine upsets your stomach, take it with solid food, milk or an antacid.

If you forget to take a dose of this medicine, take it as soon as you remember. If you do not remember a missed dose until it is almost time for you to take the next one, omit the missed dose entirely and take only the regularly scheduled dose. *Do not take a double dose to make up for the missed one.*

STORAGE

Keep fenoprofen in the container it came in, and keep it out of the reach of children. Do not allow anyone else to take your fenoprofen. If you have arthritis, you may ask your pharmacist to put this medicine in a bottle without a childproof cap.

Ibuprofen
(eye byoo′ proe fen)

PRODUCT INFORMATION
Brand names: Advil, Motrin, Nuprin

USES

Ibuprofen is used to relieve the pain, redness, tenderness, swelling and stiffness of certain types of arthritis. Ibuprofen also is used to relieve other types of mild to moderate pain including menstrual cramps.

UNDESIRED EFFECTS

The most common side effects are stomach upsets such as bloating or gas, heartburn or indigestion, nausea or vomiting, stomach cramps or stomach pain and diarrhea. To prevent these problems, take this medicine with meals, a snack, milk or an antacid. If these problems continue, contact your doctor.

Ibuprofen makes some people dizzy. Do not drive a car or operate dangerous machinery until you know how this medicine will affect you.

Other effects, which may go away as you continue to take ibuprofen, are constipation, decreased appetite, headache and nervousness.

More serious side effects, which do not occur often, will require medical attention if they do occur. Contact your doctor if you have skin rash; hives; itching; ringing or buzzing in the ears; swelling of the feet, ankles or lower legs; unusual weight gain; bloody or tarry stools; blurred or partial loss of vision; change in color in your vision; mental depression; difficult or painful urination; shortness of breath or difficult breathing, wheezing or tightness in the chest; or sore throat or fever.

PRECAUTIONS

You should not take ibuprofen if you have ever had a bad reaction to it in the past or have ever had an unusual reaction to aspirin or other salicylates, diflunisal, fenoprofen, indomethacin, meclofenamate, mefenamic acid, naproxen, oxyphenbutazone, phenylbutazone, piroxicam, sulindac or tolmetin. If you have questions, check with your doctor.

Before you start to take ibuprofen, tell your doctor if you have bleeding problems, heart disease, kidney disease, diverticulitis, a stomach ulcer or other stomach problems. Ibuprofen may make these conditions worse.

Tell your doctor what prescription or nonprescription drugs you are taking, especially anticoagulants (blood thinners), medicine for diabetes, any other medicine for arthritis, phenytoin and sulfa drugs. If you do not know the names of the drugs or why they were prescribed, bring them in their labeled containers to your doctor or pharmacist.

For ibuprofen to relieve your symptoms, it must be taken regularly and exactly as prescribed by your doctor. It may take two to three weeks before you feel the full effect of this medicine. Do not take more of it than your doctor has ordered. If you feel you need more to relieve your symptoms, contact your doctor.

Your doctor may order laboratory tests such as blood counts or tests for liver function or ask you to have your eyes examined.

Do not drink alcoholic beverages while you are taking ibuprofen. Do not take aspirin regularly while you are taking ibuprofen unless you have your doctor's permission. Alcohol or aspirin can increase the chance of stomach upset.

Before you have any surgery with a general anesthetic, including dental surgery, tell the doctor or dentist that you are taking ibuprofen.

It is not known whether this drug is safe for pregnant women or nursing mothers. Be sure to tell your doctor if you are pregnant or breast-feeding.

DOSAGE

Your doctor will determine how often you should take ibuprofen and how much you should take at each dose. Carefully follow the instructions on your prescription label, and ask your doctor or pharmacist to explain any part of the instructions you do not understand.

Ibuprofen comes in tablets. If they upset your stomach, they may be taken with solid food, milk or an antacid.

If you forget to take a dose of ibuprofen, take the missed dose as soon as you remember it. If you remember the missed dose at the time you are scheduled to take the next dose, omit it completely and take only the regularly scheduled dose. *Do not take a double dose.*

STORAGE
Keep ibuprofen in the container it came in, and keep it out of the reach of children. Do not allow anyone else to take your ibuprofen. If you have arthritis, you may ask your pharmacist to put this medicine in a bottle without a childproof cap.

Indomethacin
(in doe meth' a sin)

PRODUCT INFORMATION
Brand name: Indocin

USES
Indomethacin is used to relieve the pain, redness, tenderness, swelling and stiffness of certain types of arthritis and other joint diseases, including gout attacks. Because of its possible side effects, indomethacin usually is only used when aspirin or other drugs are not helpful.

UNDESIRED EFFECTS
Headache is the most common effect of indomethacin and may occur within an hour after you take it. If you get severe headache, contact your doctor. It may be necessary to reduce the amount of indomethacin you are taking.

Indomethacin can cause stomach upsets such as indigestion, heartburn, nausea, vomiting, stomach pain or diarrhea. To lessen stomach upset, take this medicine with meals, a snack or milk. If this does not lessen your stomach upset, ask your doctor if you may take indomethacin with an antacid.

Indomethacin makes some people drowsy, dizzy or lightheaded. Do not drive a car or operate dangerous machinery until you know how this medicine will affect you.

Other effects, which may go away as you continue to take indomethacin and as your body adjusts to it, are constipation and unusual tiredness and weakness. Contact your doctor if these effects continue or are severe.

Serious and possibly fatal effects can occur. Stop taking indomethacin and contact your doctor if you have ringing or buzzing in the ears; bloody or tarry stools; blurred vision; hearing problems; mood or mental changes; shortness of breath; wheezing; difficult breathing; tightness in the chest; skin rash or hives; sore throat; fever; swelling of the ankles, feet or lower legs; unusual bleeding or bruising; unusual weight gain; or yellowing of the eyes and skin.

PRECAUTIONS

You should not take indomethacin if you have ever had a bad reaction to it or if you have ever had an unusual reaction to aspirin or other salicylates, diflunisal, fenoprofen, ibuprofen, meclofenamate, mefenamic acid, naproxen, oxyphenbutazone, phenylbutazone, piroxicam, sulindac or tolmetin. If you have questions, check with your doctor.

Because indomethacin can make certain medical conditions worse, tell your doctor if you have bleeding problems, colitis, diverticulitis, epilepsy, kidney or liver disease, mental illness, Parkinson's disease, a stomach ulcer or other stomach problems.

Tell your doctor what prescription or nonprescription drugs you are taking, including anticoagulants (blood thinners), medicine for diabetes, diuretics, medicine for high blood pressure, lithium, probenecid, any other medicine for arthritis, phenytoin and sulfa medicines. If you do not know the names of the drugs or why they were prescribed, bring them in their labeled containers to your doctor or pharmacist.

When you take indomethacin for arthritis, you may have to take it for several weeks before you begin to feel better. It could be a month before you feel the full effects of this medicine.

Take indomethacin exactly as prescribed by your doctor. Do not take more of it, take it more often or take it for a longer period than ordered by your doctor. Do not take indomethacin for any problem other than the one for which it was prescribed.

You may be required to have tests of your urine and blood or laboratory tests for your liver function while you are taking this drug. You also may need eye examinations or tests for your hearing if you have vision or hearing problems after you begin to take indomethacin. *Be sure to keep all appointments with your doctor and at the laboratory.*

Do not drink alcoholic beverages or take aspirin regularly while you are taking indomethacin. Alcohol or aspirin can make stomach upsets worse.

Before you have any kind of surgery with a general anesthetic, including dental surgery, tell the doctor or dentist that you are taking indomethacin.

Because indomethacin can harm an unborn child or a nursing baby, tell your doctor if you are pregnant or breast-feeding.

DOSAGE

Your doctor will determine how often you should take indomethacin and how much you should take at each dose. Carefully follow the instructions on your prescription label, and ask your doctor or pharmacist to explain any part of the instructions you do not understand.

Indomethacin comes in capsules. Take them with meals, a snack or milk to lessen stomach upset.

If you forget to take a dose of this medicine, take it as soon as you remember. If you remember a missed dose when it is almost time for you to take another, omit the missed dose completely and take only the regularly scheduled dose. *Do not take a double dose to make up for the missed one.*

STORAGE

Keep indomethacin in the container it came in, and keep it out of the reach of children. Do not allow anyone else to take your indomethacin. If you have arthritis, you may ask your pharmacist to put this medicine in a bottle without a childproof cap.

Meclofenamate

(me kloe fen am' ate)

PRODUCT INFORMATION
Brand name: Meclomen

USES

Meclofenamate is used to relieve pain, redness, inflammation, swelling and stiffness caused by certain types of arthritis.

Because of its possible side effects, it is usually only used when aspirin or other drugs are not helpful.

UNDESIRED EFFECTS

The most common side effect of meclofenamate is diarrhea. If this effect is severe, contact your doctor. It may be necessary to decrease the dose that you are taking. Other common side effects include nausea, vomiting and abdominal pain. To prevent these problems you may take meclofenamate with food, milk or antacids.

Meclofenamate makes some people dizzy. Do not drive a car or operate dangerous machinery until you know how this medicine will affect you.

Other effects, which may go away as you continue to take meclofenamate, are constipation, decreased appetite, headache and nervousness.

More serious side effects, which do not occur often, will require medical attention if they do occur. Contact your doctor if you have skin rash; hives; itching; ringing or buzzing in the ears; swelling of the feet, ankles or lower legs; unusual weight gain; bloody or tarry stools; blurred or partial loss of vision; change in color in your vision; difficult or painful urination; shortness of breath or difficult breathing, wheezing or tightness in the chest; or sore throat or fever.

PRECAUTIONS

Do not take meclofenamate if you ever had a bad reaction to it in the past or ever had an unusual reaction to aspirin or other salicylates, diflunisal, fenoprofen, ibuprofen, indomethacin, mefenamic acid, naproxen, oxyphenbutazone, phenylbutazone, piroxicam, sulindac or tolmetin. If you have questions about this problem, check with your doctor.

Before you start to take meclofenamate, tell your doctor if you have bleeding problems, heart disease, kidney disease, diverticulitis, a stomach ulcer or other stomach problems. Meclofenamate may make these conditions worse.

Tell your doctor what prescription or nonprescription drugs you are taking, especially anticoagulants (blood thinners), medicine for diabetes, any other medicine for arthritis, phenytoin and sulfa drugs. If you do not know the names of the drugs or why they were prescribed, bring them in their labeled containers to your doctor or pharmacist.

For meclofenamate to relieve your symptoms, it must be taken regularly and exactly as prescribed by your doctor. It may take two to three weeks before you feel the full effect of this medicine. Do not take more of it than your doctor has ordered. If you feel you need more to relieve your symptoms, contact your doctor. Your doctor may wish to increase or decrease the amount of medication you are taking. Be sure to keep all of your appointments for checkups so you are always taking the right amount of medication.

Your doctor may order laboratory tests such as blood counts or tests for liver function or ask you to have your eyes examined.

Do not drink alcoholic beverages while you are taking this drug. Do not take aspirin regularly while you are taking meclofenamate unless you have your doctor's permission. Alcohol or aspirin can increase the chance of stomach upset.

Before you have any surgery with a general anesthetic, including dental surgery, tell the doctor or dentist that you are taking meclofenamate.

It is not known whether this drug is safe for pregnant women or nursing mothers. Be sure to tell your doctor if you are pregnant or breast-feeding.

DOSAGE
Meclofenamate comes in capsules to be taken by mouth. Your doctor will determine how often you should take meclofenamate and how much you should take at each dose. Carefully follow the instructions on your prescription label, and ask your doctor or pharmacist to explain any part of the instructions you do not understand.

If you forget to take a dose, take the missed dose as soon as you remember it. If you remember the missed dose at the time you are scheduled to take the next dose, omit it completely and take only the regularly scheduled dose. *Do not take a double dose to make up for a missed dose.*

STORAGE
Keep this medication in the container it came in and out of the reach of children. You may ask your pharmacist to put this medicine in a bottle without a childproof cap.

Mefenamic Acid
(me fe nam' ik)

PRODUCT INFORMATION
Brand name: Ponstel

USES
Mefenamic acid is used to treat many types of pain, including arthritis and menstrual pain. It is a member of the drug class known as nonsteroidal anti-

inflammatory agents. It acts to decrease inflammation and also to decrease uterine contractions.

UNDESIRED EFFECTS

Diarrhea is the most common side effect of mefenamic acid. Contact your doctor if it is severe. It may be necessary to reduce the dosage that you are taking.

Other common side effects are stomach upsets such as gas, abdominal pain, nausea and vomiting. It may help to take this medication with food.

Mefenamic acid may make some people drowsy or dizzy. Do not drive a car or operate dangerous machinery until you know how this medicine will affect you.

Other side effects, which may go away as you continue to take this drug, include headache, insomnia, nervousness, decreased appetite and constipation.

More serious side effects, which do not occur often, will require medical attention if they do occur. Contact your doctor if you have blurred vision, change in color in your vision, eye or ear pain, skin rash, hives, bloody or tarry stools, difficult breathing, sore throat or fever.

PRECAUTIONS

Do not take mefenamic acid if you ever had a bad reaction to it in the past or ever had an unusual reaction to aspirin or other salicylates, diflunisal, fenoprofen, ibuprofen, indomethacin, meclofenamate, naproxen, oxyphenbutazone, phenylbutazone, piroxicam, sulindac or tolmetin. If you have any questions about this problem, check with your doctor.

Before you start to take mefenamic acid, tell your doctor if you have bleeding problems, heart disease, kidney disease, diverticulitis, a stomach ulcer or other stomach problems. Mefenamic acid may make these problems worse.

Tell your doctor what prescription or nonprescription drugs you are taking, especially anticoagulants (blood thinners), medicine for diabetes, any other medicine for arthritis, phenytoin and sulfa drugs. If you do not know the names of the drugs or what they were prescribed for, take them in their labeled containers to your doctor or pharmacist.

Do not take aspirin while you are taking mefenamic acid unless you have your doctor's permission.

Drinking alcoholic beverages while taking this medication may make stomach upsets worse.

Before you have any surgery with a general anesthetic, including dental surgery, tell the doctor or dentist that you are taking mefenamic acid.

Your doctor may order laboratory tests such as blood counts or tests for liver function or ask you to have your eyes examined. *Be sure to keep all appointments with your doctor and the laboratory.*

Tell your doctor if you are pregnant or breast-feeding a baby. It is not known if it is safe to take mefenamic acid under these circumstances. When taken late in pregnancy, this drug may interfere with or delay labor.

DOSAGE

Mefenamic acid comes in capsules to be taken by mouth. Follow the instructions on your prescription label, and ask your doctor or pharmacist to explain any part of the instructions you do not understand.

If it upsets your stomach, take this medication with food.

STORAGE
Keep this medication in the container it came in, and keep it out of the reach of children.

Naproxen
(na prox′ en)

PRODUCT INFORMATION
Brand names: Anaprox, Naprosyn

USES
Naproxen is used to relieve the pain, redness, tenderness, swelling and stiffness of certain types of arthritis. Naproxen also is used to relieve menstrual cramps and mild to moderate pain such as that following surgery or major dental work.

UNDESIRED EFFECTS
The most common side effects of naproxen are stomach upsets such as heartburn or indigestion, stomach pain, nausea and vomiting; diarrhea also is a common side effect. To lessen these upsets, take naproxen with meals, a snack, milk or an antacid.

Naproxen makes some people dizzy, lightheaded or drowsy. Do not drive a car or operate dangerous machinery until you know how this medicine will affect you.

Other side effects are constipation, soreness of the mouth, headache, pounding heartbeat and sweating. These effects may go away as you continue to take naproxen and as your body adjusts to it. However, if they continue or are severe, contact your doctor.

More serious side effects, which do not occur often, will need medical attention if they do occur. Contact your doctor if you have bloody or tarry stools; blurred vision or any other change in vision; mental depression; ringing or buzzing in the ears; any loss of hearing; skin rash or hives; swelling of the feet, ankles or lower legs; unusual weight gain; difficult or painful urination; shortness of breath or wheezing; difficulty in breathing or tightness in the chest; sore throat; fever; unusual bleeding or bruising; or yellowing of the skin and eyes.

PRECAUTIONS
You should not take naproxen if you have ever had a bad reaction to it or if you have had an unusual reaction to aspirin or other salicylates, diflunisal, fenoprofen, ibuprofen, indomethacin, meclofenamate, mefenamic acid, oxyphenbutazone, phenylbutazone, piroxicam, sulindac or tolmetin. If you have any questions about this problem, check with your doctor.

Before you start to take naproxen, tell your doctor if you have bleeding problems, heart disease, kidney disease, a stomach ulcer or other stomach problems. Naproxen may make these conditions worse.

Tell your doctor what prescription or nonprescription drugs you are taking, including anticoagulants (blood thinners), medicine for diabetes, any other medicine for arthritis, phenytoin, probenecid and sulfa medicines. If you do not know the names of the drugs or why they were prescribed, bring them in their labeled containers to your doctor or pharmacist.

For this medicine to help you, it must be taken regularly and exactly as prescribed by your doctor. You may have to take it for several weeks before you begin to feel better and for a month before you feel the full effects.

Your doctor probably will order laboratory tests such as blood tests and tests for liver or kidney function to check on how you are reacting to this drug. You may need to have an eye examination or a hearing test if you experience vision or hearing problems after you start to take naproxen. *Be sure to keep all appointments with your doctor and at the laboratory.*

Do not drink alcoholic beverages or take aspirin regularly while you are taking naproxen. Alcohol or aspirin can make stomach upsets worse.

Before you have any surgery with a general anesthetic, including dental surgery, tell the doctor or dentist that you are taking naproxen.

Because naproxen can harm an unborn child or a nursing baby, be sure to tell your doctor if you are pregnant or are breast-feeding.

DOSAGE

Your doctor will determine how often you should take naproxen and how much you should take at each dose. Carefully follow the instructions on your prescription label, and ask your doctor or pharmacist to explain any part of the instructions you do not understand.

Naproxen comes in tablets. Take them with solid food, milk or an antacid to lessen the chance of stomach upset.

If you forget to take a dose, take it as soon as you remember. If you remember a missed dose when it is almost time for you to take another one, omit the missed dose completely and take only the regularly scheduled one. *Do not take a double dose to make up for the missed one.*

STORAGE

Keep naproxen in the container it came in, and keep it out of the reach of children. Do not allow anyone else to take your naproxen. If you have arthritis, you may ask your pharmacist to put this medicine in a bottle without a childproof cap.

Phenylbutazone
(fen ill byoo′ ta zone)

PRODUCT INFORMATION
Brand names: Azolid, Butagen, Butazolidin, Butazone

USES

Phenylbutazone is used for short-term relief of pain, redness, tenderness, swelling and stiffness of certain types of arthritis and other joint diseases, including gout attacks. Because of the possible side effects and potentially very serious blood problems caused by phenylbutazone, it usually is only used when all other drugs have not been helpful.

UNDESIRED EFFECTS

Many people have undesired effects from phenylbutazone severe enough that they cannot take it. Common side effects of phenylbutazone are nausea, vomiting, indigestion, heartburn, stomach pain and diarrhea. You can help prevent stomach problems by taking this medicine immediately before or immediately after meals, with a glass of milk or with an antacid. Contact your doctor if stomach problems continue despite these precautions.

Some people become drowsy, confused or less alert when they take phenylbutazone. Do not drive a car or operate dangerous machinery until you know how this medicine will affect you.

Phenylbutazone may cause weight gain, swelling of your feet and ankles or difficult breathing. Check with your doctor if such problems occur. Using less salt in your diet may help prevent these problems.

More serious problems, such as intestinal bleeding, kidney or liver problems, allergic reactions and eye problems, may occur. Stop taking the drug and contact your doctor immediately if you have any loss of hearing; bloody or black, tarry stools; indigestion or stomach pain; bloody or cloudy urine; difficult or painful urination; difficulty in breathing; wheezing; eye pain or any change in vision; skin rash or hives; swelling of the neck or throat; or yellowing of the eyes and skin.

Serious blood problems can occur many days or weeks after you stop taking phenylbutazone, although these effects are rare. During this period, contact your doctor immediately if you have sore throat, fever, chills, sores or white spots in your mouth, unusual bleeding or bruising or unusual tiredness or weakness.

PRECAUTIONS

Do not take phenylbutazone if you have ever had a bad reaction to it or if you have ever had an unusual reaction to aspirin or other salicylates, diflunisal, fenoprofen, ibuprofen, indomethacin, meclofenamate, mefenamic acid, naproxen, oxyphenbutazone, piroxicam, sulfinpyrazone, sulindac or tolmetin. Be sure to tell your doctor about any such reaction.

Before you start to take phenylbutazone, tell your doctor if you have or ever had asthma; diseases of the blood, heart, liver, kidneys, pancreas, salivary glands or thyroid gland; high blood pressure; a stomach ulcer or other stomach problems; or diseases characterized by muscle pain or pain in the temples. Phenylbutazone may make these conditions worse.

Tell your doctor what prescription or nonprescription drugs you are taking, especially anticoagulants (blood thinners), medicine for diabetes, isoniazid, digitoxin, any other medicine for arthritis, phenytoin, tetracyclines, iron medications and sulfa medicines. If you do not know the names of the drugs or why they were prescribed, bring them in their labeled containers to your doctor or pharmacist.

If you take phenylbutazone for a week and still have the symptoms for which it was prescribed, contact your doctor. Take phenylbutazone exactly as prescribed. Do not take more of it, take it more often or take it for a longer period of time than ordered by your doctor. Do not take phenylbutazone for any problem other than that for which it was prescribed.

You should have certain laboratory tests before you begin to take phenylbutazone, including blood tests and tests for your kidney, liver and thyroid functions. These tests should be repeated every few weeks so your doctor can check on how you are reacting to this drug. *Be sure to keep all appointments with your doctor and at the laboratory.*

Do not drink alcoholic beverages while you are taking phenylbutazone. Do not take aspirin regularly while you are taking phenylbutazone unless you first check with your doctor to find out how much to take. Alcohol or aspirin can make stomach upset more likely to occur.

Before you have surgery with a general anesthetic, including dental surgery, tell your doctor or dentist that you are taking phenylbutazone.

Because phenylbutazone may affect your baby, tell your doctor if you are pregnant or breast-feeding.

DOSAGE

Your doctor will determine how often you should take phenylbutazone and how much you should take at each dose. Carefully follow the instructions on your prescription label, and ask your doctor or pharmacist to explain any part of the instructions you do not understand.

Phenylbutazone comes in capsules and tablets. They should be taken immediately before or immediately after meals, with a full eight-ounce glass of milk or with an antacid to lessen the possibility of stomach upset.

If you forget to take a dose of this medicine, take it as soon as you remember. Then take any remaining doses for the day at evenly spaced intervals. If you remember a missed dose when it is almost time for you to take another, omit the missed dose entirely and take only the regularly scheduled dose. *Do not take a double dose to make up for the missed dose.*

STORAGE

Keep phenylbutazone in the container it came in, and keep it out of the reach of children. Do not allow anyone else to take your phenylbutazone. If you have arthritis, you may ask your pharmacist to put this medicine in a bottle without a childproof cap.

Piroxicam
(peer ox′ i kam)

PRODUCT INFORMATION
Brand name: Feldene

USES
Piroxicam is used to treat pain, redness, inflammation, swelling and stiffness caused by certain types of arthritis.

UNDESIRED EFFECTS
The most common side effects are stomach upsets such as heartburn or indigestion, nausea or vomiting, stomach pain, bloating or gas and diarrhea. To prevent these problems, take this medicine with a light snack. If symptoms continue, contact your doctor.

Other side effects include headache, rash and dizziness. Do not drive a car or operate dangerous machinery until you know how this medicine will affect you.

More serious side effects, which do not occur often, will require medical attention if they do occur. Contact your doctor if you have skin rash; hives; itching; ringing or buzzing in the ears; swelling of the feet, ankles or lower legs; unusual weight gain; bloody or tarry stools; blurred or partial loss of vision; change in color in your vision; shortness of breath or difficult breathing, wheezing or tightness in the chest; or sore throat or fever.

PRECAUTIONS
You should not take piroxicam if you ever had a bad reaction to it in the past or ever had an unusual reaction to aspirin or other salicylates, diflunisal, fenoprofen, ibuprofen, indomethacin, meclofenamate, mefenamic acid, naproxen, oxyphenbutazone, phenylbutazone, sulindac or tolmetin. If you have questions about this problem, check with your doctor.

Before you start to take piroxicam, tell your doctor if you have bleeding problems, heart disease, kidney disease, diverticulitis, a stomach ulcer or other stomach problems. Piroxicam may make these conditions worse.

Tell your doctor what prescription or nonprescription drugs you are taking, especially anticoagulants (blood thinners), medicine for diabetes, any other medicine for arthritis, phenytoin and sulfa drugs. If you do not know the names of the drugs or why they were prescribed, bring them in their labeled containers to your doctor or pharmacist.

For piroxicam to relieve your symptoms, it must be taken regularly and exactly as prescribed by your doctor. It may take two to three weeks before you feel the full effect of this medicine. Do not take more of it than your doctor has ordered. If you feel you need more to relieve your symptoms, contact your doctor.

Your doctor may order laboratory tests such as blood counts or tests for liver function or ask you to have your eyes examined. *Keep all appointments with your doctor and the laboratory.*

Do not drink alcoholic beverages while you are taking piroxicam. Do not take aspirin regularly while you are taking piroxicam unless you have your doctor's permission. Alcohol or aspirin can increase the chance of stomach upset.

Before you have any surgery with a general anesthetic, including dental surgery, tell the doctor or dentist that you are taking piroxicam.

It is not known whether this drug is safe for pregnant women or nursing mothers. Be sure to tell your doctor if you are pregnant or breast-feeding.

Your doctor may wish to increase or decrease the amount of medication you are taking. Be sure to keep all appointments for checkups so you are always taking the right amount of medication.

DOSAGE

Piroxicam comes in capsules to be taken by mouth. It is usually taken once a day. Follow the instructions on your prescription label, and ask your doctor or pharmacist to explain any part of the instructions you do not understand. If piroxicam upsets your stomach, it may be taken with food.

If you forget to take a dose of piroxicam, take the missed dose as soon as you remember it. If you remember the missed dose near the time you are scheduled to take the next dose, omit the missed dose completely and take only the regularly scheduled dose. *Do not take a double dose to make up for a missed dose.*

STORAGE

Keep this medication in the container it came in, and keep it out of the reach of children. You may ask your pharmacist to put this medicine in a container without a childproof cap.

Sulindac
(sul in' dak)

PRODUCT INFORMATION
Brand name: Clinoril

USES

Sulindac is used to relieve the pain, redness, tenderness, swelling and stiffness of certain types of arthritis. The drug also is used to relieve joint pain resulting from gout, bursitis and tendonitis.

UNDESIRED EFFECTS

The most common side effects of sulindac are stomach upsets such as indigestion, nausea, vomiting, stomach pain, constipation and diarrhea. To minimize stomach upsets, take sulindac with milk, meals, a snack or an antacid. If these effects continue or are severe, contact your doctor.

Sulindac makes some people dizzy or less alert. Do not drive a car or operate dangerous machinery until you know how this medicine will affect you.

Other effects, which may go away as you continue to take sulindac and as your body adjusts to it, include headache, loss of appetite or a bloated feeling, blurred vision, dry or sore mouth, nervousness, trembling, increased sweating and fast or pounding heartbeat. Contact your doctor if these effects continue or are bothersome.

More serious side effects can occur and may require medical attention. Contact your doctor if you have a ringing or buzzing in your ears; skin rash; hives; itching; bloody or tarry stools; partial loss of hearing; vision problems; swelling of the hands, feet, ankles or lower legs; shortness of breath or difficult breathing, wheezing or tightness in the chest; or unusual tiredness or weakness.

PRECAUTIONS

You should not take sulindac if you ever had a bad reaction to it or if you ever had an unusual reaction to aspirin or other salicylates, diflunisal, fenoprofen, ibuprofen, indomethacin, meclofenamate, mefenamic acid, naproxen, oxyphenbutazone, phenylbutazone, piroxicam or tolmetin. If you have questions about this problem, check with your doctor.

Because sulindac can make certain medical conditions worse, tell your doctor if you have asthma, blooding problems, heart disease, high blood pressure, colitis, kidney disease, liver disease, a stomach ulcer or other stomach problems.

Tell your doctor what prescription or nonprescription drugs you are taking, including anticoagulants (blood thinners), medicine for diabetes, any other medicine for arthritis, phenytoin and sulfa medicines. If you do not know the names of the drugs or why they were prescribed, bring them in their labeled containers to your doctor or pharmacist.

It may take a few days for you to feel better after you take sulindac, and you may have to take it for two to three weeks before you feel the full effects. Take sulindac exactly as prescribed. Do not take more of it, do not take it more often and do not take it for a longer period than ordered by your doctor. If you think you need more to relieve your symptoms, contact your doctor.

Laboratory tests such as blood tests or kidney and liver function tests may be required while you are taking sulindac. If you experience problems with your vision or hearing after you start to take this drug, you should tell your doctor and have your eyes examined or have your hearing tested. *Be sure to keep all appointments with your doctor and at the laboratory.*

Alcoholic beverages will increase the drowsiness caused by sulindac. Do not take aspirin regularly unless you have permission from your doctor. Alcohol or aspirin can increase the chance of stomach upset.

Before you have surgery with a general anesthetic, including dental surgery, tell the doctor or dentist that you are taking sulindac.

Because it is not known whether this medicine may be safely used by pregnant women or nursing mothers, tell your doctor if you are pregnant or breast-feeding.

DOSAGE

Your doctor will determine how often you should take sulindac and how much you should take at each dose. Carefully follow the instructions on your prescription label, and ask your doctor or pharmacist to explain any part of the instructions you do not understand.

Sulindac comes in tablets. If this medicine upsets your stomach, take it with solid food, milk or an antacid.

If you forget to take a dose of this medicine, take the missed dose as soon as you remember unless it is almost time to take the next dose. If it is almost time for your next dose, omit the missed dose entirely and take only the regularly scheduled dose. *Do not take a double dose.*

STORAGE
Keep sulindac in the container it came in, and keep it out of the reach of children. Do not allow anyone else to take your sulindac. If you have arthritis, you may ask your pharmacist to put this medicine in a bottle without a childproof cap.

Tolmetin
(tole' met in)

PRODUCT INFORMATION
Brand name: Tolectin

USES
Tolmetin is used to relieve the pain, redness, tenderness, stiffness and swelling of certain types of arthritis.

UNDESIRED EFFECTS
The most common side effects of tolmetin are stomach upsets such as indigestion, heartburn, nausea, vomiting and stomach pain; diarrhea also is a side effect. To prevent or lessen stomach upset, take this medicine with a meal or snack, milk or an antacid other than sodium bicarbonate (baking soda). If stomach upsets continue, contact your doctor.

Tolmetin may cause some people to become dizzy, lightheaded or drowsy. Do not drive a car or operate dangerous machinery until you know how this medicine will affect you. Other effects, which may disappear as you continue to take this drug and as your body adjusts to it, include headache, constipation and nervousness. Contact your doctor if these effects continue to bother you.

More serious effects, which do not occur often, will require medical attention if they do occur. Contact your doctor if you have a ringing or buzzing in the ears; skin rash or hives; swelling of the feet, ankles or lower legs; unusual weight gain; bloody or tarry stools; shortness of breath; difficulty breathing; wheezing; tightness in the chest; sore throat; or fever.

PRECAUTIONS
Do not take tolmetin if you ever had a bad reaction to it or if you ever had an unusual reaction to aspirin or other salicylates, diflunisal, fenoprofen, ibuprofen,

indomethacin, meclofenamate, mefenamic acid, naproxen, oxyphenbutazone, phenylbutazone, piroxicam or sulindac. Be sure to tell your doctor about any such reaction.

Because tolmetin can make certain medical problems worse, tell your doctor if you have bleeding problems, heart disease, kidney disease, a stomach ulcer or other stomach problems.

Tell your doctor what prescription or nonprescription drugs you are taking, especially anticoagulants (blood thinners), medicine for diabetes, any other medicine for arthritis, phenytoin, sulfa medicines and sodium bicarbonate (baking soda). If you do not know the names of the drugs or why they were prescribed, bring them in their labeled containers to your doctor or pharmacist.

Tolmetin will help you only if you take it regularly as prescribed by your doctor. You should begin to feel better within a week after you start to take tolmetin.

Your doctor probably will order laboratory tests for your kidney and liver functions as well as blood tests while you are taking this drug. If you have blurred vision or other problems with your eyes after you start to take tolmetin, you also will need an eye examination. *Be sure to keep all appointments with your doctor and at the laboratory.*

Do not drink alcoholic beverages or take aspirin regularly while you are taking tolmetin. Alcohol or aspirin can add to stomach upset. If you have questions, check with your doctor or pharmacist.

Before you have any surgery with a general anesthetic, including dental surgery, tell the doctor or dentist that you are taking tolmetin.

Although harm to an unborn child or a nursing baby has not been reported after taking tolmetin, tell your doctor if you are pregnant or breast-feeding before you start to take tolmetin.

DOSAGE

Your doctor will determine how often you should take tolmetin and how much you should take at each dose. Carefully follow the instructions on your prescription label, and ask your doctor or pharmacist to explain any part of the instructions you do not understand.

Tolmetin comes in capsules and tablets. Take the drug with milk or solid food or with an antacid (not sodium bicarbonate) if it upsets your stomach.

If you forget to take a dose of tolmetin, take it as soon as you remember. If you remember a missed dose when it is almost time for you to take another, omit the missed dose entirely and take only the regularly scheduled dose. *Do not take a double dose to make up for a missed dose.*

STORAGE

Keep tolmetin in the container it came in, and keep it out of the reach of children. Do not allow anyone else to take your tolmetin. If you have arthritis, you may ask your pharmacist to put this medicine in a bottle without a childproof cap.

CORTICOSTEROIDS
(kore ti kos' ter oids)

USES
The body produces a number of hormones that are essential to good health. When too little of these hormones (cortisones) is produced, corticosteroids may be prescribed to help make up the difference.

In addition, corticosteroids are used to reduce inflammation, redness and swelling in various parts of the body and to relieve allergic reactions.

The oral forms (capsules, tablets and liquid) are used to relieve the symptoms of arthritis, asthma, severe allergies and skin problems. There is also a form that is injected directly into the joint for the treatment of arthritis.

Included in this group of medicines are both the natural hormone (hydrocortisone) and substances made in the laboratory (dexamethasone, prednisone and triamcinolone) that act in the body like the natural hormone.

UNDESIRED EFFECTS
The most common side effect of corticosteroids is stomach upset (heartburn, indigestion and stomach pain). Take the medicine with meals or a snack, and contact your doctor if stomach upsets continue in spite of this precaution.

Other side effects, which may go away as your body adjusts to the medicine, are a false sense of well-being, an increase in appetite, nervousness, restlessness, trouble in sleeping and weight gain. Contact your doctor if these effects are severe.

Short-term therapy: Serious side effects requiring medical attention are rare. However, you should contact your doctor if you have decreased or blurred vision, frequent urination, increased thirst or skin rash.

Long-term therapy: In addition to the above side effects, a corticosteroid can cause a number of other serious problems when it is taken over a long period. Contact your doctor if you develop acne or other skin problems, back or rib pain, bloody or black stools, continuing stomach pain or burning, depression, fever or sore throat, irregular heartbeats, menstrual problems, mood or mental changes, puffiness of the face, muscle cramps or pains, muscle weakness, nausea or vomiting, seeing of halos around lights, swelling of the feet or lower legs or unusual tiredness or weakness.

If you take a corticosteroid over a long period of time, your body may need time to adjust after you stop taking this medicine. During this adjustment period be alert for side effects. Contact your doctor if you have fever, dizziness or fainting, muscle or joint pain, nausea or vomiting, loss of appetite for several days, shortness of breath, unusual tiredness or weakness or unusual weight loss.

PRECAUTIONS
Because a corticosteroid can make certain medical conditions worse, tell your doctor if you have bone disease, colitis, diabetes, diverticulitis, glaucoma, heart disease, herpes simplex of the eyes, high blood pressure, high cholesterol levels, fungal infection, kidney disease or kidney stones, liver disease, myasthenia gravis,

stomach ulcer or other stomach problems, tuberculosis (positive skin test, partially healed TB or a history of TB) or underactive thyroid.

Before you start to take a corticosteroid, tell your doctor what prescription or nonprescription drugs you are taking, including amphotericin B, anticoagulants (blood thinners), aspirin or other salicylates, oral diabetes medicine, digitalis, diuretics (water pills), medicine for high blood pressure, other arthritis medicines, insulin, phenobarbital, phenytoin, rifampin and somatropin.

If you do not know the names of the drugs you are taking or what they were prescribed for, bring them in their labeled containers to your doctor or pharmacist.

A corticosteroid must be taken regularly to be effective. Take it exactly as prescribed by your doctor. Do not take more of it, do not take it more often and do not take it for a longer period of time than your doctor has ordered.

Keep in touch with your doctor while you are taking this medicine. Your doctor may want to adjust the dose after checking your response to the corticosteroid. *Keep all your appointments with your doctor.*

Do not stop taking this medicine without first checking with your doctor. Your doctor may want you to reduce gradually the amount you are taking before you stop completely. When your doctor tells you to stop taking this medicine, throw away any unused portion.

Your doctor may instruct you to weigh yourself every day. Be sure to report any unusual weight gain, and follow instructions about cutting down on your intake of calories. Your doctor also may want you to follow a low-salt or potassium-rich diet.

Tell every doctor or dentist who treats you that you are taking a corticosteroid. You should wear a Medic-Alert bracelet or some other kind of identification in case of accident or other kind of medical emergency. Ask your pharmacist how to get this kind of identification.

Do not have a vaccination, other immunization or any type of skin test while you are taking a corticosteroid unless your doctor specifically tells you that you may.

If you have diabetes, this medicine may cause blood sugar levels to rise. If you notice a change in the results of your urine sugar test or if you have any questions, check with your doctor.

While you are taking a corticosteroid, do not take aspirin, Anacin, Bufferin or Excedrin unless you ask your doctor how many of these tablets you may take.

Because a corticosteroid can harm the growth of an unborn child and a nursing baby, be sure to tell your doctor if you are pregnant or are breast-feeding a baby before you take a corticosteroid. If you become pregnant while taking this medicine, notify your doctor immediately.

Dexamethasone
(dex a meth′ a sone)

PRODUCT INFORMATION
Brand names: Decadron, Deronil, Dexameth, Dexone, Hexadrol, SK-Dexameth-asone

USES
See the general statement titled Corticosteroids.

UNDESIRED EFFECTS
See the general statement titled Corticosteroids.

PRECAUTIONS
See the general statement titled Corticosteroids.

If you are taking the oral form of dexamethasone, do not drink alcoholic beverages. Alcohol can worsen stomach upset caused by taking dexamethasone.

If dexamethasone is injected into one of your joints, be careful not to put too much stress or strain on that joint. Ask your doctor how much you are allowed to move the joint while it is healing. If redness or swelling occurs at the place of the injection, contact your doctor.

DOSAGE
Your doctor will determine how often you should take dexamethasone. Carefully follow the instructions on your prescription label, and ask your doctor or pharmacist to explain any part of the instructions you do not understand.

If you are to take dexamethasone once a day, take it in the morning with breakfast. If you are to take this medicine more than once a day, take it at regular intervals between the time you get up in the morning and the time you go to bed at night. For example, if your doctor tells you to take it three times a day, take it at 7:00 a.m., 3:00 p.m. and 11:00 p.m.

Dexamethasone comes in liquid form and in tablets. Take this medicine with meals or a snack to decrease stomach upset.

If you forget to take a dose of dexamethasone when you are on a once-a-day schedule, take the missed dose as soon as you remember it that day. If you do not remember a missed dose until the next day, take only your regularly scheduled dose. *Do not take a double dose to make up for the missed one.*

If you are taking dexamethasone more than once a day and forget to take a dose, take it as soon as you remember. Take any remaining doses for that day at evenly spaced intervals. If you do not remember a missed dose until it is time for you to take another, you may take both doses at one time.

STORAGE
Keep dexamethasone in the container it came in. If you have arthritis, you may ask your pharmacist to put this medicine in a bottle without a childproof cap.

Keep dexamethasone out of the reach of children. Do not allow anyone else to take your dexamethasone.

Hydrocortisone
(hye droe kor′ ti sone)

PRODUCT INFORMATION
Brand names: Cortef, Hydrocortone, Panhydrosone

USES
See the general statement titled Corticosteroids.

UNDESIRED EFFECTS
See the general statement titled Corticosteroids.

PRECAUTIONS
See the general statement titled Corticosteroids.

If you are taking the oral form of hydrocortisone, do not drink alcoholic beverages. Alcohol can worsen the stomach upset caused by taking hydrocortisone.

If hydrocortisone is injected into one of your joints, be careful not to put too much stress or strain on that joint. Ask your doctor how much you are allowed to move the joint while it is healing. If redness or swelling occurs at the place of the injection, contact your doctor.

DOSAGE
Your doctor will determine how often you should take hydrocortisone. Carefully follow the instructions on your prescription label, and ask your doctor or pharmacist to explain any part of the instructions you do not understand.

If you are to take hydrocortisone once a day, take it in the morning with breakfast. If you are to take this medicine more than once a day, take it at regular intervals between the time you get up in the morning and the time you go to bed at night. For example, if your doctor tells you to take it three times a day, take it at 7:00 a.m., 3:00 p.m. and 11:00 p.m.

Hydrocortisone comes in liquid form and in tablets. Take this medicine with meals or a snack to decrease stomach upset. Shake the liquid well before each dose.

If you forget to take a dose when you are on a once-a-day schedule, take the missed dose as soon as you remember it. If you do not remember a missed dose until it is time for you to take another, omit the missed dose entirely and take only the regularly scheduled dose.

If you are taking hydrocortisone more than once a day and forget to take a dose, take the missed dose as soon as you remember it. Take any remaining doses for that day at evenly spaced intervals. If you remember a missed dose when it is time for you to take another, you may take both doses at one time.

STORAGE
Keep hydrocortisone in the container it came in, and keep it out of the reach of children. If you have arthritis, you may ask your pharmacist to put this medicine in a bottle without a childproof cap, but be sure to keep it out of the reach of children.

Do not allow anyone else to take your hydrocortisone.

Prednisone
(pred′ ni sone)

PRODUCT INFORMATION
Brand names: Delta-Dome, Deltasone, Fernisone, Meticorten, Orasone, Pan-Sone, Paracort, Pred-5, Prednicen-M, Ropred, Servisone, SK-Prednisone, Stera-pred

USES
See the general statement titled Corticosteroids.

UNDESIRED EFFECTS
See the general statement titled Corticosteroids.

PRECAUTIONS
See the general statement titled Corticosteroids.
Do not drink alcoholic beverages while you are taking this medicine. Alcohol with prednisone can cause severe stomach upset.

DOSAGE
Your doctor will determine how often you should take prednisone. Carefully follow the instructions on your prescription label, and ask your doctor or pharmacist to explain any part of the instructions you do not understand.

If you are to take prednisone every other day, take it at breakfast on the first day. Do not take it at all on the second day. Then take it at breakfast on the third day.

If you are to take prednisone once a day, take it in the morning with breakfast.

If you are to take this medicine more than once a day, take it at regular intervals between the time you get up in the morning and the time you go to bed at night. For example, if your doctor tells you to take it three times a day, take it at 7:00 a.m., 3:00 p.m. and 11:00 p.m.

Prednisone comes in tablets. Take them with meals or a snack to decrease stomach upset.

If you forget to take a dose of prednisone, do one of the following, depending on your dosage schedule:

Schedule of every other day—If you remember a missed dose on the morning of the day you should have taken it, take the missed dose as soon as you remember it. If you remember a missed dose on the afternoon of the day you should have taken it, start a new schedule. Take the missed dose on the next morning (day one), do not take it at all on day two and take the next dose on the morning of day three.

Schedule of once a day—Take the missed dose as soon as you remember it. If you do not remember a missed dose until it is time for you to take another, omit the missed dose entirely and take only the regularly scheduled dose.

Schedule of more than once a day—Take the missed dose as soon as you remember it, and take any remaining doses for that day at evenly spaced intervals. If you remember a missed dose when it is time for you to take another, you may take both doses at one time.

STORAGE

Keep prednisone in the container it came in. If you have arthritis, you may ask your pharmacist to put this medicine in a bottle without a childproof cap, but be sure to keep it out of the reach of children.

Do not allow anyone else to take your prednisone.

Triamcinolone
(trye am sin' oh lone)

PRODUCT INFORMATION

Brand names: Aristocort, Aristo-Pak, Kenacort, Rocinolone, SK-Triamcinolone, Spencort

USES

See the general statement titled Corticosteroids.

UNDESIRED EFFECTS

See the general statement titled Corticosteroids.

PRECAUTIONS

See the general statement titled Corticosteroids.

If you are taking an oral form of triamcinolone, do not drink alcoholic beverages. Alcohol can add to the stomach upset triamcinolone causes.

If triamcinolone is injected into one of your joints, be careful not to put too much stress or strain on that joint. Ask your doctor how much you are allowed to move this joint while it is healing. If redness or swelling occurs at the place of the injection, contact your doctor.

DOSAGE

Your doctor will determine how often you should take triamcinolone. Carefully follow the instructions on your prescription label, and ask your doctor or pharmacist to explain any part of the instructions you do not understand.

If you are to take triamcinolone every other day, take it at breakfast on the first day. Do not take it at all on the second day. Then take it at breakfast on the third day.

If you are to take triamcinolone once a day, take it in the morning with breakfast.

If you are to take this medicine more than once a day, take it at regular intervals between the time you get up in the morning and the time you go to bed at night.

For example, if your doctor tells you to take it three times a day, take it at 7:00 a.m., 3:00 p.m. and 11:00 p.m.

Triamcinolone comes in tablets and in liquid form. Take this medicine with meals or a snack to lessen stomach upset.

If you forget to take a dose of triamcinolone, do one of the following, depending on your dosage schedule:

Schedule of every other day—If you remember a missed dose on the morning of the day you should have taken it, take the missed dose as soon as you remember it. If you remember a missed dose on the afternoon of the day you should have taken it, start a new schedule. Take the missed dose on the next morning (day one), do not take it at all on day two and take the next dose on the morning of day three.

Schedule of once a day—Take the missed dose as soon as you remember it. If you do not remember a missed dose until it is time for you to take another, omit the missed dose entirely and take only the regularly scheduled dose.

Schedule of more than once a day—Take the missed dose as soon as you remember it and take any remaining doses for that day at evenly spaced intervals. If you remember a missed dose when it is time for you to take another, you may take both doses at one time.

STORAGE

Keep triamcinolone in the container it came in, and keep it out of the reach of children. If you have arthritis, you may ask your pharmacist to put this medicine in a bottle without a childproof cap, but be sure to keep it out of the reach of children.

Do not allow anyone else to take your triamcinolone.

Pain

DRUGS USED TO TREAT PAIN

Pain

Pain probably is the most common symptom, yet its causes are not well understood. Most of the time, pain is caused by a combination of physical and psychological factors. Anxiety and depression increase the sensation of pain. As a result, the perception of pain varies widely among individuals, making it difficult to evaluate.

Pain has a number of characteristics that provide clues to its underlying causes. These characteristics include:
- severity
- type—dull and aching or sharp
- location—in a specific place (for example, a joint) or diffuse
- time of appearance—only at certain times of the day (for example, before or after meals or upon awakening) or constant
- factors that affect its appearance—certain types of weather or particular physical activities

Drugs used to relieve pain are called analgesics. Certain analgesics, such as aspirin and other salicylates, reduce inflammation and fever as well as relieve pain. Because of their ability to decrease inflammation, they are commonly used to treat arthritis.

Acetaminophen relieves pain and fever but does not reduce inflammation. All nonprescription analgesics are used for headache and other minor aches and pains, and they are safe and effective when used according to instructions. The biggest danger associated with these medications is accidental overdosage. Because of its widespread use, aspirin causes more accidental poisonings in children than any other drug. It is important to store these products out of the reach of children and to keep them in childproof containers.

The narcotic analgesics are reserved for treating severe pain. They are usually prescribed in small quantities following tooth extractions, treatment of fractures or surgery. Although narcotics are very effective pain relievers, they have other effects that make them unsuitable for long-term use. These effects include depression of the central nervous system and high potential for addiction.

NONPRESCRIPTION ANALGESICS

Acetaminophen

(a seat a mee' noe fen)

PRODUCT INFORMATION
Brand names: Anacin-3, Datril, Liquiprin, Panadol, Phenaphen, SK-Apap, Tempra, Tylenol, Valadol and others

Brand names of some combination products containing acetaminophen: Darvocet N-100, Empracet, Excedrin, Percocet-5, Tylox

USES
Acetaminophen is used to relieve pain and reduce fever. It does *not* relieve the stiffness, redness and swelling of arthritis.

Acetaminophen and preparations containing acetaminophen are available without a prescription. Many cough and cold products also contain acetaminophen. *Carefully read the label on the container for a nonprescription medicine to determine if the medicine contains acetaminophen.*

UNDESIRED EFFECTS
When taken as directed for short periods, acetaminophen is almost free of side effects. Rarely, this medicine can cause dizziness, which tends to disappear as your body adjusts to the drug.

Liver problems, allergic reactions and blood disorders are rare side effects, but they require medical attention. If you experience unusual weakness or tiredness, yellowing of the skin and eyes (symptoms of liver problems), itching or skin rash (symptoms of an allergic reaction), sore throat and fever or unusual bleeding or bruising (symptoms of blood problems), contact your doctor.

Large doses of this medicine can cause acetaminophen poisoning. Some signs of overdose are diarrhea, nausea or vomiting and stomach cramps or pain. Contact your doctor immediately if any of these problems occur.

PRECAUTIONS
Before you start to take acetaminophen or a product containing it, tell your doctor or pharmacist if you ever had an unusual reaction to this medicine or to phenacetin, if you have kidney disease or if you have liver disease or cirrhosis of the liver.

Take only as much acetaminophen as directed by your doctor or as recommended on the package label. Taking too much of this medicine for too long a time can cause liver damage.

Children up to 12 years of age should not take acetaminophen for more than five days in a row. Adults should not take it for more than 10 days in a row. If the symptoms of the condition for which acetaminophen was prescribed still exist after five days in children or 10 days in adults, contact your doctor.

If you take acetaminophen to lower a fever, contact your doctor if the fever lasts for more than three days or if it returns.

Check the labels on all the prescription or nonprescription medicines you are taking. If any of them contains acetaminophen, ask your doctor or pharmacist about taking more than one medicine containing acetaminophen. You will avoid taking an overdose this way.

DOSAGE

Acetaminophen comes in tablets, in liquid form and in rectal suppositories. The liquid should be measured in a specially marked spoon to be sure of an accurate dose. Liquid drops for infants and children should be measured with the dropper that comes with the bottle. Drops may be placed directly into the child's mouth or mixed with water or juice.

To use a rectal suppository, remove the wrapper and dip the tip of the suppository in water. Then lie on your side, draw your top knee up to your chest and insert the suppository well into the rectum with your finger. Hold it there for a few moments; then get up and resume your usual activities. Try not to have a bowel movement for at least an hour after inserting the suppository.

STORAGE

Keep acetaminophen in the container it came in. Be sure to keep this medicine out of the reach of children. An overdose of acetaminophen is very dangerous in young children.

Aspirin

(as′ pir in)

Aspirin belongs to the group of medicines known as salicylates. Aspirin is also called acetylsalicylic acid. It is used to relieve mild to moderate pain, to reduce fever caused by infection and to relieve redness and swelling caused by arthritis. Aspirin also helps to prevent blood from clotting. See the section titled Aspirin/Salicylates (page 297) under Drugs Used to Treat Arthritis.

PRESCRIPTION ANALGESICS
Codeine
(koe′ deen)

PRODUCT INFORMATION

Brand names of some cough medicines containing codeine: Actifed-C, Ambenyl Expectorant, Cerose, Cetro-Cirose, Cheracol, Colrex Compound, Copavin, Cosanyl Cough Syrup, Cotussis, Dimetane Expectorant DC, Ephedrol with Codeine, Histadyl EC Syrup, Isoclor Expectorant, Mercodol, Novahistine DH, Pediacof, Phenergan Expectorant with Codeine, Robitussin A-C, Tolu-Sed, Tussar, Tussi-Organidin

Brand names of some pain medicines containing codeine: A.P.C. with Codeine, Aceta with Codeine, Acetaminophen with Codeine, Anexsia with Codeine, Ascriptin with Codeine, Bancap with Codeine, Capital with Codeine, Codalan, Empirin with Codeine, Empracet with Codeine, Fiorinal, G-2, G-3, Maxigesic, Phenaphen with Codeine, SK-Apap with Codeine, Soma Compound with Codeine, Tabloid brand A.P.C. with Codeine, Tylenol with Codeine

USES

Codeine is a narcotic which acts on the cough center in the brain to decrease coughing. It is used alone or with other cough medicines, expectorants, decongestants and antihistamines to relieve cough and cold symptoms. It is used in higher doses to relieve pain and is available by prescription.

UNDESIRED EFFECTS

When you first start to take codeine, you may become nauseated. If you lie down for awhile, this effect usually will go away. Codeine also can cause vomiting or constipation. Drink plenty of fluids; if these effects continue or are severe, contact your doctor.

While taking codeine, you may be dizzy or lightheaded or you may faint when getting up from a lying or sitting position. If you get up slowly, this problem will be less bothersome. However, if it continues in spite of your precautions, contact your doctor.

A more serious problem is the effect codeine can have on the central nervous system (brain and spinal cord). If you experience shortness of breath, have difficulty breathing or notice that your heartbeat is unusually slow, contact your doctor. In children, a central nervous system problem can have the opposite effect and cause unusual excitement. Contact your doctor if your child behaves in this way after taking codeine.

Codeine makes some people drowsy or less alert than usual. Do not drive a car or operate dangerous machinery until you know what effect this medicine will have on you.

PRECAUTIONS

Codeine can make certain medical conditions worse. Be sure to tell your doctor if you have colitis; emphysema, asthma or chronic lung disease; enlarged prostate or problems with urination; gallbladder disease or gallstones; kidney or liver disease; underactive adrenal glands (Addison's disease); underactive thyroid; or unusually slow or irregular heartbeat.

Other medicines that slow down function of the central nervous system should not be taken with codeine. Tell your doctor what other prescription or nonprescription drugs you are taking, including antihistamines, medicine for allergy or colds, barbiturates, other narcotics, prescription medicine for pain, sedatives, tranquilizers, medicine to help you sleep, medicine for seizures and medicine for depression. Also tell your doctor if you are taking prescription medicine for stomach cramps or spasms and if you are now taking or have taken MAO inhibitors (isocarboxazid, pargyline, phenelzine or tranylcypromine) within the past two weeks.

If you do not know the names of the drugs you are taking or what they were prescribed for, bring them in their labeled containers to your doctor or pharmacist. Contact your doctor or pharmacist before you start to take any of the above drugs while you are taking codeine.

You should not consume alcohol while you are taking codeine because of the possibility of side effects. If you have any questions, check with your doctor or pharmacist.

Do not take codeine if you ever had problems with it in the past.

Before having any kind of surgery with general anesthesia, including dental surgery, tell the doctor or dentist that you are taking codeine.

To select the best treatment for you and your baby, tell your doctor if you are pregnant or are breast-feeding.

DOSAGE

Your doctor will determine how often you should take codeine or a product containing codeine and how much you should take at each dose. Carefully follow the instructions on your prescription label, and ask your doctor or pharmacist to explain any part of the instructions you do not understand.

Codeine and products containing codeine come in tablets, capsules and liquid form. Codeine often is prescribed to be taken as needed for pain or for coughing. However, if this medicine has been prescribed for you, do not take more of it or take it more often or for a longer period than your doctor has instructed. Products containing codeine can be habit-forming.

If you are taking codeine on a schedule and forget to take a dose, take the missed dose as soon as you remember, unless you remember it when you are scheduled to take another dose. Then take only the regularly scheduled dose. Omit the missed dose completely; *do not take a double dose*.

STORAGE

Keep codeine in the container it came in, and keep it out of the reach of children. Do not allow anyone else to take your codeine.

Oxycodone
(ox i koe' done)

PRODUCT INFORMATION
Brand names of products containing oxycodone with acetaminophen: Percocet-5, Tylox

Brand names of products containing oxycodone with aspirin: Percodan, Percodan-Demi

USES
Oxycodone is a narcotic used to relieve moderate pain, such as that associated with bursitis, dislocations, simple fractures and nerve problems. Oxycodone also is used to relieve pain following surgery, tooth extraction and childbirth.

Oxycodone is also available in combination with aspirin or acetaminophen. Oxycodone can be obtained only with a doctor's prescription, and the prescription cannot be refilled. You must get another prescription if you continue to take a product containing oxycodone.

UNDESIRED EFFECTS
Oxycodone can cause nausea and vomiting, especially after the first few doses. You may take the medicine with food or milk, or lie down for awhile to relieve nausea or vomiting. If these precautions do not make you more comfortable or if these effects are very bothersome, contact your doctor.

Some people become drowsy or less alert than usual when they take oxycodone. Do not drive a car or operate dangerous machinery until you know what effect this medicine will have on you.

If you experience dizziness, lightheadedness or fainting when you get up from a lying or sitting position, get up slowly. This precaution should help decrease these effects. If they continue or are severe, contact your doctor.

When you start to take oxycodone, you may have redness or flushing of the face, unusual increase in sweating, blurred vision, constipation, difficult urination or a frequent urge to urinate, dry mouth, unusual tiredness or weakness or unusually fast or pounding heartbeat. These effects may decrease as you continue to take oxycodone and as your body adjusts to it; if they do not decrease, contact your doctor.

More serious side effects of oxycodone are shortness of breath, difficult breathing and an unusually slow heartbeat. These signs indicate that the medicine is having a bad effect on your central nervous system, and they require medical attention. Inform family members or alert some other person who is likely to be nearby to call your doctor immediately if you have difficulty breathing.

Be sure to check the side effects of aspirin (see Aspirin/Salicylates, page 297) if you are taking a preparation that combines oxycodone with aspirin. Side effects for acetaminophen (page 332) should be checked if you are taking a combination of oxycodone and acetaminophen.

PRECAUTIONS
Before you start to take oxycodone, tell your doctor if you have a history of

emphysema, asthma, chronic lung disease, enlarged prostate, problems with urination, gallbladder disease, gallstones, kidney disease, liver disease, underactive adrenal gland (Addison's disease), underactive thyroid, or unusually slow or irregular heartbeat. Oxycodone can make these conditions worse.

Certain medications, when taken with oxycodone, can increase the possibility and severity of side effects. These medications include antihistamines or other medicine for hay fever, allergies or colds; sedatives, tranquilizers or medicine to help you sleep; barbiturates, other narcotics or other prescription medicine for pain; medicine for seizures; medicine for depression; prescription medicine for stomach cramps or spasms; and MAO inhibitors (isocarboxazid, pargyline, phenelzine or tranylcypromine).

Tell your doctor what prescription or nonprescription medicines you are taking (or, in the case of MAO inhibitors, have taken within the past two weeks). If you do not know the names of the drugs or what they were prescribed for, bring them in their labeled containers to your doctor or pharmacist.

Do not drink alcoholic beverages while taking oxycodone, and do not take any of the drugs listed above without first checking with your doctor or pharmacist.

Oxycodone can be habit-forming. Do not take more of it, do not take it more often and do not take it for a longer time than directed by your doctor.

Before you have any kind of surgery with a general anesthetic, including dental surgery, tell the doctor or dentist in charge that you are taking oxycodone.

The safe use of oxycodone during pregnancy has not been established. Be sure to tell your doctor if you are pregnant so the best treatment for you and your baby can be selected.

Check the precautions for aspirin (see Aspirin/Salicylates, page 297) and acetaminophen (page 332) when you are taking oxycodone combined with any of these drugs.

DOSAGE
Preparations containing oxycodone come in capsules and tablets. Your doctor will determine how often you should take this medicine and how much you should take at each dose. Carefully follow the instructions on your prescription label, and ask your doctor or pharmacist to explain any part of the instructions you do not understand.

STORAGE
Keep oxycodone in the container it came in, and keep it out of the reach of children. Do not allow anyone else to take your oxycodone.

Pentazocine
(pen taz' oh seen)

PRODUCT INFORMATION
Brand name: Talwin

Brand name of a product containing pentazocine combined with aspirin: Talwin Compound

USES

Pentazocine is used to relieve moderate to severe pain caused by many types of medical problems. The injectable form of this medicine is used to supplement anesthesia during surgery, to treat pain following surgery and to relieve the pain of childbirth.

Pentazocine is available only with a doctor's prescription, and a prescription for pentazocine may not be refilled. If you continue to take this medicine, you will need a new prescription each time.

UNDESIRED EFFECTS

With the first few doses of pentazocine, you may experience nausea or vomiting. If you lie down, these effects usually will disappear.

Some people who take pentazocine become drowsy, dizzy or lightheaded or get a false sense of well-being. Do not drive a car or operate dangerous machinery until you know how this drug will affect you.

Other effects that may occur when you start to take pentazocine are flushing, sweating, itching, constipation, difficulty urinating, headache, tremor or shakiness, numbness, blurred vision and ringing in the ears. These effects tend to decrease or disappear as your body adjusts to the medicine. However, contact your doctor if they continue or are severe.

Contact your doctor if you have any signs of an allergic reaction to pentazocine such as hives, skin rash, chills or fever.

More serious side effects also can occur and will require medical attention. Stop taking this medicine and contact your doctor if you have difficulty breathing, changes in mood, mental confusion, a feeling that something wrong is about to happen, depression or hallucinations (seeing, hearing or feeling things that are not there).

PRECAUTIONS

Before you start to take pentazocine, tell your doctor if you have emphysema, asthma, chronic lung disease, enlarged prostate, problems with urination, gallbladder disease, gallstones, history of convulsions or seizures, kidney disease, liver disease or dependence on or addiction to narcotics. Pentazocine may make these medical problems worse.

Certain other medications, when taken with pentazocine, can increase the possibility and severity of side effects. Tell your doctor if you are taking any of the following: meperidine; methadone or other narcotics to treat dependence on or addiction to narcotics; morphine; prescription medicine for stomach cramps or spasm; antihistamines or other medicine for hay fever, allergies or colds; barbiturates, narcotics or other prescription medicine for pain; sedatives, tranquilizers or medicine to help you sleep; medicine for seizures; medicine for depression; or MAO inhibitors (isocarboxazid, pargyline, phenelzine or tranylcypromine), even if you stopped taking them recently.

If you do not know the names of the drugs you are taking or what they were prescribed for, bring them in their labeled containers to your doctor or pharmacist.

Do not drink alcoholic beverages while you are taking pentazocine. Do not start taking any of the medicines listed above without first checking with your doctor or pharmacist.

Pentazocine can be habit-forming. Therefore, do not take more of it, do not take it more often and do not take it for a longer time than directed by your doctor. If the amount prescribed does not relieve your pain, contact your doctor. Your doctor may want to adjust your dose or change your medication.

If you will be taking pentazocine for several weeks or months, your doctor will want to check your progress at regular intervals. *Be sure to keep all appointments with your doctor.*

Do not have surgery with general anesthesia, including dental surgery, unless you tell the doctor or dentist in charge that you are taking pentazocine.

Pentazocine should not be taken by children under 12 years of age or by pregnant women. Before you start taking pentazocine, tell your doctor if you are pregnant. If you become pregnant while taking this medicine, stop taking it and contact your doctor immediately.

DOSAGE
Your doctor will determine how often you should take pentazocine and how much you should take at each dose. Carefully follow the instructions on your prescription label, and ask your doctor or pharmacist to explain any part of the instructions you do not understand.

Pentazocine comes in tablets to be taken orally. If you are taking a combination of pentazocine and aspirin, see Aspirin/Salicylates (page 297) for side effects, precautions and special instructions on the use of aspirin.

STORAGE
Keep pentazocine in the container it came in. Keep it out of the reach of children. Do not allow anyone else to take your pentazocine.

Propoxyphene
(proe pox′ i feen)

PRODUCT INFORMATION
Brand names: Darvon, Dolene, Profene, SK-65

Brand names of products containing propoxyphene with acetaminophen: Darvocet N-50, Darvocet N-100, Dolene AP-65, Dolocet, SK-65 APAP, Wygesic

Brand names of products containing propoxyphene with aspirin: Darvon Compound, Darvon Compound-65, Darvon with A.S.A., Dolene Compound-65, SK-65 Compound

USES
Propoxyphene is used for the relief of mild to moderate pain. Propoxyphene is prescribed alone or in combination with aspirin or acetaminophen. If you are taking one of these combination preparations, see Aspirin/Salicylates (page 297) and Acetaminophen (page 332) for additional side effects and precautions.

UNDESIRED EFFECTS
Nausea and vomiting may occur, particularly after the first few doses. If you lie down, these effects usually will disappear. Contact your doctor if these effects continue after taking this precaution.

Propoxyphene makes some people drowsy, dizzy or lightheaded or gives a false sense of well-being. Do not drive a car or operate dangerous machinery until you know how this medicine will affect you.

Other effects, which tend to decrease or disappear as your body adjusts to propoxyphene, include blurred vision, constipation, headache, stomach pain and unusual weakness or tiredness. If these effects continue or are severe, contact your doctor.

Itching or skin rash indicates that you are allergic to this medicine. If you have either of these effects, stop taking propoxyphene and contact your doctor.

Taking more propoxyphene than prescribed or taking it with alcohol or other narcotics can cause symptoms of overdosage, including weakness, difficult breathing, confusion, anxiety and severe drowsiness and dizziness. You may become unconscious. If any of these symptoms occur, call your doctor or arrange to have someone call your doctor immediately to obtain help.

PRECAUTIONS
Certain medications should not be taken with propoxyphene, including carbamazepine (medicine for seizures); antihistamines or medicine for hay fever, other allergies or colds; barbiturates, narcotics and other prescription medicine for pain; sedatives, tranquilizers or medicine to help you sleep; medicine for seizures; and medicine for depression. Anyone who is taking MAO inhibitors (isocarboxazid, pargyline, phenelzine or tranylcypromine) or who has taken them within the past two weeks should not take propoxyphene.

Before you start to take propoxyphene, tell your doctor what prescription or nonprescription medicines you are taking. If you do not know the names of the drugs or what they were prescribed for, bring them in their labeled containers to your doctor or pharmacist.

Take propoxyphene only as directed by your doctor. Do not take more of it, do not take it more often and do not take it for a longer time than your doctor has ordered. If you take too much of this medicine, it can be habit-forming or result in an overdose.

Do not drink alcoholic beverages while taking propoxyphene because you may have serious side effects. Do not start taking any of the drugs listed above unless you have your doctor's permission.

If you will be taking this medicine for several weeks or months, your doctor will want to check your response at regular intervals. *Be sure to keep all appointments with your doctor.*

If you are going to have surgery with a general anesthetic, including dental surgery, be sure the doctor or dentist in charge knows you are taking propoxyphene.

Tell your doctor if you are pregnant or think you may become pregnant while taking this medicine. Propoxyphene is passed by the mother to her unborn child and may lead to withdrawal symptoms in the newborn baby.

DOSAGE

Propoxyphene comes in tablets and capsules. Your doctor will choose the form best for you and will determine how often you should take this medicine and how much you should take at each dose. Carefully follow the instructions on your prescription label, and ask your doctor or pharmacist to explain any part of the instructions you do not understand.

STORAGE

Keep propoxyphene in the container it came in. Keep this medicine out of the reach of children. Overdose is very serious in young children. Do not allow anyone else to take your propoxyphene.

MUSCLE RELAXANTS

Muscle ache or pain is a frequent problem in our society, where many people do not regularly perform strenuous work or exercise. Muscles that are unaccustomed to vigorous activity become strained easily, resulting in pain and stiffness in them. Muscle pain also can follow prolonged periods of staying in one position or result from anxiety or exposure to dampness and cold.

In most cases, the discomfort of muscle strain will disappear within a few days. Nonprescription analgesics, such as aspirin and acetaminophen, and topical liniments, gels and lotions are helpful in relieving pain during that time. When muscle strains are more severe, the prescription drugs described in this section are used to help relax the muscles.

In addition to drug therapy, application of heat is an effective means of relaxing muscles. Moist heat is more effective than dry heat because it penetrates to muscles better than dry heat does. To apply moist heat, use towels soaked in hot water. Steam packs and moist electric heating pads also are available.

Dry heat can be applied with a heating pad, heat lamp or hot water bottle. Any heat treatment, dry or moist, should be used cautiously to avoid burns. Never go to sleep while using a heating pad or heat lamp.

Baclofen
(bak′ loe fen)

PRODUCT INFORMATION
Brand name: Lioresal

USES
Baclofen is used to treat the spasticity and muscle rigidity caused by multiple sclerosis or spinal cord diseases. It decreases the number and severity of spasms, relieves pain and improves mobility.

UNDESIRED EFFECTS
The most common side effect of baclofen is drowsiness. Use caution when driving a car or operating dangerous machinery until you know how this drug will affect you.

Other side effects that may occur are fatigue, nausea, dizziness, muscle weakness, mental depression, headache and frequent urination. Contact your doctor if these effects are bothersome. It may be necessary to decrease the dose you are taking.

PRECAUTIONS
If you ever had a bad reaction to baclofen, you should not take it. Discuss this problem with your doctor. Baclofen can make some medical conditions worse. Tell your doctor if you have epilepsy, kidney disease or a history of ulcers.

Tell your doctor what other prescription or nonprescription drugs you are taking, including sedatives, tranquilizers, sleeping pills and muscle relaxants. Contact your doctor before you start to take any of these drugs because they add to the drowsiness caused by baclofen. If you do not know the names of the drugs you are taking or what they were prescribed for, bring them in their labeled containers to your doctor or pharmacist.

It may take two months to feel the full effect of baclofen. Do not stop taking this medication abruptly because you may experience hallucinations (seeing, hearing or feeling things that are not there), nervousness, convulsions and worsening of spasticity. If you wish to stop taking baclofen, contact your doctor. Your doctor will want to reduce the amount you are taking gradually.

Alcohol may add to the drowsiness caused by baclofen. Ask your doctor for advice concerning how much alcohol is safe to drink.

Keep all appointments so that your doctor can monitor your response to baclofen. It may be necessary to increase the dose you are taking.

Tell your doctor if you are pregnant or are breast-feeding a baby. It is not known if it is safe to take baclofen during pregnancy or while breast-feeding.

DOSAGE
Baclofen comes in tablets. Your doctor has determined how often you should take this medication and how much you should take at each dose. Carefully follow the instructions on your prescription label, and ask your doctor or pharmacist to explain any part of the instructions you do not understand.

If you forget to take a dose of this medicine, take it as soon as you remember. Take any remaining doses for that day at evenly spaced intervals. If you remember a missed dose at the time you are scheduled to take another, omit the missed dose entirely and take only the scheduled dose. *Do not take a double dose.*

STORAGE
Keep this medication in the container it came in, and keep it out of the reach of children.

Cyclobenzaprine
(sye kloe ben′ za preen)

PRODUCT INFORMATION
Brand name: Flexeril

USES
Cyclobenzaprine is a muscle relaxant used to relieve pain and stiffness caused by muscle strains or sprains.

UNDESIRED EFFECTS
The most common side effects of cyclobenzaprine are dry mouth, drowsiness and dizziness. Dry mouth can be relieved by sucking hard candies or lozenges.

Other side effects that are less common include blurred vision, fast heartbeat and insomnia.

PRECAUTIONS
Because cyclobenzaprine may cause drowsiness, do not drive a car or do anything requiring alertness until you know how this drug will affect you. Do not drink alcoholic beverages or take tranquilizers or sleeping pills while taking this medication. Tell your doctor if you have an overactive thyroid gland, heart disease (congestive heart failure, abnormal heart rhythm or a recent heart attack), glaucoma or difficulty urinating.

Tell your doctor about all prescription and nonprescription medications you are taking. Take the labeled containers to your doctor or pharmacist if you do not know the names of these medications or what they were prescribed for.

Tell your doctor if you are pregnant or are breast-feeding a baby. It is not known if cyclobenzaprine is safe under these circumstances or for children younger than 15 years of age.

DOSAGE
Cyclobenzaprine comes in tablets to be taken by mouth. Follow the instructions on your prescription label, and ask your doctor or pharmacist to explain any part you do not understand.

Follow your doctor's instructions for rest and exercise. This conduct is as important as remembering to take your medicine. If you forget to take a dose of cyclobenzaprine, take it as soon as you remember. Take the remaining doses for that day at evenly spaced intervals. *Do not take a double dose.*

STORAGE
Keep this medication in the container it came in, and keep it out of the reach of children.

Diazepam

Diazepam (brand name: Valium) is used primarily to treat patients who are anxious or tense. However, diazepam also acts as a muscle relaxant and frequently is used for this purpose. For a complete description, see Diazepam (page 445) in the section Drugs Used to Treat Psychiatric Problems.

Methocarbamol
(meth oh kar′ ba mole)

PRODUCT INFORMATION
Brand names: Delaxin, Metho-500, Robaxin
Brand name of a combination product containing aspirin: Robaxisal

USES
Methocarbamol relaxes certain muscles. Methocarbamol is used along with rest, physical therapy, medicine for pain and other measures to relieve the pain and discomfort of strains, sprains, injury, bursitis or surgery.

UNDESIRED EFFECTS
The most common side effects of methocarbamol are blurred or double vision, dizziness, drowsiness and lightheadedness. Do not drive a car or operate dangerous machinery until you know how this medicine will affect you. These effects tend to decrease or disappear as you continue to take methocarbamol and as your body adjusts to it. However, if they continue or are severe, contact your doctor.

Less often, methocarbamol will cause a fever, headache or nausea. Contact your doctor if these effects bother you.

The most serious side effect of methocarbamol is an allergic reaction. Stop taking this medicine and contact your doctor at once if you get a skin rash, itching, stuffy nose and red or bloodshot eyes.

Do not be concerned if your urine has a brown, black or green color. This effect is harmless.

PRECAUTIONS
Before you start to take methocarbamol, tell your doctor if you have epilepsy or

kidney disease. The injectable form of this medicine may make these conditions worse.

Tell your doctor what prescription or nonprescription drugs you are taking, including antihistamines or medicine for hay fever, allergies or colds; barbiturates, narcotics or prescription medicine for pain; sedatives, tranquilizers or medicine to help you sleep; medicine for seizures; medicine for depression and MAO inhibitors (isocarboxazid, pargyline, phenelzine or tranylcypromine), even if you stopped taking them two weeks ago. If you do not know the names of the drugs or what they were prescribed for, bring them in their labeled containers to your doctor or pharmacist.

Do not drink alcoholic beverages while taking methocarbamol. Do not start taking any of the drugs listed above unless you have your doctor's permission. All of them can increase the possibility and severity of side effects. If you have any questions, ask your doctor or pharmacist.

To help your doctor select the best treatment for you and your baby, tell your doctor if you are pregnant or are breast-feeding. Safe use in pregnancy and during breast-feeding has not been established.

Children under the age of 12 years should not take methocarbamol. Safe use in this age group has not yet been established.

DOSAGE

Your doctor will determine how often you should take methocarbamol and how much you should take at each dose. Carefully follow the instructions on your prescription label, and ask your doctor or pharmacist to explain any part of the instructions you do not understand.

If you forget to take a dose of this medicine, take it as soon as you remember. If you remember a missed dose at the time you are scheduled to take another, omit the missed dose entirely and take only the regularly scheduled dose. *Do not take a double dose.*

STORAGE

Keep methocarbamol in the container it came in. Keep it out of the reach of children. Do not allow anyone else to take your methocarbamol.

Diabetes

DRUGS USED TO TREAT DIABETES

Diabetes

Diabetes is caused by the inability of the pancreas to produce sufficient insulin for the body's needs. Insulin is required to regulate the metabolism of glucose (sugar). It has been estimated that two to four percent of the U.S. population have diabetes. It is caused by hereditary and environmental factors.

Diabetes varies according to the degree of insulin deficiency. "Type I insulin dependent" diabetes (formerly known as juvenile-onset diabetes) is a condition where almost no insulin is produced. In this situation, insulin injections are required to maintain normal glucose metabolism. "Type II noninsulin dependent" (formerly known as adult-onset diabetes) refers to a less severe deficiency of insulin. In many cases, this form of diabetes can be treated with diet alone or with a combination of diet and oral medications.

The symptoms of diabetes include excessive hunger, thirst and urination. Individuals with severe insulin deficiency will develop high blood sugar, leading to dehydration and collapse unless insulin is administered. In contrast, individuals with a milder condition may experience minimal or no symptoms; their diabetes may be diagnosed only upon results from laboratory tests.

Diabetes can cause damage to many organs throughout the body, especially the eyes (blindness), kidneys and skin. Damage results from a buildup of sugar deposits in blood vessels and impairment of circulation. To minimize or prevent such damage, it is essential that you take your medication regularly, as prescribed by your doctor. Urine sugar measurements are used to determine appropriate dosages. In addition to medication, special diets often are prescribed. It is very important to follow your doctor's instructions on diet and exercise.

Acetohexamide
(a set oh hex' a mide)

PRODUCT INFORMATION
Brand name: Dymelor

USES
Acetohexamide is used to treat type II (noninsulin dependent) diabetes mellitus (formerly known as adult-onset), particularly in people whose diabetes cannot be controlled by diet alone or who cannot tolerate insulin injections.

Acetohexamide helps to lower blood sugar by stimulating the pancreas to secrete insulin. The pancreas must be capable of producing insulin before this medicine can work. Acetohexamide is not used in the treatment of type I (insulin dependent) diabetes (formerly known as juvenile-onset).

People who are taking acetohexamide or any other oral medicine for diabetes may have to switch to insulin injections if they develop diabetic coma or ketoacidosis, have a severe injury or burn, develop a severe infection, need surgery or become pregnant.

UNDESIRED EFFECTS

Drowsiness, nervousness, headache, excessive hunger, warmth, sweating or numbness of the fingers, lips and nose may indicate that your blood sugar is too low (hypoglycemia). If you experience any of these effects, drink orange juice or eat something containing sugar and contact your doctor immediately. If you think you are going to faint, instruct someone to take you to your doctor or to a hospital right away.

Other side effects include stomach upset, heartburn, diarrhea and headache. Contact your doctor if these side effects persist. It may be necessary to reduce the dosage that you are taking.

An allergic skin rash and itching may occur but will usually disappear as you continue to take acetohexamide. If this problem does not go away, stop taking this medication and contact your doctor immediately.

Acetohexamide also may make you sunburn more easily than usual. Be careful about exposing yourself to sunlight or sunlamps.

PRECAUTIONS

Before you start to take this medicine, tell your doctor what prescription or nonprescription drugs you are taking, particularly anticoagulants (blood thinners); aspirin, salsalate or other salicylates; nonsteroidal anti-inflammatory drugs (diflunisal, fenoprofen, ibuprofen, indomethacin, meclofenamate, mefenamic acid, naproxen, oxyphenbutazone, phenylbutazone, piroxicam, sulindac and tolmetin); phenytoin (medicine for seizures); probenecid; sulfonamides (e.g., sulfamethoxazole, sulfasalazine and sulfisoxazole); thiazide diuretics (water pills); and thyroid medicine. If you do not know the names of the drugs or what they were prescribed for, bring them in their labeled containers to your doctor or pharmacist.

Because acetohexamide can make some medical conditions worse, tell your doctor if you have kidney disease, liver disease, thyroid disease or a severe infection.

Diet is extremely important in the treatment of diabetes. Acetohexamide will work properly only if you follow your doctor's instructions concerning diet and exercise.

Skipping or delaying meals or exercising much more than usual can cause your blood sugar to drop (hypoglycemia). Maintaining a proper diet and exercise schedule will help you avoid this problem.

Drinking alcoholic beverages may cause nausea or symptoms of hypoglycemia (low blood sugar). Ask your doctor for advice if you have questions regarding alcohol consumption.

Pregnant women should not take acetohexamide. During pregnancy, insulin is required to control diabetes properly. If you become pregnant while taking acetohexamide, contact your doctor immediately. Tell your doctor if you are breast-feeding a baby. It is not known if acetohexamide is passed to a breast-fed baby through the milk.

DOSAGE
Your doctor will determine how often you should take acetohexamide and at what time of day you should take it. Carefully follow the instructions on the prescription label, and ask your doctor or pharmacist to explain any part you do not understand.

Acetohexamide comes in tablets. Your doctor may need to adjust your dose to your particular needs. Keep in close touch with your doctor, particularly during the first few weeks that you are taking this medicine.

Ask your doctor what you should do if you occasionally forget to take a dose. Write down these instructions so you can refer to them later if you forget a dose.

STORAGE
Keep this medication in its original container, and keep it out of the reach of children. Do not allow anyone else to take it.

Chlorpropamide
(klor proe' pa mide)

PRODUCT INFORMATION
Brand name: Diabinese

USES
Chlorpropamide is used to treat type II (noninsulin dependent) diabetes mellitus (formerly known as adult-onset), particularly in people whose diabetes cannot be controlled by diet alone or who cannot tolerate insulin injections.

Chlorpropamide helps to lower blood sugar by increasing the output of insulin by the pancreas. The pancreas must be capable of producing insulin before this medicine can work. Chlorpropamide is not used in the treatment of type I (insulin dependent) diabetes (formerly known as juvenile-onset).

People who are taking chlorpropamide or any other oral medicine for diabetes may have to switch to insulin injections if they develop diabetic coma or ketoacidosis, have a severe injury or burn, develop a severe infection, need surgery or become pregnant.

UNDESIRED EFFECTS
Chlorpropamide may cause diarrhea, headache, heartburn, loss of appetite, nausea, vomiting or general stomach upset. Check with your doctor about taking less of this medicine or taking it in several small doses rather than in a singe daily dose to decrease these effects.

If chlorpropamide gives you a skin rash, stop taking the medicine and contact your doctor immediately. Chlorpropamide also may make you sunburn more easily than usual. Be careful about exposing yourself to sunlight or sunlamps.

Rarely, chlorpropamide may cause liver or blood problems that require medical attention. Contact your doctor if you have dark urine, itching of the skin, light-colored stools, yellowing of the eyes or skin, fatigue, fever and sore throat or unusual bleeding or bruising.

Some people who take chlorpropamide retain more body water than usual. Symptoms of this problem are drowsiness; muscle cramps; seizures; swelling or puffiness of the face, hands or ankles; tiredness and weakness. Contact your doctor if you experience any of these effects.

Drowsiness, nervousness, headache, excessive hunger, warmth, sweating or numbness of the fingers, lips and nose may indicate that your blood sugar is too low (hypoglycemia). If you experience any of these effects, drink orange juice or eat something containing sugar and contact your doctor immediately. If you think you are going to faint, instruct someone to take you to your doctor or to a hospital right away.

PRECAUTIONS

Because chlorpropamide may make some medical conditions worse, tell your doctor if you have kidney disease, liver disease, thyroid disease or a severe infection.

Before you start to take this medicine, tell your doctor what prescription or nonprescription drugs you are taking, particularly anticoagulants (blood thinners), aspirin, salsalate or other salicylates, chloramphenicol, cortisone-like medicines, dextrothyroxine, epinephrine, guanethidine, insulin, MAO inhibitors (isocarboxazid, pargyline, phenelzine or tranylcypromine), oxyphenbutazone, oxytetracycline, phenylbutazone, phenytoin (medicine for seizures), probenecid, propranolol, sulfonamides (e.g., sulfamethoxazole, sulfasalazine and sulfisoxazole), thiazide diuretics (water pills) and thyroid medicine.

If you do not know the names of the drugs or what they were prescribed for, bring them in their labeled containers to your doctor or pharmacist.

Do not take any other medicine, including nonprescription medicine, while you are taking chlorpropamide unless you have your doctor's permission.

Before having any kind of surgery, including dental surgery, tell the doctor or dentist in charge that you are taking chlorpropamide.

Diet is extremely important in the treatment of diabetes. Chlorpropamide will work properly only if you follow your doctor's instructions concerning diet and exercise.

If you drink alcoholic beverages while taking chlorpropamide, your blood sugar may drop and you may experience nausea or the symptoms of hypoglycemia described earlier (see Undesired Effects). If you have any of these symptoms, contact your doctor. It is better not to drink alcohol while you are taking chlorpropamide. If you have any questions, contact your doctor or pharmacist.

Skipping or delaying meals or exercising much more than usual can cause your blood sugar to drop. (See symptoms of low blood sugar under Undesired Effects.) Maintaining a proper diet and exercise schedule will help you avoid this problem.

Women who are pregnant or who are nursing babies should not take chlorpropamide. During pregnancy, insulin is required to control diabetes properly. If you become pregnant while taking chlorpropamide, contact your doctor immediately.

DOSAGE
Your doctor will determine how often you should take chlorpropamide and at what time of day you should take it. Carefully follow the instructions on your prescription label, and ask your doctor or pharmacist to explain any part of the instructions you do not understand.

Chlorpropamide comes in tablets and should be taken exactly as prescribed by your doctor. This medicine begins to work after the first dose, but you may have to take chlorpropamide every day for a week or two before it is fully effective in controlling your diabetes. In addition, your doctor may need to adjust your dose to your particular needs. Keep in close touch with your doctor, particularly during the first few weeks you are taking this medicine.

Before you start to take chlorpropamide, ask your doctor what you should do if you forget to take a dose at the right time. Write down these instructions so you will be able to refer to them later if you forget a dose.

STORAGE
Keep chlorpropamide in the container it came in, and store the container in a cool, dry place. Keep this medicine out of the reach of children. Do not allow anyone else to take your chlorpropamide.

Glipizide
(glip′ i zide)

PRODUCT INFORMATION
Brand name: Glucotrol

USES
Glipizide is used to treat type II (noninsulin dependent) diabetes mellitus (formerly known as adult-onset), particularly in people whose diabetes cannot be controlled by diet alone or who cannot tolerate insulin injections.

Glipizide helps to lower blood sugar by increasing the secretion of insulin by the pancreas and increasing the action of insulin in the body. For this medicine to work, the pancreas must be capable of producing insulin. Glipizide is not used in the treatment of type I (insulin dependent) diabetes (formerly known as juvenile-onset).

People who are taking glipizide or any other oral medicine for diabetes may have to switch to insulin injections if they develop diabetic coma or ketoacidosis, have a severe injury or burn, develop a severe infection, require surgery or become pregnant.

Glipizide may help to control blood sugar in people in whom other oral diabetes medication is not effective. It may also be used with insulin injections to lower blood sugar.

UNDESIRED EFFECTS
Glipizide may cause nausea, loss of appetite, vomiting, diarrhea, constipation, heartburn and stomach pain. Contact your doctor if these symptoms do not decrease or if they are bothersome. Your doctor may decrease your dose or have you take this medicine in two or three small doses rather than a single daily dose to avoid these effects.

Glipizide may cause an allergic skin reaction. If you develop a red, itching or burning skin rash, contact your doctor. The rash should disappear as you continue to take the drug.

Glipizide may make you sunburn more easily than usual. Be careful about exposing yourself to sunlight and sunlamps.

Drowsiness, nervousness, headache, excessive hunger, warmth, sweating or numbness of the fingers, lips and nose may indicate that your blood sugar is too low (hypoglycemia). If you experience any of these effects, drink orange juice or eat something containing sugar and contact your doctor immediately. If you think you are going to faint, instruct someone to take you to your doctor or to a hospital right away.

Rarely, glipizide may cause liver or blood problems that require medical attention. Contact your doctor immediately if you have dark urine, itching of the skin, light-colored stools, yellowing of the eyes or skin, fatigue, fever and sore throat or unusual bleeding or bruising.

PRECAUTIONS
Because glipizide can make some medical conditions worse, tell your doctor if you have kidney disease, liver disease, thyroid disease or a severe infection.

Before you start to take this medicine, tell your doctor what prescription and nonprescription drugs you are taking, particularly anticoagulants (blood thinners); aspirin, salsalate and other salicylates; beta blockers (atenolol, metoprolol, nadolol, pindolol, propranolol or timolol); calcium channel blockers (diltiazem, nifedipine or verapamil); cimetidine; corticosteroids; furosemide; ethacrynic acid; estrogens; isoniazid; MAO inhibitors (isocarboxazid, pargyline, phenelzine or tranylcypromine); nicotinic acid; oral contraceptives (birth-control pills); phenobarbital; phenylbutazone; phenytoin; probenecid; rifampin; thiazide diuretics (chlorthalidone, chlorothiazide, hydrochlorothiazide or methyclothiazide); and thyroid (levothyroxine, liothyronine, liotrix or thyroglobulin).

If you do not know the names of the drugs or what they were prescribed for, bring them in their labeled containers to your doctor or pharmacist. Do not take any other medicine, including nonprescription medicine, without your doctor's permission.

Before having surgery, including dental surgery, tell the doctor or dentist in charge that you are taking glipizide.

If you drink alcoholic beverages while taking glipizide, your blood sugar may decrease and you may experience drowsiness, nervousness, headache, excessive hunger, warmth, sweating or numbness of the fingers, lips and nose. If you experience any of these symptoms of hypoglycemia, contact your doctor. It is better not to drink alcohol while taking glipizide. If you have any questions, contact your doctor or pharmacist.

Diet is extremely important in the treatment of diabetes. Follow your doctor's instructions concerning diet and exercise. Your doctor will give you instructions for a diet that restricts calories and may result in weight loss (particularly if you are overweight). Regular physical activity is also important. Ask you doctor for advice on exercise.

Skipping or delaying meals or exercising much more than usual can cause your blood sugar to drop (hypoglycemia) and you may experience symptoms of hypoglycemia (see Undesired Effects). Maintaining a proper diet and exercise schedule will help you avoid this problem.

Keep in touch with your doctor so that your response to the medication can be monitored. Keep all appointments with your doctor and the laboratory. Contact your doctor if glipizide is not effective in lowering your blood sugar. You may need a larger dose or a different drug.

If you are switching from insulin injections to glipizide, test your urine for glucose and ketones at least three times a day while you are switching.

If you are switching from chlorpropamide (another oral medication for diabetes) to glipizide, you may experience symptoms of hypoglycemia (see Undesired Effects) during the first two weeks. Contact your doctor if this problem occurs.

Tell your doctor if you are pregnant, plan to become pregnant or are breast-feeding. Usually, insulin is required to control diabetes during pregnancy. It is not known if glipizide is passed from a mother to a nursing baby through the milk.

DOSAGE

Glipizide comes in tablets. Your doctor will determine how much, how often, and at what time of day you should take the drug. Glipizide is usually taken once a day in the morning 30 minutes before breakfast. Glipizide is sometimes taken two or three times a day (30 minutes before meals) in small doses to decrease side effects. Carefully follow the instructions on your prescription label, and ask your doctor or pharmacist to explain any part you do not understand.

Keep in touch with your doctor. It may be necessary to adjust the dose you are taking.

Before you start to take glipizide, ask your doctor what you should do if you forget to take a dose. Write down these instructions so you will be able to refer to them later if you forget a dose.

STORAGE

Keep this medication in the container it came in, and store the container in a cool, dry place. Keep it out of the reach of children. Do not allow anyone else to take your glipizide.

Glyburide
(glye' byoor ide)

PRODUCT INFORMATION
Brand names: Diabeta, Micronase

USES
Glyburide is used to treat type II (noninsulin dependent) diabetes mellitus (formerly known as adult-onset), particularly in people whose diabetes cannot be controlled by diet alone or who cannot tolerate insulin injections.

Glyburide helps to lower blood sugar by increasing the secretion of insulin by the pancreas and increasing the action of insulin in the body. For this medicine to work, the pancreas must be capable of producing insulin. Glyburide is not used in the treatment of type I (insulin dependent) diabetes (formerly known as juvenile-onset).

People who are taking glyburide or any other oral medicine for diabetes may have to switch to insulin injections if they develop diabetic coma or ketoacidosis, have a severe injury or burn, develop a severe infection, require surgery or become pregnant.

Glyburide may help to control blood sugar in people in whom other oral diabetes medication is not effective. It may also be used with insulin injections to lower blood sugar.

UNDESIRED EFFECTS
Glyburide may cause nausea, heartburn and a feeling of fullness in the stomach. If these symptoms are bothersome, contact your doctor. It may be necessary to decrease the dose you are taking.

Glyburide may cause severe hypoglycemia (low blood sugar). Drowsiness, nervousness, headache, excessive hunger, warmth, sweating or numbness of the fingers, lips and nose may indicate that your blood sugar is too low. If you experience any of these effects, drink orange juice or eat something containing sugar and contact your doctor immediately. If you think you are going to faint, instruct someone to take you to your doctor or to a hospital right away.

Glyburide may cause an allergic skin reaction. If you develop a red, itching or burning skin rash, contact your doctor. The rash may go away as you continue to take the drug.

Glyburide may make you sunburn more easily than usual. Be careful about exposing yourself to sunlight and sunlamps.

Rarely, glyburide may cause liver or blood problems that require medical attention. Stop taking glyburide and contact your doctor immediately if you have dark urine, itching of the skin, light-colored stools, yellowing of the eyes or skin, fatigue, fever and sore throat or unusual bleeding or bruising.

PRECAUTIONS
Because glyburide can make some medical conditions worse, tell your doctor if

you have kidney disease, liver disease, thyroid disease, hormone problems, adrenal insufficiency, severe infection or pituitary disease.

Before you start to take this medicine, tell your doctor what prescription and nonprescription drugs you are taking, particularly anticoagulants (blood thinners); aspirin, salsalate and other salicylates; beta blockers (atenolol, metoprolol, nadolol, pindolol, propranolol or timolol); calcium channel blockers (diltiazem, nifedipine or verapamil); corticosteroids; furosemide; ethacrynic acid; estrogens; isoniazid; MAO inhibitors (isocarboxazid, pargyline, phenelzine or tranylcypromine); nicotinic acid; oral contraceptives (birth-control pills); phenobarbital; phenylbutazone; phenytoin; probenecid; rifampin; thiazide diuretics (chlorthalidone, chlorothiazide, hydrochlorothiazide or methyclothiazide); and thyroid (levothyroxine, liothyronine, liotrix or thyroglobulin).

If you do not know the names of the drugs or what they were prescribed for, bring them in their labeled containers to your doctor or pharmacist. Do not take any other medicine, including nonprescription medicine, without your doctor's permission.

Before having surgery, including dental surgery, tell the doctor or dentist in charge that you are taking glyburide.

If you drink alcoholic beverages while taking glyburide, your blood sugar may decrease and you may experience nausea, drowsiness, nervousness, headache, excessive hunger, warmth, sweating or numbness of the fingers, lips and nose. If you experience any of these symptoms of hypoglycemia, contact your doctor. It is better not to drink alcohol while taking glyburide. If you have any questions, contact your doctor or pharmacist.

Diet is extremely important in the treatment of diabetes. Follow your doctor's instructions concerning diet and exercise. Your doctor will give you instructions for a diet that restricts calories and may result in weight loss (particularly if you are overweight). Regular physical activity is also important. Ask your doctor for advice on exercise.

Skipping or delaying meals or exercising much more than usual can cause your blood sugar to drop (hypoglycemia) and you may experience symptoms of hypoglycemia (see Undesired Effects). Maintaining a proper diet and exercise schedule will help you avoid this problem.

Keep in touch with your doctor so that your response to the medication can be monitored. Keep all appointments with your doctor and the laboratory.

Contact your doctor if glyburide is not effective in lowering your blood sugar. You may need a larger dose or a different drug. Once a year, your doctor may ask you to stop taking glyburide for two or three days and have a blood test to determine whether the drug is controlling your blood sugar properly.

If you are switching from insulin injections to glyburide, test your urine for glucose and acetone at least three times a day while you are switching.

If you are switching from chlorpropamide (another oral medication for diabetes) to glyburide, you may experience symptoms of hypoglycemia (see Undesired Effects) during the first two weeks. Contact your doctor if this problem occurs.

Tell your doctor if you are pregnant, plan to become pregnant or are breast-feeding. Usually, insulin is required to control diabetes during pregnancy. Glyburide is passed from a mother to her unborn baby, but it is not known what effect this may have. Do not take this drug within two weeks of your expected delivery date. It is not known if glyburide is passed from a mother to a nursing baby through the milk.

DOSAGE
Glyburide comes in tablets. Your doctor will determine how much, how often and what time of day you should take this medicine. It is usually taken once a day with breakfast or twice a day (when a large daily dose is required). If you are taking glyburide more than once a day, take any morning or mid-day doses 30 minutes before meals for best blood sugar control. Carefully follow the instructions on your prescription label, and ask your doctor or pharmacist to explain any part you do not understand.

Keep in touch with your doctor. It may be necessary to adjust your dose.

Before you start to take glyburide, ask your doctor what you should do if you forget to take a dose. Write down these instructions so you will be able to refer to them later if you forget a dose.

STORAGE
Keep this medication in the container it came in, and store the container in a cool, dry place. Keep it out of the reach of children. Do not allow anyone else to take your glyburide.

Insulin
(in′ sul in)

PRODUCT INFORMATION
Brand names: Actrapid, Humulin, Iletin, Insulatard, Lentard, Lente, Mixtard, Monotard, Novolin, Protophane, Semilente, Semitard, Ultralente, Ultratard, Velosulin

USES
Insulin is a hormone produced in the pancreas. Insulin is necessary to move sugar from the blood into other body tissues, where it produces energy. In people with diabetes, the pancreas does not produce enough insulin for the body's needs, so injection of additional insulin is necessary. It must be injected because stomach acids would destroy it if it was taken orally.

Insulin comes from cattle (beef) and pigs (pork) or may be synthesized in a laboratory. Synthetic insulin is identical to human insulin and is purer than beef or pork insulin. Synthetic human insulin may be preferred for people who have allergic reactions to beef or pork insulin and for pregnant women.

UNDESIRED EFFECTS
Undesired effects from insulin use usually result from too much or too little insulin, resulting in low or high blood sugar. This problem can occur even though

your doctor has carefully determined your needs. Your body's need for insulin is affected by diet, exercise, drugs and other diseases.

Symptoms are as follows:

1. Low blood sugar (hypoglycemia). Giving yourself too much insulin or performing too much strenuous exercise can result in low blood sugar. This condition is often called an "insulin reaction." The symptoms may be weakness, tiredness, nervousness, anxiety, trembling, headache, sweating and dizziness. Drinking orange juice or eating a candy bar will stop these reactions quickly. Always carry a candy bar or other sugar candy with you when you are not at home. These reactions may happen at anytime but are most common late in the afternoon or during the night. They usually happen when insulin is working hardest.

2. High blood sugar (hyperglycemia). By forgetting to use your insulin or by not using enough, you may develop high blood sugar. Some signs of high blood sugar are frequent urination, thirst, headache, weakness, nausea, dizziness and even loss of consciousness and coma.

Often it is difficult to tell if your level of blood sugar is too high or too low; call your doctor if you are not sure. You can keep tabs on your level of blood sugar by measuring the amount of sugar in your urine. Several methods are available, such as the use of a tape, tablet or plastic stick that changes color according to how much sugar is in the urine. If your doctor wishes you to test your urine, discuss which method is best for you. You will be shown how to measure, read and record the amount of your urine sugar accurately.

PRECAUTIONS

Your doctor will prescribe a diet for you to follow while using insulin. It is extremely important that you *stick to this diet*, because your insulin dose is based in part on your intake of calories from food.

Tell your doctor if you ever had an allergic reaction to beef or pork insulin, are pregnant or have any medical problems such as thyroid, liver or kidney disease or infection.

Many types of medications will affect your body's response to insulin. Be sure to tell your doctor what medications you are taking, including nonprescription medications. Do not begin taking any medications unless you first check with your doctor.

You should obtain either a Medic-Alert necklace or keep a card in your wallet that indicates you have diabetes. Write on the card your doctor's name and phone number and the current dose of insulin you are taking. Ask your doctor or pharmacist how you may get one of these cards.

It is a good idea to carry an extra prescription for insulin syringes with you at all times.

DOSAGE

Your doctor will tell you how often and at what time of day to inject your insulin. Insulin usually is given by subcutaneous injection. The amount you need depends on several things, such as other diseases you may have, how much you exercise and your diet, and may change with time.

There are several different types of insulin. The differences among them mostly involve how long they work to lower the sugar in the blood. For example, short-acting insulins, such as regular insulin or Semilente, work for six to 12 hours; long-acting insulins, such as Ultralente, work for over a day. Regular human insulin is rapid acting, and both isophane insulin human and insulin human zinc are inter-mediate acting. Your doctor will determine which insulin or insulin combination will best control the level of sugar in your blood.

All bottles for insulin are marked with large black letters to remind you which insulin they contain. For example, R is Regular and N is NPH. It is very important that you know which one you use.

All types of insulin are measured in units. No matter what type you use, you always must know how many units you take with each injection. Although most diabetics use U-100 insulin (100 units in one milliliter), some may still be using the red-capped bottle of U-40 insulin. If you are using U-40 insulin, it is important that you let all your doctors and your pharmacist know this fact.

Different syringes must be used with U-40 insulin. Be sure you have the right kind of syringe for your type of insulin.

Use a new syringe each time you take your insulin. Never reuse a syringe. Used needles will be dull, will hurt more and may cause an infection.

Be sure you fill the syringe to the correct number of units. If you have trouble seeing the small markings, have a friend or family member help you, and tell your doctor and pharmacist about this problem. They can provide syringes that are easier to read or special tools to help you fill the syringe more easily.

Do not inject cold insulin. Take it out of the refrigerator and allow it to reach room temperature before you administer it. Never heat the bottle of insulin to warm it.

Some doctors recommend storing the bottle you are using at room temperature.

Do not use the insulin if it looks as though it has changed color or if the expiration date has passed. Regular insulin should be a clear solution. Discard the vial if the solution is cloudy or seems to have thickened. Other forms of insulin should be cloudy in appearance; do not use the insulin if it has clumped or if it is clear. Roll the bottle between the palms of your hands to mix it before preparing the dose. Do not shake the bottle.

It is easier to withdraw insulin from the bottle if you first inject air into the bottle. Inject the same number of units of air as insulin you will be taking. If you are taking two types of insulin at the same time—Regular and NPH, for example—draw up the Regular (the clear solution) first.

You will be shown how to inject the insulin correctly. It is important that you do not use the same injection site on your body repeatedly. Change sites frequently. You can inject insulin into your stomach, thighs and arms. Clean the skin at the injection site with an alcohol pad or rubbing alcohol before injection. For the zinc and isophane forms of human insulin, it is important to inject the entire dose quickly (less than five seconds) to prevent the needle from clogging.

You do not need a prescription to buy insulin—just ask your pharmacist for the right kind. It's best if you bring an empty bottle to the pharmacy. You may need a prescription for the syringes, depending on the state you live in. Check with your pharmacist.

Ask your doctor ahead of time what to do if you forget to take a dose of insulin at the correct time.

STORAGE
Unopened vials of insulin should be stored in the refrigerator; however, the vial in use may be stored at room temperature. Avoid exposure to extreme heat and direct sunlight. Never allow insulin to freeze, and do not use insulin that has been frozen and thawed. If you are traveling, you do not need to refrigerate the insulin. It is a good idea to make sure insulin bottles are protected from bumps or other rough handling (if you are traveling, keep them wrapped in clothes in the middle of a suitcase). Do not keep insulin in hot parts of a car, such as the glove compartment or trunk.

Tolazamide
(tole az' a mide)

PRODUCT INFORMATION
Brand name: Tolinase

USES
Tolazamide helps to lower blood sugar by increasing the amount of insulin produced by the pancreas. Tolazamide is used to treat type II (noninsulin dependent) diabetes mellitus (formerly known as adult-onset), particularly in people whose diabetes cannot be controlled by diet alone or who cannot tolerate insulin injections. Tolazamide is not used to treat type I (insulin dependent) diabetes (formerly known as juvenile-onset).

UNDESIRED EFFECTS
Tolazamide may cause diarrhea, headache, heartburn, loss of appetite, nausea, vomiting or general stomach upset. If you experience any of these problems and they are severe, contact your doctor. Decreasing the dose or taking this medicine in several small doses rather than in a single daily dose may decrease these effects.

Stop taking tolazamide and contact your doctor immediately if you develop a skin rash or itching. This medicine also makes some people more sensitive to sunlight than they normally are. Be careful about exposing yourself to sunlight and sunlamps.

Although they are not common with tolazamide, liver or blood problems will require medical attention. Contact your doctor if you have dark urine, itching of the skin, light-colored stools, yellowing of the eyes or skin, fatigue, fever and sore throat or unusual bleeding or bruising.

Tolazamide may cause your blood sugar level to drop too low, particularly if you skip or delay meals, exercise more than usual or drink significant amounts of alcohol.

Symptoms of low blood sugar (hypoglycemia) are drowsiness, nervousness, headache, excessive hunger, warmth, sweating and numbness of the fingers, lips and nose. If you experience any of these symptoms, drink orange juice or eat something containing sugar and contact your doctor immediately. If you think you are going to faint, instruct someone with you to take you to your doctor or to a hospital right away.

PRECAUTIONS

Before you start to take tolazamide, tell your doctor if you have kidney disease, liver disease, thyroid disease or a severe infection. Tolazamide may make these conditions worse or may not have the desired effect when these conditions are present.

Tolazamide may affect the way your body responds to certain other drugs. Tell your doctor what prescription or nonprescription drugs you are taking, particularly anticoagulants (blood thinners), aspirin or other salicylates, chloramphenicol, cortisone-like medicines, dextrothyroxine, epinephrine, guanethidine, insulin, MAO inhibitors (isocarboxazid, pargyline, phenelzine or tranylcypromine), oxyphenbutazone, oxytetracycline, phenytoin (medicine for seizures), probenecid, propranolol, sulfonamides (e.g., sulfamethoxazole, sulfasalazine and sulfisoxazole), thiazide diuretics (water pills) and medicine for your thyroid. If you do not know the names of the drugs or what they were prescribed for, bring them in their labeled containers to your doctor or pharmacist.

While you are taking tolazamide, do not take any other medicine, including nonprescription medicine, unless you have your doctor's permission.

Before having any kind of surgery, including dental surgery, tell the doctor or dentist in charge that you are taking tolazamide

Diet is extremely important in the treatment of diabetes. Tolazamide will work properly only if you follow your doctor's instructions concerning diet and exercise. Maintaining a proper diet and exercise schedule also will help you avoid the problems of a severe drop in blood sugar.

It is better not to drink alcoholic beverages while you are taking tolazamide. Alcohol can cause a severe drop in blood sugar and produce the symptoms described earlier. Contact your doctor if you have any of these symptoms.

You may have to take insulin rather than tolazamide if you develop diabetic coma or ketoacidosis, have a severe injury or burn, develop a severe infection or need surgery. If you have any questions, check with your doctor or pharmacist.

Women who are pregnant or who are nursing babies should not take tolazamide. During pregnancy, insulin is required to control a woman's diabetes properly. If you become pregnant while taking tolazamide, contact your doctor immediately.

DOSAGE

Your doctor will determine how often you should take tolazamide and at what time of day you should take it. Carefully follow the instructions on your prescription label, and ask your doctor or pharmacist to explain any part of the instructions you do not understand.

Tolazamide comes in tablets and should be taken exactly as prescribed by your doctor. This medicine begins to work about four to six hours after it is taken. However, it may be necessary for you to take it every day for one to two weeks before it is fully effective in controlling your diabetes. Keep in close touch with your doctor, particularly during the first few weeks you are taking this medicine. Your doctor may need to adjust your dose to your particular needs.

Before you start to take tolazamide, ask your doctor what you should do if you forget to take a dose at the right time. Write down the instructions so you can refer to them later.

STORAGE
Keep tolazamide in the container it came in, and store it in a cool, dry place. Keep this medicine out of the reach of children. Do not allow anyone else to take your tolazamide.

Tolbutamide
(tole byoo' ta mide)

PRODUCT INFORMATION
Brand name: Orinase

USES
Tolbutamide is used to treat type II (noninsulin dependent) diabetes mellitus (formerly known as adult-onset), particularly in people who cannot tolerate insulin or whose problem cannot be controlled by diet. Tolbutamide helps to lower the blood sugar by stimulating the secretion of insulin from the pancreas and will not work unless the pancreas is functioning. Tolbutamide is not used to treat type I (insulin dependent) diabetes (formerly known as juvenile-onset). People using tolbutamide or any other oral medication for diabetes may be switched to insulin injections if they develop ketoacidosis, have a severe injury or infection, need surgery or become pregnant.

UNDESIRED EFFECTS
Tolbutamide may cause diarrhea, headache, heartburn, loss of appetite, nausea, vomiting or general stomach upset. If you experience any of these effects, check with your doctor. Decreasing the dose or taking this medicine in several small doses rather than in a single daily dose may decrease these effects.

If tolbutamide gives you a skin rash, stop taking the medicine and contact your doctor. Tolbutamide also may make you more sensitive to sunlight than you usually are. Be careful about exposing yourself to sunlight and sunlamps.

Tolbutamide may cause liver or blood problems. Although these effects are rare, they will require medical attention. Contact your doctor if you have dark urine, itching of the skin, light-colored stools, yellowing of the eyes or skin, fatigue, fever and sore throat or unusual bleeding or bruising.

Be alert for signs of low blood sugar (hypoglycemia), such as drowsiness, nervousness, headache, excessive hunger, warmth, sweating and numbness of the fingers, lips and nose. If you experience any of these effects, drink orange juice or eat something containing sugar and contact your doctor immediately. If you think you are going to faint, instruct someone to take you to your doctor or to a hospital right away.

PRECAUTIONS

Before you start to take tolbutamide, tell your doctor if you have kidney disease, liver disease, thyroid disease or a severe infection. Tolbutamide can make these conditions worse or may not have the desired effect when these conditions are present.

Tell your doctor what prescription or nonprescription medicine you are taking, including anticoagulants (blood thinners), aspirin or other salicylates, chloramphenicol, cortisone-like medicines, dextrothyroxine, epinephrine, guanethidine, insulin, MAO inhibitors (isocarboxazid, pargyline, phenelzine or tranylcypromine), oxyphenbutazone, oxytetracycline, phenylbutazone, phenytoin (medicine for seizures), probenecid, propranolol, sulfonamides (e.g., sulfamethoxazole, sulfasalazine and sulfisoxazole), thiazide diuretics (water pills) and medicine for your thyroid. If you do not know the names of the drugs or what they were prescribed for, bring them in their labeled containers to your doctor or pharmacist.

Do not take any other medicine, including nonprescription medicine, while taking tolbutamide unless you have your doctor's permission.

Diet is extremely important in the treatment of diabetes. Be sure to follow your doctor's instructions concerning diet and exercise so that tolbutamide can work properly. If you skip meals, delay meals or exercise much more than usual, your blood sugar may drop. (See Undesired Effects for symptoms of low blood sugar.)

Drinking alcoholic beverages while you are taking tolbutamide may cause a severe drop in blood sugar with the symptoms of hypoglycemia described earlier. Contact your doctor if you have any of these effects. If you have any questions about your consumption of alcohol, check with your doctor or pharmacist.

Before having any kind of surgery, including dental surgery, tell the doctor or dentist in charge that you are taking tolbutamide.

Women who are pregnant or who are nursing babies should not take tolbutamide. During pregnancy, insulin is required to control a woman's diabetes properly. If you become pregnant while taking tolbutamide, contact your doctor immediately.

DOSAGE

Your doctor will determine how often you should take tolbutamide and at what time of day you should take it. Carefully follow the instructions on your prescription label, and ask your doctor or pharmacist to explain any part of the instructions you do not understand.

Tolbutamide comes in tablets and should be taken exactly as prescribed by your doctor. This medicine begins to work about three to six hours after you take it.

However, you may have to take this medicine every day for one to two weeks before it is fully effective in controlling your diabetes.

Keep in close touch with your doctor while taking tolbutamide, particularly during the first few weeks of therapy. Your doctor may need to adjust your dose to fit your particular needs.

Ask your doctor what you should do if you forget to take a dose at the right time. Write down these instructions and refer to them if you forget to take a dose.

STORAGE

Keep tolbutamide in the container it came in, and store the container in a cool place. Keep this medicine out of the reach of children. Do not allow anyone else to take your tolbutamide.

Glaucoma

DRUGS USED TO TREAT GLAUCOMA

Glaucoma

Glaucoma is a disease in which the pressure inside the eyeball is greatly increased. This is the result of a fluid buildup inside the eyeball caused by infection, injury or other unknown factors.

This increased pressure inside the eyeball damages the retina and the optic nerve. For this reason, glaucoma is one of the most common causes of blindness.

Glaucoma has two major forms. Open-angle glaucoma is a chronic hereditary disease that progresses slowly and often is not diagnosed until significant damage to the eyes causes changes in vision. Open-angle glaucoma is the most common type of glaucoma and occurs predominantly in people over 40. Because this type of glaucoma produces no symptoms until significant damage has already occurred, it is important to have periodic eye exams, particularly if you have a family history of glaucoma.

Closed-angle glaucoma is a rapid increase in pressure inside the eyeball. Closed-angle glaucoma causes severe pain, nausea, vomiting and visual disturbances.

People with such symptoms (particularly if there is a family history of glaucoma) should seek treatment at once. This form of glaucoma is treated with drugs or surgery.

Acetazolamide
(a set a zole' a mide)

PRODUCT INFORMATION
Brand name: Diamox

USES
Acetazolamide is used to remove excess fluid from body tissues in order to help the heart work more efficiently in the treatment of heart failure and may be used in some patients with chronic lung disease. It is also used for glaucoma to decrease pressure in the eyeball and for certain kinds of epilepsy. Sometimes acetazolamide is used to change the acidity of the urine for short periods of time.

UNDESIRED EFFECTS
Acetazolamide can cause nausea, vomiting or loss of appetite. To decrease the chance of stomach upset, take this medicine with food or after meals.

Some people become dizzy or less alert than normal when they take acetazolamide. Be sure you know how this drug will affect you before you drive a car or operate dangerous machinery.

Other side effects, which tend to decrease or disappear as your body adjusts to acetazolamide, include tingling of the fingers and toes, increased urination, rash, confusion, fatigue and dryness of the mouth. If these effects are severe or give you great discomfort, contact your doctor. Your doctor may want to decrease the amount of acetazolamide you are taking.

Serious side effects do not happen often, but they require medical attention when they do occur. Contact your doctor at once if you develop a severe headache, blurred vision or other disturbances of vision, convulsions, fever, itching, blood in your urine or black stools.

PRECAUTIONS

If you are allergic to sulfa drugs, you should not take acetazolamide because you may be allergic to this medicine also. Before you start to take acetazolamide, tell your doctor if you ever had an unusual reaction to a sulfa drug.

Acetazolamide makes the urine alkaline, and this may affect the way other drugs are cleared from your body. Tell your doctor what prescription or nonprescription drugs you are taking, including lithium, amphetamines, medicine for irregular heartbeat, medicine for depression, methenamine compounds, diuretics (water pills), medicine for diabetes, digitalis, cortisone-like medicine, amphotericin B, phenytoin and primidone. If you do not know the names of the drugs or what they were prescribed for, bring them in their labeled containers to your doctor or pharmacist.

Because acetazolamide can make some medical conditions worse, tell your doctor if you have liver disease, cirrhosis of the liver, kidney disease, a breathing disorder or lung disease or diabetes.

Take acetazolamide exactly as prescribed by your doctor. If you think you need more acetazolamide to relieve your symptoms, contact your doctor.

Your doctor will want to determine how you are responding to this medicine. *Remember to keep all your appointments for checkups and for blood tests.*

Acetazolamide may have a bad effect on the fetus during the first few months of pregnancy. Be sure to tell your doctor if you are pregnant or think you may become pregnant while you are taking this drug.

DOSAGE

Your doctor will determine how much acetazolamide you should take and how often you should take it. Carefully follow the instructions on your prescription label, and ask your doctor or pharmacist to explain any part of the instructions you do not understand.

Acetazolamide comes in tablets and in long-acting capsules. It is taken several times a day at evenly spaced intervals.

If you forget to take a dose of acetazolamide, take it as soon as you remember and then take any remaining doses for that day at evenly spaced intervals. If you do not remember a missed dose until it is time for you to take another, omit the missed dose entirely and take only the regularly scheduled dose. *Do not take a double dose to make up for a missed dose.*

STORAGE
Keep acetazolamide in the container it came in, and keep it out of the reach of children. Do not allow anyone else to take your acetazolamide.

Carbachol
(kahr′ bah coal)

PRODUCT INFORMATION
Brand names: Isopto Carbachol, Miostat

USES
Carbachol is applied directly to the eye to treat glaucoma, an eye disease that increases the intraocular pressure. This medicine reduces the pressure and helps to prevent loss of vision and damage to the optic nerve.

UNDESIRED EFFECTS
The most common side effects of carbachol are eye pain, blurred vision, decreased vision for distance and poor vision in dim light (night blindness). Do not drive a car or operate dangerous machinery until you know how carbachol will affect you.

Other side effects are twitching of the eyelids, stinging or burning of the eyes, production of tears, eye pain or headache, unusual sensitivity to light and seeing floating shapes before the eyes. Contact your doctor if these effects are severe or give you great discomfort.

When you use carbachol for a long period of time, it can be absorbed into the body. Stop using this medicine and contact your doctor if you develop nausea, vomiting, diarrhea, abdominal pain and cramps, frequent urination, unusual paleness or difficulty breathing.

PRECAUTIONS
Before you start to take carbachol, tell your doctor if you have asthma, intestinal disease, obstruction of the urinary tract, an ulcer, heart or blood vessel disease, overactive thyroid, high blood pressure, seizures or Parkinson's disease.

Because some drugs can affect the way carbachol works, tell your doctor what prescription or nonprescription drugs you are taking, including other medicine for glaucoma, cortisone medications, antihistamines, medicines for allergies and colds, medicine for Parkinson's disease, prescription medicine for pain, medicine for ulcers and medicine for depression. If you do not know the names of the drugs or what they were prescribed for, bring them in their labeled containers to your doctor or pharmacist.

Use carbachol exactly as prescribed by your doctor. Do not use more or less; do not use it more often or for a longer period of time than instructed by your doctor.

Do not stop using this medicine until your doctor tells you to. If you still have the symptoms of glaucoma after you begin using carbachol, contact your doctor.

Tell your doctor if you are pregnant or think you may be. The safe use of carbachol in pregnant women has not been established.

DOSAGE

Your doctor will determine how often you should use carbachol. To be effective, this medicine should be used at regularly spaced intervals. Carefully follow the instructions on your prescription label, and ask your doctor or pharmacist to explain any part of the instructions you do not understand.

Carbachol comes as eyedrops. First, check the eyedrops in the bottle. The solution should be clear, and the end of the dropper should not be cracked or chipped. Next, wash your hands thoroughly with soap and water.

Stand in front of a mirror, and tilt your head back until you are looking at the ceiling. With one hand, pull the lower lid of your eye downward to form a kind of pocket. Hold the eyedropper in your other hand, as close as possible to your eye without touching it, and drop the prescribed number of drops into the pocket. Try to keep the eyedropper pointed downward all the time you are using it so that the drops do not flow back into the bulb of the eyedropper.

Put the eyedropper back into the bottle. Now press your finger against the inner corner of your eye (the corner next to your nose) for one minute. This is important because it prevents the drops from going into your nose and throat, where they might be absorbed into your system and cause problems.

Close your eye gently, and wipe away any liquid around the eye with a tissue. Wash your hands again with soap and water.

STORAGE

Keep carbachol in the container it came in, and store the container in a cool place. Keep this medicine out of the reach of children. Do not allow anyone else to use your carbachol.

Physostigmine
(fye so stig' meen)

PRODUCT INFORMATION

Brand name: Isopto Eserine

USES

Physostigmine, in the form of eyedrops or ointment, is applied to the eye to treat glaucoma. Physostigmine helps relieve the excess pressure in the eye and, therefore, helps prevent the eye damage glaucoma can cause.

UNDESIRED EFFECTS

Eye pain, blurred vision, decreased vision for distance and poor vision in dim light (night blindness) are common side effects of physostigmine. Until you know how this medicine will affect you, do not drive a car or operate dangerous machinery.

Other side effects, which usually do not require medical attention, include twitching of the eyelids, stinging or burning of the eyes, tearing, headache, unusual sensitivity to light and seeing floating shapes before the eyes. However, if you experience these effects and they are severe or give you great discomfort, contact your doctor.

More serious side effects result from the absorption of physostigmine into your body. If you develop nausea, vomiting, diarrhea, abdominal pain, stomach pain and cramps, frequent urination, unusual paleness or difficulty breathing, stop using this medicine and contact your doctor.

PRECAUTIONS

Tell your doctor what prescription or nonprescription drugs you are taking, including other medicine for glaucoma, cortisone-like medicine, antihistamines, medicines for allergies and colds, medicine for Parkinson's disease, prescription medicine for pain, medicine for ulcers and medicine for depression. If you do not know the names of the drugs or what they were prescribed for, bring them in their labeled containers to your doctor or pharmacist.

Your doctor will want to examine your eyes periodically to make sure that physostigmine is controlling your glaucoma. *Be sure to keep all your appointments for these checkups.*

Use physostigmine exactly as prescribed by your doctor. Do not use more or less of it, and do not use it more often or for a longer time than instructed by your doctor.

Do not stop using this medicine until your doctor tells you to. If you still have the symptoms of glaucoma after you begin using this medicine, contact your doctor.

Before you have any kind of surgery, including dental surgery, tell the doctor or dentist in charge that you are taking physostigmine.

If you are pregnant or think you may become pregnant while taking this medicine, tell your doctor. The safe use of physostigmine in pregnant women has not been established.

DOSAGE

Your doctor will determine how often you should use physostigmine. Carefully follow the instructions on your prescription label, and ask your doctor or pharmacist to explain any part of the instructions you do not understand. This medicine should be used at regularly spaced intervals to be effective.

Physostigmine comes in eyedrops to be used during the day and in ointment form, which usually is put into the eye at night.

Before you use the eyedrops, check the color of the solution. If it has turned red, blue or brown, throw away the solution. It is no longer effective and may irritate your eyes.

To apply the eyedrops, follow the instructions with your medicine or proceed in the following way. First, check the end of the eyedropper to make sure it is not chipped or cracked. Next, wash your hands thoroughly with soap and water.

Stand in front of a mirror, and tilt your head back until you are looking at the ceiling. With one hand, pull the lower eyelid downward to form a kind of pocket. Hold the eyedropper in your other hand, as close as possible to your eye without touching it. Drop the prescribed number of drops into the pocket. Try to keep the eyedropper pointed downward all the time you are using it so that the drops do not flow back into the bulb of the eyedropper.

Put the eyedropper back into the bottle. Now press your finger against the inner corner of your eye (the corner next to your nose) for one minute. This is important because it prevents the drops from going into your nose and throat, where they might be absorbed into your body and cause problems.

Close your eye gently, and wipe away any liquid around the eye with a tissue. Wash your hands again with soap and water.

STORAGE

Keep this medicine in the container that it came in, and store the container in a cool place. Keep physostigmine out of the reach of children. Do not allow anyone else to use your physostigmine.

Pilocarpine
(pie low car' peen)

PRODUCT INFORMATION
Brand names: Adsorbocarpine, Almocarpine, Isopto Carpine, Ocusert, Pilocar, Pilomiotin, Pilo-M, P.V. Carpine

USES
Pilocarpine is one of the primary drugs used in the treatment of glaucoma because pilocarpine is relatively free of side effects, particularly serious side effects. It is applied directly to the eye to reduce the pressure.

Pilocarpine also is used prior to certain types of eye surgery.

UNDESIRED EFFECTS
Pilocarpine affects the ability of some patients to see well, especially at night. Do not drive a car or operate dangerous machinery until you know how this medicine will affect you.

Other side effects that may occur after you use pilocarpine are twitching of the eyelids, stinging, burning, tearing, headache and eye pain. These effects usually are mild. However, if they are severe or cause you great discomfort, contact your doctor.

Contact your doctor if you experience excessive sweating, nausea, fainting or confusion.

PRECAUTIONS
Before you start to use pilocarpine, tell your doctor if you have asthma, intestinal

disease, obstruction of the urinary tract, ulcers, heart or blood vessel disease, an overactive thyroid, high blood pressure, seizures or Parkinson's disease.

Tell your doctor what prescription or nonprescription drugs you are taking, including other medicines for glaucoma, cortisone-like medicines, antihistamines, medicines for allergies and colds, medicine for Parkinson's disease, prescription medicine for pain, medicine for ulcers and medicine for depression. If you do not know the names of the drugs or what they were prescribed for, bring them in their labeled containers to your doctor or pharmacist.

Use pilocarpine exactly as prescribed by your doctor. Do not use more or less of it, and do not use it more often or for a longer time than instructed by your doctor. Do not stop using this medicine until your doctor tells you to.

If you still have the symptoms of glaucoma after you begin using pilocarpine, contact your doctor. The amount of pilocarpine you use and the frequency with which you use it may need to be adjusted.

Tell your doctor if you are pregnant or think you may become pregnant while you are using pilocarpine. Safe use of this medicine in pregnant women has not been established.

DOSAGE

Your doctor will determine how often you should use pilocarpine. To be effective, this medicine should be used at regularly spaced intervals. Carefully follow the instructions on your prescription label, and ask your doctor or pharmacist to explain any part of the instructions you do not understand.

Pilocarpine comes in eyedrops and in controlled-release systems, which put the drug into your eye over a seven-day period. If your doctor has prescribed the controlled-release system, be sure you understand exactly how to use it. Check with your doctor or pharmacist if you have questions.

Directions for the use of eyedrops usually are included with the prescription. The eyedrops should be used in this way. First, check the eyedrops in the bottle. The solution should be clear, and the end of the eyedropper should not be cracked or chipped.

Next, wash your hands thoroughly with soap and water.

Stand in front of a mirror, and tilt your head back until you are looking at the ceiling. With one hand, pull the lower lid of your eye downward to form a kind of pocket. Hold the eyedropper in your other hand, as close as possible to your eye without touching it, and drop the prescribed number of drops into the pocket. Try to keep the eyedropper pointed downward all the time you are using it so that the drops do not flow back into the bulb of the eyedropper.

Put the eyedropper back into the bottle. Now press your finger against the inner corner of your eye (the corner next to your nose) for one minute. This is important because it prevents the drops from going into your nose and throat, where they might be absorbed into your body and cause problems.

Close your eye gently, and wipe away any liquid around the eye with a tissue. Wash your hands again with soap and water.

Try to keep the eyedropper from touching anything. If it does touch the eye or any other surface, rinse the eyedropper thoroughly with tap water before you put it back into the bottle.

STORAGE
Keep pilocarpine in the container it came in, and store the container in a cool place. Keep this medicine out of the reach of children, and do not allow anyone else to use your pilocarpine.

Timolol Ophthalmic
(tye′ moe lole)

PRODUCT INFORMATION
Brand name: Timoptic

USES
Timolol ophthalmic drops are used to reduce pressure within the eyeball. It is used to treat various forms of glaucoma and other eye diseases in which increased pressure can lead to gradual loss of vision.

UNDESIRED EFFECTS
Timolol ophthalmic drops may cause eye irritation, mental confusion, weakness, difficulty in breathing or unusually slow heartbeat. If any of these effects occurs, contact your doctor at once.

PRECAUTIONS
Timolol may be absorbed through the eye and can make certain medical conditions worse. Therefore, before you begin to use timolol, tell your doctor if you have asthma or other breathing problems, heart disease or any other chronic medical conditions. You should also tell your doctor about any other medications you are taking, including nonprescription medications.

Timolol controls increased pressure in the eye but does not cure it. Timolol only works as long as you continue to use it. Therefore, do not stop using timolol unless your doctor tells you to do so. *Be sure to keep all your appointments for checkups* so that your doctor can monitor your response to timolol.

It has not been determined whether timolol is safe for use by women who are pregnant or breast-feeding. Therefore, tell your doctor if you are or intend to become pregnant while using this drug or if you are breast-feeding.

DOSAGE
Your doctor will determine how often you should use timolol drops. Follow the instructions on your prescription label, and ask your doctor or pharmacist to explain any part you do not understand. If you are also using other eyedrops, use them at least several minutes apart.

Apply eyedrops in the following way:

1. Use a mirror or have someone else put the drops in your eye.
2. Before using the drops, wash your hands thoroughly with soap and water.
3. Make sure there are no chips or cracks at the end of the dropper.
4. Avoid touching the dropper against the eye or against anything else.
5. Hold the dropper tip down at all times. This prevents the drops from flowing back into the bulb, where they may become contaminated.
6. Lie down or tilt your head back.
7. Holding the bulb of the dropper between your thumb and index finger, place the dropper as near as possible to your eyelid without touching it.
8. Brace the remaining fingers of this hand against your cheek or nose to steady your hand.
9. With the index finger of your other hand, pull the lower lid of the eye down to form a pocket.
10. Drop the prescribed number of drops into the pocket made by the lower lid and the eye. Placing drops on the surface of the eyeball can cause stinging.
11. Replace and tighten the cap or dropper right away. Do not wipe or rinse it off.
12. Press your finger against the inner corner of your eye for one minute. This prevents medication from entering the tear duct.
13. Close your eye gently, and wipe off any excess liquid with a clean tissue.
14. Wash your hands again to remove any medicine.

STORAGE

Keep timolol in the container it came in, and store it at room temperature in a dark place. Keep timolol out of the reach of children.

Do not allow anyone else to use your timolol.

Seizures and Epilepsy

DRUGS USED TO TREAT SEIZURES AND EPILEPSY

Seizures and Epilepsy

The two most common types of epilepsy are grand mal epilepsy and petit mal epilepsy. Both types are caused by excessive electrical activity in the brain. The difference between them is primarily the degree to which the excessive activity spreads over the brain and nervous system.

In grand mal seizures, excessive activity spreads throughout the brain and even to the spinal cord. This produces a loss of consciousness and muscle rigidity, which is followed by uncontrollable rhythmic jerking movements. Usually, a grand mal seizure is followed by a feeling of severe fatigue lasting up to several hours.

Petit mal seizures (also called absence seizures) are brief periods (five to 20 seconds) of loss of consciousness. During this period, the individual shows a blank, staring expression and may have some minor twitching. Usually, the person is unaware of the seizure and resumes previous activities as if nothing happened.

Other types of seizures include psychomotor and psychosensory seizures. These disorders vary quite a bit, depending on the portion of the brain involved. In some cases, several types of seizures may occur at once, and diagnosis often is difficult.

Carbamazepine
(kar ba maz' e peen)

PRODUCT INFORMATION
Brand name: Tegretol

USES
Carbamazepine is used to treat certain types of convulsions and seizures. However, since this medicine has dangerous side effects, it usually is prescribed only when other anticonvulsant drugs have been unable to control the seizures. Carbamazepine also is used to treat facial nerve pain (trigeminal neuralgia).

UNDESIRED EFFECTS
Carbamazepine can cause dizziness, blurred vision, drowsiness and poor coordination. Do not drive a car, operate dangerous machinery or do anything that requires you to be mentally and physically alert until you know how this medicine will affect you.

Nausea and vomiting, common side effects of carbamazepine, can be avoided if you take this medicine with meals or immediately after eating.

Serious side effects, such as blood problems, liver problems, kidney problems and heart and blood vessel problems, can occur when you are taking carbamazepine.

Contact your doctor immediately if you develop fever, sore throat, mouth ulcers, unusual bleeding or bruising, purple-colored spots on the skin, yellowing of the eyes or skin, frequent or difficult urination, swelling of the feet and legs, irregular heartbeat or skin rash or hives.

PRECAUTIONS

If you ever had a bad reaction to any of the tricyclic antidepressant drugs (amitriptyline, desipramine, imipramine, protriptyline, nortriptyline, etc.), you should not take carbamazepine.

Because carbamazepine can make certain medical conditions worse, tell your doctor if you have a history of blood disease such as bone marrow depression, heart disease, liver disease, high blood pressure, thrombophlebitis (blood clots), kidney disease or thyroid disease.

Before you start to take carbamazepine, tell your doctor what prescription or nonprescription drugs you are taking, including barbiturates, tranquilizers, other anticonvulsant drugs, doxycycline, coumarin-type anticoagulants (blood thinners), MAO inhibitors (isocarboxazid, pargyline, phenelzine and tranylcypromine), even if you stopped taking them in the past two weeks, and oral contraceptives (birth-control pills). If you do not know the names of the drugs or what they were prescribed for, bring them in their labeled containers to your doctor or pharmacist.

While you are taking carbamazepine, do not take any other medicines unless your doctor specifically tells you that you may. Take carbamazepine exactly as your doctor has prescribed, and do not take more of it or take it more often than your doctor tells you to.

Do not stop taking carbamazepine until your doctor tells you that you may. You can have problems if you abruptly stop taking this medicine. Your doctor probably will want you to reduce the amount gradually before you stop taking the medicine completely.

Keep in touch with your doctor while you are taking carbamazepine so your doctor can check your response to it and adjust the amount you take. Your doctor also will want to check how this medicine is affecting you by doing complete blood counts (usually once a week when you start therapy), tests for liver function and tests of your urine. Your doctor also may want you to have your eyes checked. *Be sure to keep all your appointments for checkups.*

If you are pregnant or are nursing a baby, tell your doctor. Pregnant women and breast-feeding mothers should not take this medicine. If you become pregnant while you are taking carbamazepine, inform your doctor immediately.

DOSAGE

Your doctor will determine how much carbamazepine you should take and how often you should take it. Carefully follow the instructions on your prescription label, and ask your doctor or pharmacist to explain any part of the instructions you do not understand.

Carbamazepine comes in tablets, which may be taken with milk or solid food to decrease the chance of stomach upset.

If you forget to take a dose of carbamazepine, take it as soon as you remember and take any remaining doses for that day at evenly spaced intervals. If you do not remember a missed dose until it is almost time for you to take another, omit the missed dose entirely. Take only the regularly scheduled dose. *Do not take a double dose to make up for a missed dose.*

STORAGE
Keep carbamazepine in the container it came in, and keep it out of the reach of children. Do not allow anyone else to take your carbamazepine, which was prescribed for your particular condition.

Ethosuximide
(eth oh sux′ i mide)

PRODUCT INFORMATION
Brand name: Zarontin

USES
Ethosuximide is used to treat petit mal seizures, the form of epilepsy that makes a person lose consciousness for very short periods.

UNDESIRED EFFECTS
The most common side effects of ethosuximide are nausea, vomiting, stomach cramps and loss of appetite. If you take this medicine after meals, you will decrease the chance of stomach upset. These effects should disappear as you continue to take ethosuximide and as your body adjusts to it. If they do not, contact your doctor.

Ethosuximide makes some people dizzy or drowsy. Do not drive a car or operate dangerous machinery until you know how this medicine will affect you. Less often, this medicine may cause headache, tiredness or irritability. If these effects bother you, contact your doctor.

More serious side effects of ethosuximide are allergic reactions or blood problems. Contact your doctor if you develop a skin rash or itching, sore throat and fever, hiccups, unusual bruising or bleeding or swollen lymph glands.

PRECAUTIONS
If you ever had an unusual reaction to an anticonvulsant (seizure medicine) in the past, you should not take ethosuximide.

Because this medicine can make some medical conditions worse, tell your doctor if you have blood disease, kidney disease or liver disease.

Tell your doctor what prescription or nonprescription medicines you are taking, including medicine for mental illness or depression and any other anticonvulsant drugs. If you do not know the names of the drugs or what they were prescribed for, take them in their labeled containers to your doctor or pharmacist.

Your doctor will want to check on your response to this medicine so that he or she can prescribe more or less of it, depending on your need. Keep in touch with your doctor, and *keep all your appointments for checkups* so that your doctor can do blood counts and other tests to be sure this medicine is not affecting you badly.

Take ethosuximide exactly as prescribed by your doctor. Do not take more of it or take it more often than your doctor has ordered. Do not stop taking this medicine unless your doctor tells you to do so. Your doctor may want you to reduce the amount gradually before you stop taking this medicine completely.

Tell your doctor if you are pregnant or are nursing a baby. Pregnant women and women who are breast-feeding should not take ethosuximide. If you become pregnant while taking ethosuximide, contact your doctor immediately.

DOSAGE
Your doctor will determine how much ethosuximide you should take and how often you should take it. Carefully follow the instructions on your prescription label, and ask your doctor or pharmacist to explain any part of the instructions that you do not understand.

Ethosuximide comes in capsules and in liquid form. Your doctor will choose the form best for you.

If you forget to take a dose of this medicine, take it as soon as you remember. Take any remaining doses for the day at evenly spaced intervals. If you do not remember a missed dose until it is almost time for you to take another, omit the missed dose completely and take only the regularly scheduled dose. *Do not take a double dose.*

STORAGE
Keep ethosuximide in the container it came in, and store the tightly closed container away from extreme heat and sunlight. Keep this medicine out of the reach of children. Do not allow anyone else to take your ethosuximide.

Methsuximide
(meth sux′ i mide)

PRODUCT INFORMATION
Brand name: Celontin

USES
Methsuximide is used to control petit mal seizures, the form of epilepsy that involves brief periods of loss of consciousness and/or jerking of the eyelids and muscles of the face and arms. Methsuximide also may be used in combination with other drugs to treat medical conditions that result in convulsions.

UNDESIRED EFFECTS
The most common side effect of methsuximide is stomach upset. Take this medicine with food or a glass of milk to avoid this problem.

Methsuximide makes some people dizzy or drowsy. Do not drive a car or operate dangerous machinery until you know how this medicine will affect you.

Some effects that may decrease or disappear as your body adjusts to methsuximide are headache, irritability, tiredness, loss of appetite, nausea and vomiting. If you experience any of these effects and they are severe or continue, contact your doctor.

Less often, methsuximide will cause allergic reactions and, rarely, blood problems. Contact your doctor immediately if you have a skin rash or itching, sore throat and fever, swollen lymph glands, unusual bruising or bleeding or mood changes.

PRECAUTIONS

If you ever had an unusual reaction to another type of medicine for seizures, you should not take methsuximide. Your doctor should know if you have certain medical problems, such as blood disease, kidney disease or liver disease, before you start to take methsuximide.

Tell your doctor what prescription or nonprescription drugs you are taking, including medicine for mental illness or depression and any other anticonvulsant drugs. If you do not know the names of the drugs or what they were prescribed for, bring them in their labeled containers to your doctor or pharmacist.

While you are taking methsuximide, do not drink alcoholic beverages, because they may make the side effects worse. If you have questions, check with your doctor or pharmacist.

Your doctor will want to adjust the amount of methsuximide you take according to the way you respond to it. *Be sure to keep all appointments for checkups with your doctor.* Your doctor also will want to do blood counts and other tests to determine how this medicine is affecting you.

Take this medicine exactly as prescribed by your doctor. Do not stop taking it unless your doctor tells you to do so. Your doctor may want you to reduce the amount gradually before you stop taking methsuximide completely.

Be sure you have enough medicine on hand to take all the doses prescribed for you. Check your supply before vacations, holidays and other times when you might have difficulty getting more.

Tell your doctor if you are pregnant or are nursing a baby. Pregnant women and women who are breast-feeding should not take this medicine. If you become pregnant while taking methsuximide, contact your doctor immediately.

DOSAGE

Your doctor will determine how much methsuximide you should take and how often you should take it. Carefully follow the instructions on your prescription label, and ask your doctor or pharmacist to explain any part of the instructions you do not understand.

Methsuximide comes in capsules. It can be taken with solid food or milk to decrease the chance of stomach upset.

If you forget to take a dose of methsuximide, take it as soon as you remember it. Then take any remaining doses for the day at evenly spaced intervals. If you do not remember a missed dose until it is almost time for you to take another, omit the missed dose entirely and take only the regularly scheduled dose. *Do not take a double dose to make up for a missed dose.*

STORAGE
Keep methsuximide in the container it came in, and keep it out of the reach of children. Do not allow anyone else to take your methsuximide.

Phenobarbital
(fee noe bar' bi tal)

Phenobarbital is a member of the drug class known as the barbiturates. It is used to control epileptic seizures as well as to help people fall asleep and to relieve anxiety and tension. For a complete description of phenobarbital, see the section Barbiturates (page 424) under Drugs Used to Treat Sleep Disturbances.

Phenytoin
(fen' itoe in)

PRODUCT INFORMATION
Brand names: Dilantin, Diphenylan

USES
Phenytoin is used alone or in combination with other medicines to control various types of convulsions or seizures.

UNDESIRED EFFECTS
Phenytoin can cause redness, swelling or bleeding of the gums, usually after you have been taking it for two to three months. Be sure to brush your teeth carefully and regularly, to use dental floss and to see your dentist on a regular basis for checkups. If you have any questions about how to care for your teeth and gums, check with your doctor or dentist. Contact your doctor or dentist if you develop problems as a result of taking phenytoin.

Nausea and vomiting can occur when you take phenytoin. Take this medicine with meals or immediately after eating to help prevent upset stomach.

Other effects, which require medical attention if they occur, include skin rash, blurred vision, slurred speech, difficulty walking, mental confusion, pain in the joints, unexplained fever, enlarged lymph glands, unusual bleeding or bruising and yellowing of the eyes or skin. Contact your doctor if you experience any of these effects.

Phenytoin may color your urine pink, red or brown. This effect is harmless and should not concern you.

PRECAUTIONS

If you ever had an unusual reaction to any anticonvulsant medicine, you should not take phenytoin. If you have questions, check with your doctor.

If you have high blood sugar, liver disease or alcoholism, tell your doctor. Phenytoin may make these conditions worse.

Certain medications should not be taken with phenytoin. Tell your doctor what prescription or nonprescription drugs you are taking, particularly barbiturates, chloramphenicol, coumarin-type anticoagulants (blood thinners), dexamethasone or other cortisone-like medicines, oral medicine for diabetes, disulfiram (medicine for alcoholism), doxycycline, folic acid (found in many vitamin formulas), isoniazid, medicine for mental illness, oxyphenbutazone, phenylbutazone, sulfa drugs and medicine for depression.

If you do not know the names of the drugs you are taking or what they were prescribed for, bring them in their labeled containers to your doctor or pharmacist.

Keep in touch with your doctor while you are taking phenytoin. Your doctor may want to adjust your dose or change your medication schedule, depending on your response to phenytoin.

Take phenytoin exactly as prescribed by your doctor. Do not take more of it, and do not take it more often than your doctor has prescribed. If you have been taking phenytoin regularly for several weeks, do not stop taking it without your doctor's permission. Your doctor may want you to reduce the amount gradually before you stop taking it completely.

Be sure you have enough of this medicine on hand at all times so that you can take all doses that have been prescribed for you. Check your supply before vacations, holidays and other occasions when it may be difficult for you to get more.

Alcoholic beverages may alter the way phenytoin works. Check with your doctor before drinking alcoholic beverages while you are taking this medicine.

If you have diabetes, phenytoin may affect your blood sugar level. If you notice a change in the results of your urine sugar tests, check with your doctor.

Before you have any surgery, including dental surgery, tell the doctor or dentist in charge that you are taking phenytoin.

Be sure to tell your doctor if you are pregnant or are breast-feeding. Pregnant women and breast-feeding mothers should not take phenytoin. If you become pregnant while you are taking this medicine, contact your doctor at once.

DOSAGE

Your doctor will determine how much phenytoin you should take and how often you should take it. Carefully follow the instructions on your prescription label, and ask your doctor or pharmacist to explain any part of the instructions you do not understand.

Phenytoin comes in capsules, chewable tablets and liquid form. Your doctor will choose the form best for you. If you are taking the liquid form, be sure to shake it well before each use. Chewable tablets should be chewed well before they are swallowed. All forms of this medicine may be taken with milk or solid food to prevent stomach upset.

If you forget to take a dose of phenytoin, take the missed dose as soon as you remember it. Take the remaining doses for that day at regularly spaced intervals. If you remember a missed dose when it is almost time for you to take another, omit the missed dose entirely and take only the regularly scheduled dose. *Do not take two doses at one time.*

STORAGE
Keep phenytoin in the container it came in, and store the container at room temperature. Keep this medicine out of the reach of children. Do not allow anyone else to take your phenytoin.

Primidone
(pri′ mi done)

PRODUCT INFORMATION
Brand name: Mysoline

USES
Primidone is an anticonvulsant chemically related to phenobarbital. Primidone acts on the brain and central nervous system to control certain types of muscular convulsions or seizures. When used with other drugs, it also helps control grand mal epilepsy seizures.

UNDESIRED EFFECTS
Among the most common side effects of primidone are nausea and vomiting. These effects may occur when you start to take this medicine and then disappear as your body adjusts to the medicine. If you take primidone with meals, you may decrease the chance of stomach upset.

Primidone may make some people dizzy, drowsy or less alert than they usually are. Even when taken at bedtime, it can cause these effects the next morning. Do not drive a car or operate dangerous machinery until you know how this medicine will affect you.

Occasionally, children and older people may show signs of restlessness and excitement after taking primidone. If this occurs, contact your doctor.

More serious side effects with primidone are rare. However, contact your doctor if you experience skin rash, pain in the joints, unexplained fever, swelling of the eyelids or wheezing or tightness in the chest.

An overdose of or intolerance to primidone can cause symptoms similar to barbiturate poisoning. Contact your doctor immediately if you have changes in vision, mental confusion, shortness of breath or difficulty breathing.

PRECAUTIONS
If you ever had an unusual reaction to any barbiturate (such as amobarbital,

butabarbital, pentobarbital, phenobarbital or secobarbital), you should not take primidone. If you have questions, check with your doctor or pharmacist.

To help your doctor select the best treatment for you, tell your doctor if you have asthma, emphysema, chronic lung disease, hyperactivity (in children), kidney disease, liver disease or porphyria.

Before you start to take primidone, tell your doctor what prescription or nonprescription drugs you are taking. Some drugs that will affect the way your body responds to primidone are antihistamines, medicine for allergies and colds, narcotics, other barbiturates, other medicine for seizures, prescription medicine for pain, sedatives, tranquilizers, medicine to help you sleep, medicine for depression, MAO inhibitors (isocarboxazid, pargyline, phenelzine and tranylcypromine), even if you stopped taking them two weeks ago, anticoagulants (blood thinners), corticosteroids (cortisone-like medicine), digitalis, digitoxin, doxycycline, griseofulvin and phenytoin. If you do not know the names of the drugs you are taking or what they were prescribed for, bring them in their labeled containers to your doctor or pharmacist.

Do not drink alcoholic beverages while you are taking primidone. Alcohol can increase the possibility of or severity of side effects. Do not start to take any of the drugs listed above unless you first check with your doctor.

Take primidone exactly as prescribed by your doctor. Do not take more of it, and do not take it more often than your doctor has indicated. Be sure you have enough of this medicine to take all doses prescribed. Check your supply before vacations, holidays and other occasions on which you may not be able to get more.

Do not stop taking this medicine unless your doctor tells you to do so. Your doctor probably will want you to reduce the amount of primidone gradually before you stop taking it entirely.

While you are taking this medicine, keep in touch with your doctor. Your doctor will want to check your response to primidone and may adjust your dose, depending on your needs.

Before you have any kind of surgery, including dental surgery, be sure to tell the doctor or dentist in charge that you are taking primidone.

If you are pregnant or breast-feeding a baby, be sure to tell your doctor before you begin to take primidone. If you become pregnant while you are taking this medicine, contact your doctor immediately.

DOSAGE

Your doctor will determine how much primidone you should take and how often you should take it. Carefully follow the instructions on your prescription label, and ask your doctor or pharmacist to explain any part of the instructions you do not understand.

Primidone comes in tablets and in liquid form. It may be taken with meals to decrease the chance of stomach upset. The liquid should be shaken well before each use.

If you forget to take a dose of primidone, take it as soon as you remember. Take any remaining doses for that day at evenly spaced intervals. If you do not remember a missed dose until it is almost time for you to take another, omit the missed dose completely. Take only the regularly scheduled dose. *Do not take a double dose.*

STORAGE

Keep primidone in the container it came in, and store it at room temperature. Keep this medicine out of the reach of children. Do not allow anyone else to take your primidone.

Gout

DRUGS USED TO TREAT GOUT

Gout

Gout is caused by excess uric acid in the blood. The excess uric acid accumulates in different tissues throughout the body to produce pain and inflammation. Although arthritis is the most common form of gout, gout can appear in skin and also in the kidneys to produce kidney stones.

Most frequently, gout causes inflammation, swelling and pain in the joints, particularly in the feet and ankles. A gout attack can be precipitated by factors such as surgery, excessive alcohol consumption, dietary excess, emotional stress or even excessive walking.

Several different types of medications are used to treat gout. Colchicine and phenylbutazone are used to relieve pain and inflammation. Usually these drugs begin to relieve these symptoms within six to 12 hours. Other medications such as probenecid and sulfinpyrazone are used to increase the amount of uric acid passed in the urine, thereby preventing or relieving a buildup of uric acid in the bloodstream.

Another drug used to treat gout is allopurinol. It acts to prevent the formation of uric acid in the blood.

The choice of these medications depends on a variety of factors, including your response to particular medication, other health problems and other medication you may be taking.

With any treatment, it is important that you continue to take the medications as prescribed. They control gout only as long as they are taken regularly. Your doctor probably will want to perform some blood tests periodically to measure your response to treatment. *Be sure to keep all such appointments.*

Allopurinol
(al oh pure′ i nole)

PRODUCT INFORMATION
Brand name: Zyloprim

USES
Allopurinol is used to treat chronic gout. Allopurinol also is used to keep the body from producing too much uric acid, which could lead to or aggravate various medical problems.

UNDESIRED EFFECTS
Skin rash is the most common side effect of allopurinol. If you develop a rash, stop taking the medicine and contact your doctor.

Allopurinol makes some people drowsy or dizzy. Do not drive a car or operate dangerous machinery until you know how this medicine will affect you. Allopurinol also can cause stomach upset, stomach pain or diarrhea. If allopurinol upsets your stomach, you may take it after meals. Contact your doctor if stomach upsets continue.

Rarely, allopurinol will cause nerve, blood or liver problems, which will require medical attention. Contact your doctor if you have numbness, tingling, pain or weakness in the hands or feet; sore throat and fever; unusual bruising or bleeding; unusual weakness or tiredness; or yellowing of the eyes or skin.

PRECAUTIONS

Before you start to take allopurinol, tell your doctor if you have kidney disease or if you or any member of your immediate family has a disease known as idiopathic hemochromatosis.

Tell your doctor what prescription or nonprescription drugs you are taking, particularly ampicillin, anticoagulants (blood thinners), azathioprine, cyclophosphamide, diuretics (water pills), medicine to make the urine more acid or mercaptopurine. If you do not know the names of the drugs or what they were prescribed for, bring them in their labeled containers to your doctor or pharmacist.

Do not drink alcoholic beverages and do not take vitamin C while you are taking allopurinol. Too much alcohol can lessen the effect of allopurinol, and too much vitamin C can increase the chance of your developing kidney stones. If you have any questions about this, check with your doctor or pharmacist.

To help prevent kidney stones, you should drink at least 10 to 12 full (eight-ounce) glasses of fluids a day while you are taking allopurinol. If you are giving this medicine to a child, ask your doctor how much water or other fluids the child should drink every day.

Allopurinol is used to help prevent gout attacks, but it will not relieve a gout attack that has already started. Even if you take another medicine for gout attacks, continue to take allopurinol as well. Check with your doctor if you have any questions.

Be sure to keep in touch with your doctor while you are taking allopurinol so that your doctor can check on the way this medicine is affecting you.

Your doctor should be told if you are pregnant or are nursing a baby, although no harm to the fetus or nursing baby has been reported as a result of using allopurinol. This will help your doctor choose the best and safest treatment for you and your baby.

DOSAGE

Your doctor will determine how often you should take allopurinol and how much you should take at each dose. Carefully follow the instructions on your prescription label, and ask your doctor or pharmacist to explain any part of the instructions you do not understand.

Allopurinol comes in tablets that are usually taken once a day. They should be taken with meals if this medicine upsets your stomach.

Allopurinol only controls the conditions for which it is prescribed; it does not cure them. Therefore, it is important to follow the schedule prescribed by your doctor. Do not stop taking allopurinol unless your doctor tells you to.

If you forget to take a dose of allopurinol, take it as soon as you remember it. Take any remaining doses for that day at evenly spaced intervals. If you miss two or more doses in a row, contact your doctor.

STORAGE
Keep allopurinol in the container it came in, and keep it out of the reach of children. Do not allow anyone else to take your allopurinol.

Colchicine
(kol′ chi seen)

PRODUCT INFORMATION
Brand names of preparations containing colchicine: Acetycol, ColBenemid, Colsalide, Darth with Colchicine, Neocylate, Salamide with Colchicine, Salpaba, Tolsylate-K

USES
Colchicine relieves inflammation, pain and swelling caused by attacks of gout and gouty arthritis. Colchicine is used to treat and to prevent these attacks. It is prescribed alone or in combination preparations with medicine for pain.

UNDESIRED EFFECTS
The most common effects of colchicine are diarrhea, nausea, vomiting and stomach pain. These effects are signs the medicine is beginning to poison your body. If any of them occur, stop taking colchicine immediately and contact your doctor.

If you take this medicine over a long period of time, you may develop skin rash or numbness, tingling, pain or weakness in your hands or feet; you may have symptoms of serious blood problems, such as sore throat and fever, unusual bruising or bleeding or unusual tiredness or weakness. Stop taking colchicine and contact your doctor if you have any of these effects.

PRECAUTIONS
Because colchicine may make some medical problems worse, tell your doctor if you have blood disease, heart disease, intestinal disease, kidney disease, liver disease, stomach ulcers or other stomach problems.

Before you start to take colchicine, tell your doctor what other prescription or nonprescription drugs you are taking. If you do not know the names of the drugs or what they were prescribed for, bring them in their labeled containers to your doctor or pharmacist.

Do not drink alcoholic beverages while you are taking colchicine, unless you have your doctor's permission to do so. Drinking too much alcohol can lessen the effectiveness of this medicine.

Colchicine may affect the results of certain urine tests. If you are to have a urine test while you are taking this medicine, tell the doctor or laboratory personnel that you are taking colchicine.

If you take this medicine for a long time, your doctor will want to check your progress with complete blood counts and other tests at regular intervals. *Be sure to keep all appointments with your doctor.*

DOSAGE

Colchicine comes in tablets to be taken orally and in an injectable form. Your doctor will prescribe the form best for you and will determine how often you should take this medicine and how much you should take at each dose. Carefully follow the instructions on your prescription label, and ask your doctor or pharmacist to explain any part of the instructions you do not understand.

If you are taking colchicine to relieve symptoms of gout attack, take colchicine at the first sign of pain. For this medicine to be fully effective, you must begin to take it when you first start to feel pain. Relief usually will be felt in 24 to 48 hours. Take a dose of colchicine every two hours until the pain is relieved or until you begin to have nausea, vomiting or diarrhea.

If you are taking colchicine regularly to reduce the number and severity of attacks, follow your doctor's instructions for taking this medicine.

When you are taking colchicine to relieve symptoms of a gout attack, the medicine should be taken according to the dosage schedule your doctor has recommended. If you forget to take a dose, take it as soon as you remember it. However, if you do not remember it until it is almost time for you to take another dose, omit the missed dose entirely and take only the regularly scheduled dose. *Do not take a double dose.*

If you are taking colchicine to prevent a gout attack and you forget to take a dose, omit that dose completely. *Do not take an extra dose the next day to make up for the missed dose.* If you take this medicine every day or once every few days, you may find it easier to remember to take your doses if you take them at the same time you do something else every day, such as brushing your teeth in the morning or going to bed at night.

STORAGE

Keep colchicine in the container it came in, and keep it out of the reach of children. Do not allow anyone else to take your colchicine.

Probenecid
(proe ben' e sid)

PRODUCT INFORMATION
Brand names: Benemid, Probalan, Probenimead, Robenecid

USES
Probenecid is used to prevent attacks of gout and to treat other medical problems that cause too much uric acid to be produced by the body. Probenecid acts on the kidneys to help the body eliminate uric acid by passing it in the urine. Probenecid also is used to make certain antibiotics more effective because it prevents the body from passing them in the urine.

UNDESIRED EFFECTS
The most common side effects of probenecid are headache, loss of appetite, nausea and vomiting. To help prevent stomach upset, take probenecid with solid food or milk. If this is not effective, take it with an antacid. Contact your doctor if stomach upsets continue in spite of your precautions.

Other effects, which may disappear as you continue to take probenecid and as your body adjusts to it, are dizziness, flushing or redness of the face, a frequent urge to urinate and sore gums. If these effects continue or are severe, contact your doctor.

Probenecid can cause the formation of uric acid stones. Contact your doctor if you have bloody urine, pain in the lower back or painful urination.

Rarely, probenecid will cause an allergic reaction or blood problems, which will require medical attention. Contact your doctor if you have difficulty breathing, skin rash or itching, unexplained fever, sore throat and fever, unusual bleeding or bruising or unusual tiredness or weakness.

PRECAUTIONS
Because probenecid can make certain medical conditions worse, tell your doctor if you have blood disease, kidney stones, stomach ulcers or a history of stomach ulcers.

Tell your doctor what prescription or nonprescription drugs you are taking, including aminosalicylic acid, antibiotics, aspirin or other salicylates, dapsone, diuretics (water pills), indomethacin, methotrexate, nitrofurantoin, oral medicine for diabetes and sulfa drugs.

While you are taking probenecid, drink at least six to eight eight-ounce glasses of water or fruit juice each day, unless your doctor tells you to limit the amount of fluids you drink.

Do not drink alcoholic beverages or take aspirin or any medication containing aspirin while you are taking probenecid. Both alcohol and aspirin can affect the way your body responds to probenecid. If you need to take something to relieve minor pain or fever, ask your doctor or pharmacist to recommend a substitute for aspirin.

Take probenecid exactly as prescribed by your doctor. This medicine must be taken regularly to be effective. Do not stop taking it unless your doctor tells you to.

Your doctor may want you to start with a small dose and then gradually increase the amount you take. Keep in touch with your doctor so your doctor can adjust your dose of probenecid to meet your needs.

Be sure you have enough probenecid on hand at all times to permit you to take all the doses prescribed for you. Check your supply before vacations, holidays and other occasions when you may not be able to obtain more.

If you have diabetes, probenecid can cause inaccurate results in certain tests for urine sugar. Check with your doctor or pharmacist if you have any questions.

Children under the age of two years should not take probenecid.

Probenecid has been used in pregnant women with no reported problems. However, it is best to tell your doctor if you are pregnant or are nursing a baby.

DOSAGE
Your doctor will determine how often you should take probenecid and how much you should take at each dose. Carefully follow the instructions on your prescription label, and ask your doctor or pharmacist to explain any part of the instructions you do not understand.

Probenecid comes in tablets. Probenecid should be taken at meals or with a snack to avoid stomach upset.

If you forget to take a dose of probenecid, take it as soon as you remember. If you do not remember a missed dose until it is almost time for you to take another, omit the missed dose entirely and take only the regularly scheduled dose. *Do not take a double dose to make up for a missed one.*

STORAGE
Keep probenecid in the container it came in, and keep it out of the reach of children. Do not allow anyone else to take your probenecid, which was prescribed for your particular problem.

Sulfinpyrazone
(sul fin pye' ra zone)

PRODUCT INFORMATION
Brand name: Anturane

USES
Sulfinpyrazone acts on the kidneys to help the body eliminate uric acid by passing it in the urine. Sulfinpyrazone is used to prevent attacks of gout and to treat other medical conditions that cause the body to produce too much uric acid.

UNDESIRED EFFECTS
Sulfinpyrazone frequently causes indigestion, nausea or pain in the stomach or intestines. To lessen stomach upset, take this medicine with solid food or milk; contact your doctor if stomach upsets continue in spite of your taking this precaution.

Other side effects, which may go away as you continue to take sulfinpyrazone and as your body adjusts to it, are dizziness, fainting, ringing or buzzing in the ears and swelling of the feet or legs. If these effects continue or are severe, contact your doctor.

Sulfinpyrazone may cause the formation of uric acid stones. Contact your doctor if you have bloody urine, pain in the lower back or painful urination.

Although serious side effects from sulfinpyrazone are rare, they require medical attention if they do occur. Contact your doctor if you have difficulty breathing, skin rash or itching, unexplained fever, sore throat and fever, unusual bleeding or bruising or unusual tiredness or weakness.

PRECAUTIONS

You should not take sulfinpyrazone if you ever had an unusual reaction to oxyphenbutazone or to phenylbutazone. Check with your doctor or pharmacist if you have questions about this problem. Before you start to take sulfinpyrazone, tell your doctor if you have blood disease, kidney disease, a stomach ulcer or a history of stomach ulcer or inflammation or ulceration of the intestines. Sulfinpyrazone may make these conditions worse.

Tell your doctor what prescription or nonprescription drugs you are taking, including aminosalicylic acid, antibiotics, anticoagulants (blood thinners), aspirin or other salicylates, colchicine, dapsone, diuretics (water pills), indomethacin, insulin, methotrexate, nitrofurantoin, oral medicine for diabetes and sulfonamides. If you do not know the names of the drugs or what they were prescribed for, bring them in their labeled containers to your doctor or pharmacist.

While you are taking sulfinpyrazone, drink at least six to eight eight-ounce glasses of water or fruit juice each day, unless your doctor tells you to limit the amount of fluids you drink.

Do not drink alcoholic beverages or take aspirin or any medication containing aspirin while you are taking sulfinpyrazone. Both alcohol and aspirin can affect the way your body responds to sulfinpyrazone. If you must take something to relieve minor pain or fever, ask your doctor or pharmacist to recommend a substitute for aspirin.

Take this medicine exactly as prescribed by your doctor. Sulfinpyrazone must be taken regularly to be effective. Do not stop taking it unless your doctor tells you to. Your doctor may want you to start with a small dose and then gradually increase the amount you take.

Keep in touch with your doctor while you are taking this medicine so your doctor can adjust the amount you take to meet your needs and can check on your response to the medicine.

Be sure you have enough sulfinpyrazone on hand at all times to permit you to take all the doses prescribed for you. Check your supply before vacations, holidays and other occasions when you may not be able to obtain more.

Although sulfinpyrazone has been used in pregnant women with no reported problems, it is best to tell your doctor if you are pregnant.

DOSAGE

Your doctor will determine how often you should take sulfinpyrazone and how much you should take at each dose. Carefully follow the instructions on your prescription label, and ask your doctor or pharmacist to explain any part of the instructions you do not understand.

Sulfinpyrazone comes in tablets and capsules. Sulfinpyrazone should be taken at meals or with a snack to avoid stomach upset.

If you forget to take a dose of this medicine, take it as soon as you remember. If you do not remember a missed dose until it is almost time for you to take another, omit the missed dose entirely and take only the regularly scheduled dose. *Do not take a double dose to make up for a missed one.*

STORAGE

Keep sulfinpyrazone in the container it came in, and keep it out of the reach of children. Do not allow anyone else to take your sulfinpyrazone.

Parkinson's Disease

DRUGS USED TO TREAT PARKINSON'S DISEASE

Parkinson's Disease

Parkinson's disease is caused by chemical imbalances in portions of the brain. The reasons for developing these imbalances are not known. Since the disease usually begins between the ages of 50 and 65, it is assumed that the aging process is partially responsible. Parkinson's disease affects both men and women of all races and does not appear to be hereditary.

The symptoms of Parkinson's disease usually begin as muscle tremors in one or both hands. This problem is followed by stiffness of the arms and legs, a general slowing of movements and increasing difficulty in performing routine activities. As the disease progresses facial muscles are affected so that facial expressions and eye blinking are decreased and speech is slowed.

Some types of medications, particularly certain tranquilizers, can cause symptoms similar to those of Parkinson's disease. Although these symptoms usually disappear within a few days after you stop taking the medication, they may last considerably longer in susceptible individuals.

Parkinson's disease is treated with a variety of medications that correct the chemical imbalances responsible. In addition to these medications, physical therapy often is used to keep muscles in tone and to slow progression of the disease.

Amantadine
(a man' ta deen)

PRODUCT INFORMATION
Brand name: Symmetrel

USES
Amantadine is used to treat Parkinson's disease and symptoms similar to those of Parkinson's disease that can result from disease, injury or certain drugs. Amantadine also is used to prevent influenza caused by type A virus.

UNDESIRED EFFECTS
Amantadine can cause loss of appetite, nausea or vomiting. To decrease the chance of stomach upset, take it after meals or with food.

Amantadine makes some people dizzy, drowsy or less alert than usual. Do not drive a car or operate dangerous machinery until you know how this medicine will affect you.

Other effects that may occur are double vision, mental confusion, difficulty sleeping, tiredness and hallucinations (seeing, hearing or feeling things that are not there). Contact your doctor if any of these effects continue or cause you a great deal of discomfort.

More serious side effects will require medical attention if they occur. Contact your doctor if you develop a skin rash, swelling of the feet and legs, a feeling of depression, difficulty in urinating or convulsions.

PRECAUTIONS

Because amantadine can make some medical conditions worse, tell your doctor if you have epilepsy or any other form of seizures, heart disease, kidney disease, liver disease, recurring skin rash or mental illness.

Before you start to take amantadine, tell your doctor what prescription or nonprescription drugs you are taking, including benztropine, trihexyphenidyl, other medicine for Parkinson's disease, ulcer medicine, medicine for seizures and medicine for spasms of the intestines. If you do not know the names of the drugs or what they were prescribed for, bring them in their labeled containers to your doctor or pharmacist.

Do not stop taking this medicine unless your doctor tells you that you may. If you stop taking amantadine abruptly, your condition may get worse. Your doctor will want you to decrease the amount you take gradually before you stop taking this medicine entirely.

Tell your doctor if you are pregnant or are nursing a baby. Amantadine can be passed to a baby through the mother's milk. Safe use of this medicine in pregnant women has not been established.

DOSAGE

Your doctor will determine how much amantadine you should take and how often you should take it. Carefully follow the instructions on your prescription label, and ask your doctor or pharmacist to explain any part of the instructions you do not understand.

Amantadine comes in capsules and in liquid form. It can be taken after meals or with food to lessen stomach upset. This medicine usually is taken once or twice a day.

If you forget to take a dose of amantadine, take it as soon as you remember the missed dose. However, if you do not remember a missed dose until it is time for you to take another, take only the regularly scheduled dose. Omit the missed dose entirely. *Do not take a double dose to make up for a missed dose.*

STORAGE

Keep amantadine in the container it came in, and keep it out of the reach of children. Do not allow anyone else to take your amantadine.

Benztropine
(benz′ troe peen)

PRODUCT INFORMATION
Brand name: Cogentin

USES
Benztropine is used alone or with other drugs to treat Parkinson's disease or "shaking palsy." Benztropine improves muscle control and allows more normal movement of the body. It is also used to control side effects resembling Parkinson's disease that are brought about by some drugs used to treat mental illness.

UNDESIRED EFFECTS
One of the most common effects of benztropine is dry mouth. To relieve it, suck hard candies, chew gum or dissolve bits of ice in your mouth.

Other effects, which usually are mild when they occur, include blurred vision, nervousness, heart palpitation, loss of appetite, nausea and difficulty urinating. If you experience any of these effects and they are severe or cause you great discomfort, contact your doctor.

Benztropine will cause some people to become drowsy, dizzy or less alert than usual. Do not drive a car or operate dangerous machinery until you know how this medicine will affect you.

While you are taking benztropine, your eyes may be more sensitive to light than they normally are. Wear sunglasses to decrease the discomfort from bright light.

Because benztropine causes you to sweat less, you may easily become overheated while you are taking this medicine. To prevent heat prostration or sunstroke, be careful not to exert yourself to excess on a hot day, in a heated place or in the sunlight.

Although they do not occur often, more serious side effects will require medical attention if they do occur. Contact your doctor if you develop a skin rash or become constipated. Intestinal problems, such as constipation, can be serious if they are not corrected.

PRECAUTIONS
Because benztropine can make some medical conditions worse, tell your doctor if you have asthma, bronchitis, difficulty urinating, emphysema, enlarged prostate, glaucoma, hiatal hernia, high blood pressure, intestinal blockage, kidney disease, liver disease, myasthenia gravis, overactive thyroid or ulcerative colitis.

To help your doctor select the best treatment for you, tell your doctor what prescription or nonprescription drugs you are taking, including amantadine, antacids, antihistamines, medicine for allergy or colds, haloperidol, medicine for your heart, medicine for diarrhea, other medicine for Parkinson's disease, medicine for sleep, medicine for your nerves, sedatives, tranquilizers, medicine for ulcers and MAO inhibitors (isocarboxazid, pargyline, phenelzine and tranylcypromine), even if you stopped taking them within the past two weeks. If you do not know the names of the drugs you are taking or what they were prescribed for, bring them in their labeled containers to your doctor or pharmacist.

Do not drink alcoholic beverages while you are taking benztropine. Alcohol can increase the chance of and severity of side effects. Do not start to take any of the drugs listed above unless you have permission from your doctor.

Do not take this medicine within one hour of taking antacids or medicine for diarrhea. Taking these medications close together may decrease the effect of benztropine.

Before you start to take benztropine, tell your doctor if you are pregnant. The safety of this medicine in pregnant women has not been established.

DOSAGE
Your doctor will determine how much benztropine you should take and how often you should take it. Carefully follow the instructions on your prescription label, and ask your doctor or pharmacist to explain any part of the instructions you do not understand.

Benztropine comes in tablets, which can be taken immediately after meals or with a snack to decrease stomach upset. Benztropine also is given by injection.

What to do if you forget to take a dose of benztropine depends on when you remember the missed dose. If your next scheduled dose is more than four hours away, take the missed dose when you remember it and then continue with your regular dosing schedule. If your next scheduled dose is less than four hours away, take the missed dose when you remember it but do not take another dose for four hours. Take any remaining doses for that day at least four hours apart. If you miss two or more doses in a row, take only one dose when you remember the missed doses. *Do not take more than one dose at a time.*

STORAGE
Keep benztropine in the container it came in, and keep it out of the reach of children. Do not allow anyone else to take your benztropine.

Levodopa
(lee voe doe' pa)

PRODUCT INFORMATION
Brand names: Bendopa, Bio-Dopa, Dopar, Larodopa; Sinemet (a combination of levodopa and carbidopa)

USES
Levodopa is used to relieve the shaking, stiffness and slowness of movement that are some of the symptoms of Parkinson's disease. Levodopa is given alone or in combination with other medicines for Parkinson's disease.

Levodopa also is used to relieve the severe pain caused by some kinds of tumors.

UNDESIRED EFFECTS

Nausea, vomiting, stomach pain and loss of appetite are among the most common side effects of levodopa. Take this medicine with solid food to decrease the chance of stomach upset. Usually these effects occur when you start to take levodopa and then disappear as your body adjusts to the medicine. If they continue or are severe, contact your doctor; your doctor may want to change the amount you are taking.

Other common but mild effects include dry or watery mouth, increased shaking of the hands, inability to walk straight, difficulty falling asleep, headache, dizziness, nightmares, fatigue, depression, constipation and diarrhea. Contact your doctor if any of these effects cause you great discomfort.

Levodopa causes some people to become dizzy or drowsy. Do not drive a car or operate dangerous machinery until you know how this medication will affect you.

Levodopa may cause your urine, saliva and sweat to change color, becoming pinkish-red to almost black. This effect is not important and can be expected during treatment with this medicine.

More serious side effects can occur, and they require medical attention when they do. Contact your doctor if you experience unusual behavior; abnormal and uncontrollable movements of the mouth, tongue, face, neck, arms or legs; difficulty urinating; dizziness when arising quickly from a sitting or lying position; or rapid heartbeat.

PRECAUTIONS

Because levodopa may make some medical conditions worse, tell your doctor if you have diabetes, emphysema, asthma, bronchitis or other chronic lung disease, glaucoma, heart or blood vessel disease, hormone problems, kidney disease, liver disease, mental illness, skin cancer or a stomach ulcer.

Before you start to take levodopa, tell your doctor what prescription or nonprescription drugs you are taking, including medicine for asthma or bronchitis (such as epinephrine, ephedrine or isoproterenol), haloperidol, medicine for appetite control, medicine for high blood pressure, methyldopa, papaverine, phenytoin, pyridoxine (vitamin B_6) and reserpine. If you do not know the names of the drugs or what they were prescribed for, bring them in their labeled containers to your doctor or pharmacist.

If you are taking any of the phenothiazine medicines (chlorpromazine, fluphenazine, perphenazine, prochlorperazine, trifluoperazine or triflupromazine) or MAO inhibitors (isocarboxazid, pargyline, phenelzine and tranylcypromine), tell your doctor.

Vitamin B_6 has been shown to reduce the effects of levodopa. Do not take vitamin products containing vitamin B_6 or eat large amounts of food that have a lot of vitamin B_6 in them. These foods include avocado, bacon, beans, beef liver, dry skim milk, oatmeal, peas, pork, sweet potatoes, tuna fish and certain health foods. If you have questions about choosing vitamin products or about your diet, check with your doctor or pharmacist.

Take levodopa exactly as directed. Do not take more or less of it, and do not take it more often than your doctor tells you to. Do not stop taking this medicine unless your doctor tells you to do so.

As your condition improves and it is easier for you to move about, be careful not to overdo physical activities. It is important that you increase your activity gradually so you can avoid falls and injuries from falling.

Before having any kind of surgery, including dental surgery, tell the doctor or dentist in charge that you are taking levodopa.

If you have diabetes, levodopa may cause inaccurate test results for sugar and ketones in your urine. Check with your doctor before changing your medicine for diabetes on the basis of tests done by the paper-strip or tablet methods.

Be sure to tell your doctor if you are pregnant or are nursing a baby. Levodopa may cause your milk to dry up, and levodopa can be passed to the baby through the milk. Safe use of levodopa in pregnant women has not been established.

DOSAGE

Your doctor will determine how much levodopa you should take and how often you should take it. Carefully follow the instructions on your prescription label, and ask your doctor or pharmacist to explain any part of the instructions you do not understand.

Levodopa comes in tablets and capsules and usually is taken several times a day. This medicine should be taken with solid food or a glass of milk to prevent stomach upset.

Your doctor may have you take only a small amount of levodopa when you first start treatment and then increase the amount gradually so your body can adjust to the medicine. Be sure to keep in touch with your doctor while you are taking levodopa, and carefully follow instructions concerning the amount you should take.

Levodopa takes time to work. Some people do not obtain relief from their symptoms until they have been taking it for several months. If you have any questions, check with your doctor or pharmacist.

If you forget to take a dose of levodopa, take it as soon as you remember. Take any remaining doses for the day at evenly spaced intervals. *Do not take a double dose to make up for a missed dose.*

STORAGE

Keep levodopa in the container it came in. Store the container away from direct sunlight and excessive heat and out of the reach of children. Keep the container tightly closed.

Do not allow anyone else to take your levodopa, which was prescribed for your particular condition.

Trihexyphenidyl

(trye hex ee fen' i dill)

PRODUCT INFORMATION

Brand names: Artane, Pipanol, Tremin

USES

Trihexyphenidyl is used to treat Parkinson's disease and the palsy-like side effects of certain other drugs. Trihexyphenidyl improves muscle control and relieves stiffness to allow more normal body movements.

UNDESIRED EFFECTS

Trihexyphenidyl may cause excess saliva in the mouth or stomach upset. To relieve stomach upset, take the medicine after meals or with food.

Dry mouth is a common effect of trihexyphenidyl. Chewing gum, sucking hard candy or dissolving bits of ice in your mouth will help relieve this effect.

Trihexyphenidyl causes some people to become drowsy or dizzy. Do not drive a car or operate dangerous machinery until you know how trihexyphenidyl will affect you. These effects often are mild and tend to disappear as your body adjusts to the medicine. However, if they continue or are severe, contact your doctor.

More serious side effects will require medical attention if they occur. Contact your doctor if you have difficulty urinating, constipation, blurred vision, fast heartbeat or pulse, fever, skin rash, extreme confusion or agitation.

PRECAUTIONS

To help your doctor select the best treatment for you, tell your doctor if you have difficulty urinating, enlarged prostate, glaucoma, high blood pressure, intestinal blockage, kidney disease, liver disease or myasthenia gravis. Trihexyphenidyl may make these medical conditions worse.

Before you start to take trihexyphenidyl, tell your doctor what prescription or nonprescription drugs you are taking, including amantadine, antacids, antihistamines, medicines for allergies or colds, haloperidol, medicine for your heart, medicine for diarrhea, medicine to help you sleep, medicine for your nerves, other medicine for Parkinson's disease, sedatives, tranquilizers, medicine for ulcers and MAO inhibitors (isocarboxazid, pargyline, phenelzine and tranylcypromine), even if you stopped taking them in the past two weeks. If you do not know the names of the drugs you are taking or what they were prescribed for, bring them in their labeled containers to your doctor or pharmacist.

Take trihexyphenidyl exactly as prescribed by your doctor. Your doctor may want you to start with a small dose and increase it gradually after determining your response to it. *Keep all your appointments for checkups with your doctor.*

Because trihexyphenidyl may cause you to sweat less, you may easily become overheated while you are taking this medicine. To prevent heat prostration or sunstroke, be careful not to exert yourself excessively on hot days or in heated places.

Do not drink alcoholic beverages while you are taking trihexyphenidyl. Alcohol can increase the chance of and severity of side effects. If you have questions, check with your doctor or pharmacist. Do not start to take any of the medicines listed above unless you have your doctor's permission.

Do not take trihexyphenidyl within an hour of taking an antacid or a medicine for diarrhea. If these two medicines are taken too close together, trihexyphenidyl may be less effective.

DOSAGE

Your doctor will determine how much trihexyphenidyl you should take and how often you should take it. Carefully follow the instructions on your prescription label, and ask your doctor or pharmacist to explain any part of the instructions you do not understand.

Trihexyphenidyl comes in tablets and in liquid form and usually is taken three or four times a day. Both forms may be taken after meals or with food to lessen the chance of stomach upset.

If you forget to take a dose of trihexyphenidyl, take it as soon as you remember. Then take any remaining doses for that day at evenly spaced intervals. However, if you remember the missed dose when it is time for you to take another, take only the regularly scheduled dose. Omit the missed dose entirely. *Do not take a double dose to make up for a missed dose.*

STORAGE

Keep this medicine in the container it came in, and keep it out of the reach of children. Do not allow anyone else to take your trihexyphenidyl.

Thyroid Disease

DRUGS USED TO TREAT
THYROID DISEASE

Thyroid Disease

The thyroid gland is located in the neck just below the voice box. The thyroid gland produces hormones that regulate all the metabolism in the body.

When the thyroid gland is overactive (hyperthyroidism), excessive hormone levels cause the body's metabolism to speed up. This results in weight loss, excessive growth (particularly in children), rapid heartbeat, increased blood pressure and respiratory rate, diarrhea, excitement and muscle tremors. An underactive thyroid (hypothyroidism) causes just the opposite.

The causes of thyroid disease are, for the most part, unknown. Hyperthyroidism occurs more commonly in young adult women and in cold climates and is hereditary. In addition to the symptoms mentioned earlier, hyperthyroidism causes the thyroid gland to increase in size; in most people it causes the eyes to bulge.

Hypothyroidism also increases the size of the thyroid gland. In severe cases, the body retains additional fluid and the result is a swollen, bloated appearance.

Treatment of hyperthyroidism is aimed at decreasing the amount of thyroid hormone produced. This is accomplished by using drugs that decrease thyroid hormone output or through surgery. Hypothyroidism is corrected by administering additional thyroid, which is produced from animals or made synthetically.

DRUGS FOR OVERACTIVE THYROID

Methimazole

(meth im′ a zole)

PRODUCT INFORMATION
Brand name: Tapazole

USES

Methimazole is used to treat hyperthyroidism, a condition that occurs when the thyroid gland produces too much thyroid hormone. Methimazole also may be given to people before they have surgery for goiter.

UNDESIRED EFFECTS

Methimazole can cause skin rash. Rashes over a small area of skin may disappear without treatment. However, if the rash lasts more than a few days or covers a lot of your body, contact your doctor.

Other side effects, which tend to disappear as your body adjusts to methimazole, are itching, dizziness, pain in joints, loss of taste and stomach pain. If you experience these effects and they are severe or cause you great discomfort, contact your doctor.

More serious side effects, when they occur, will require medical attention. Stop taking this medicine and contact your doctor immediately if you have fever and chills, sore throat, loss of hearing, swelling of the lymph nodes in the neck, severe skin rash, unusual bleeding or bruising, unusual increase or decrease in urination, backache, swelling of the feet and lower legs or yellowing of the eyes and skin.

PRECAUTIONS

Before you start to take methimazole, tell your doctor if you have blood disease, any kind of infection or liver disease.

Tell your doctor what prescription or nonprescription drugs you are taking, including anticoagulants (blood thinners). If you do not know the names of the drugs or what they were prescribed for, bring them in their labeled containers to your doctor or pharmacist.

Take methimazole exactly as prescribed. Do not take more or less of it, and do not take it more often or for a longer period of time than your doctor has ordered.

To work properly, methimazole must be taken every day in regularly spaced doses. Be sure you have enough of this medicine on hand at all times to permit you to take all doses that have been prescribed for you. Check your supply before vacations, holidays and other times when it may be difficult for you to get more. You must take this medicine as often as your doctor tells you to, even if you have to get up during the night to take it.

Food in your stomach affects the way methimazole works. To be sure that you always get the same effect from each dose, take the prescribed doses *always* with meals or *always* on an empty stomach.

Your dosage of methimazole may have to be increased or decreased to obtain the desired effect. *Be sure to keep all your appointments for checkups* so that your doctor can monitor the effect this medicine is having on you.

Before you have any kind of surgery, including dental surgery, be sure to tell the doctor or dentist in charge that you are taking methimazole. Check with your doctor right away if you have an injury, infection or illness of any kind; your doctor may want you to stop taking this medicine.

If you are pregnant or are nursing a baby, you should not take methimazole. Be sure to tell your doctor if you are pregnant or think you may be. If you get pregnant while taking this medicine, contact your doctor at once.

DOSAGE

Your doctor will determine how much methimazole you should take and how often you should take it. Carefully follow the instructions on your prescription label, and ask your doctor or pharmacist to explain any part of the instructions you do not understand.

Methimazole comes in tablets. You may need to take this medicine for one or two weeks before you feel that it is working. Even if you do not see benefits immediately, continue to take this medicine as instructed.

If you forget to take a dose of methimazole, take it as soon as you remember and then take any remaining doses for that day at evenly spaced intervals. If you do not remember a missed dose until it is time for you to take another, omit the missed dose completely and take only the regularly scheduled dose. *Do not take two doses at one time.*

STORAGE

Keep methimazole in the container it came in, and store the container away from direct sunlight. Keep this medicine out of the reach of children. Do not allow anyone else to take your methimazole.

Propylthiouracil
(proe pill thye oh yoor' a sill)

PRODUCT INFORMATION
Brand name: Propacil

USES

Propylthiouracil is used to treat conditions in which the thyroid gland produces too much thyroid hormone. Propylthiouracil also may be used in preparation for surgery for goiter. When given before surgery, this medicine is usually combined with a strong iodine solution.

UNDESIRED EFFECTS

Propylthiouracil can cause skin rash, which may disappear in a few days without treatment if only a small area of the skin is involved. However, contact your doctor if you have a rash that lasts more than a few days or covers a lot of your body.

Side effects, which tend to disappear as your body adjusts to propylthiouracil, include itching, dizziness, joint pain, loss of taste and stomach pain. If these effects are severe or cause you great discomfort, contact your doctor.

More serious side effects include blood problems, severe allergic reactions, kidney problems and liver problems. Stop taking propylthiouracil and contact your doctor immediately if you have fever and chills, sore throat, loss of hearing, swelling of the lymph nodes in the neck, severe skin rash, unusual bleeding or bruising, unusual increase or decrease in urination, backache, swelling of the feet and lower legs or yellowing of the eyes and skin.

PRECAUTIONS

To help your doctor select the treatment best for you, tell your doctor if you have blood disease, any kind of infection or liver disease. Propylthiouracil can make these conditions worse.

Before you start taking propylthiouracil, tell your doctor what prescription or nonprescription drugs you are taking, particularly anticoagulants (blood thinners). If you do not know the names of the drugs or what they were prescribed for, bring them in their labeled containers to your doctor or pharmacist.

Take propylthiouracil exactly as prescribed. Do not take more or less of it, and do not take it more often or for a longer period of time than your doctor has ordered.

This medicine must be taken every day in regularly spaced doses to work properly. Be sure you have enough propylthiouracil on hand at all times to permit you to take all doses that have been prescribed for you. Check your supply before holidays, vacations and other times when it may be difficult for you to get more. You must take this medicine as often as your doctor tells you to, even if you have to get up during the night to take it.

Food in your stomach affects the way propylthiouracil works. To be sure you always get the same effect from each dose, take the prescribed doses *always* with meals or *always* on an empty stomach.

Your dosage of this medicine may have to be increased or decreased to obtain the desired effect. *Be sure to keep all your appointments for checkups* so that your doctor can monitor this medicine's effect on you.

Before you have any kind of surgery, including dental surgery, be sure to tell the doctor or dentist in charge that you are taking propylthiouracil. If you get an injury, infection or illness of any kind, check with your doctor right away; your doctor may want you to stop taking this medicine.

If you are pregnant or are nursing a baby, you should not take propylthiouracil. Be sure to tell your doctor if you are pregnant or think that you may be. If you get pregnant while taking ths medicine, contact your doctor at once.

DOSAGE

Your doctor will determine how much propylthiouracil you should take and how often you should take it. Carefully follow the instructions on your prescription label, and ask your doctor or pharmacist to explain any part of the instructions you do not understand.

Propylthiouracil comes in tablets to be taken orally. You may need to take this medicine for one or two weeks before you feel that it is working. Even if you do not see benefits immediately, continue to take propylthiouracil as instructed.

If you forget to take a dose of propylthiouracil, take it as soon as you remember. Then take the remaining doses for that day at evenly spaced intervals. If you do not remember a missed dose until it is time for you to take another, omit the missed dose entirely and take only the regularly scheduled dose. *Do not take two doses at one time*.

STORAGE

Keep this medicine in the container it came in, and keep it out of the reach of children. Store propylthiouracil away from direct sunlight. Do not allow anyone else to take your propylthiouracil.

DRUGS FOR UNDERACTIVE THYROID

Iodine
(eye′ o dyne)

PRODUCT INFORMATION
Other names: Lugol's solution, potassium iodide, saturated solution of potassium iodide, SSKI, strong iodine

USES
Iodine, also called strong iodine solution, is used alone or with other antithyroid medicine to treat certain types of goiter or in preparation for goiter surgery. Potassium iodide solution has also been used as an expectorant in people with asthma to make the mucus in the air passages easier to cough up.

UNDESIRED EFFECTS
Strong iodine solution can cause allergic reactions. Stop taking the medicine and contact your doctor immediately if you experience swelling of the larynx (voice box), skin rash, swelling of the salivary glands or increased salivation.

PRECAUTIONS
If you have ever reacted to strong iodine solution in any of the ways described above, you should not take this medicine. Before you start to take iodine, tell your doctor if you have tuberculosis or kidney disease; strong iodine solution can make these conditions worse.

Tell your doctor what prescription or nonprescription drugs you are taking. If you do not know the names of the drugs or what they were prescribed for, bring them in their labeled containers to your doctor or pharmacist.

DOSAGE
Your doctor will determine how much of this medicine you should take and how often you should take it. Carefully follow the instructions on your prescription label, and ask your doctor or pharmacist to explain any part of the instructions you do not understand.

Strong iodine solution comes in liquid form and usually is taken mixed with water three times a day after meals. If you forget to take a dose of this medicine, take it as soon as you remember. If you do not remember a missed dose until it is almost time for you to take another, take both doses together and return to your regular schedule. If you have any questions, check with your doctor or pharmacist.

STORAGE
Keep this medicine in the container it came in. Store it in a cool, dark place, but

do not refrigerate it. If the liquid turns yellowish-brown, discard it and get a fresh supply. Do not allow anyone else to take your iodine.

Thyroid Hormone Preparations
(thye' roid)

PRODUCT INFORMATION
Brand names for thyroid USP: Armour Thyroid, S-P-T, Thyrar
Brand names for levothyroxine: Letter, Levoid, Levothroid, Synthroid, Titroid
Brand name for liothyronine: Cytomel
Brand names for liotrix: Euthroid, Thyrolar
Brand name for thyroglobulin: Proloid

USES
Thyroid is a hormone produced by the body that regulates the body's metabolism. When too little of this important hormone is produced by the thyroid gland, the result usually is poor growth, slow speech, lack of energy, weight gain, hair loss, dry and thick skin or increased sensitivity to cold. To treat these symptoms, your doctor will prescribe thyroid hormone, either that extracted from the thyroid glands of animals or made in the laboratory. Thyroid hormone, when taken correctly, can reverse all symptoms of hypothyroidism.

UNDESIRED EFFECTS
Side effects of thyroid hormone preparations include rapid heart rate, weight loss, chest pain, tremor, headache, diarrhea, nervousness, insomnia, sweating and heat intolerance. If any of these effects occur, stop taking the medicine and contact your doctor immediately. In most cases, a reduction in dose is all that is necessary.

Thyroid hormone preparations may take a few weeks to begin relieving the symptoms of hypothyroidism that were described earlier (see section on Uses). If these symptoms persist longer than a few weeks or if they become worse after you begin to take a thyroid hormone preparation, contact your doctor.

When you begin to take a thyroid hormone preparation, it may take several weeks to get your dosage correctly adjusted. If your dose is too low, some symptoms of hypothyroidism (see section on Uses) will remain. If, on the other hand, your dose is too high, you may experience nervousness, diarrhea, weight loss, fever, muscle tremors or cramps and insomnia. Check with your doctor if any of these effects occur.

PRECAUTIONS
Because thyroid hormone preparations can make certain medical conditions worse, tell your doctor if you have diabetes, hardening of the arteries, heart disease, high blood pressure, history of an overactive thyroid gland, kidney disease, liver disease, underactive adrenal gland or underactive pituitary gland.

Tell your doctor what prescription or nonprescription drugs you are taking, including anticoagulants (blood thinners), cholestyramine, cough syrup or cold medicine, medicine for diabetes, phenytoin and medicine for depression. If you do not know the names of the drugs or what they were prescribed for, bring them in their labeled containers to your doctor or pharmacist.

Take this medicine exactly as prescribed. Do not take more or less of it, and do not take it more often than your doctor has ordered. For the best effect, try to take your thyroid hormone preparation at the same time each day.

Since your condition is due to a lack of thyroid hormone, you may have to take this medicine for the rest of your life. However, your doctor may have to adjust the dose from time to time to fit your body's needs. *Be sure to keep all appointments with your doctor for checkups.*

Do not stop taking your thyroid hormone preparation without your doctor's permission. Be sure you have enough medicine on hand at all times to take the doses you need. Check your supply before vacations, holidays and other times when it may not be possible to get more.

Before you have any kind of surgery, including dental surgery or emergency treatment, tell the doctor or dentist in charge that you are taking this medicine.

Before you start to take any other medicine, particularly an ''over the counter'' medicine, check with your doctor or pharmacist to make sure the other medicine will not interfere with the way your thyroid hormone preparation works.

DOSAGE

Your doctor will determine how much thyroid hormone preparation you should take and how often you should take it. Carefully follow the instructions on your prescription label, and ask your doctor or pharmacist to explain any part of the instructions you do not understand.

If your doctor tells you to take this medicine once a day, it may be easier for you to remember to take it if you take it at the same time you do something else each day, such as brushing your teeth in the morning or eating dinner at night.

Thyroid hormone preparations come in tablets and capsules. If you forget to take a dose of this medicine, take it as soon as you remember. However, if you do not remember a missed dose until it is time for you to take another, omit the missed dose completely and take only the regularly scheduled dose. *Do not take two doses at one time.*

STORAGE

Keep this medicine in the container it came in. Keep it out of the reach of children. Do not let anyone else take your thyroid hormone preparation.

Sleep Disturbances

DRUGS USED TO TREAT
SLEEP DISTURBANCES

Sleep Disturbances

One national health survey showed that about one-third of the U.S. population experienced some type of sleep problem at some time. The exact nature and severity of sleep problems are difficult to evaluate because sleep needs vary from person to person.

Usually, trouble in sleeping is minor and only lasts for a few nights. Jet lag, ache and pain from minor illness and emotional upsets are common causes of such problems.

The following measures sometimes are helpful in avoiding sleep problems:
- avoiding the consumption of large meals before bedtime
- avoiding taking daytime naps
- avoiding the consumption of coffee and soft drinks that contain caffeine
- performing light exercise in the early evening
- keeping the bedroom dark and quiet

In some cases, trouble in sleeping can be severe enough to cause problems with normal daytime activities. If such trouble continues for weeks, you may have to consult your doctor to determine the cause. A number of medical conditions can cause insomnia, including thyroid malfunction, diabetes, depression and respiratory problems. Your doctor will want to determine if any of these conditions is the cause of your sleeping problem.

Your doctor may prescribe a medication to help you sleep. Several types of medications are available, but they all encourage sleep by depressing the central nervous system. These medications are used only for short periods because they can be habit-forming and can disrupt sleep patterns. It is important that you carefully follow your doctor's instructions. Do not take more of these medications or take them more often than your doctor has instructed.

All medications to help you sleep cause drowsiness that may linger into the daytime. Do not drive a car or operate dangerous machinery until you know how they will affect you.

Alcohol, tranquilizers, muscle relaxants, antihistamines, antidepressants and some medicines for pain will increase the effect of sleeping medications. Be sure to tell your doctor or pharmacist what medicines you are taking before you begin to use medications to help you sleep.

Medications to help you sleep are called sedatives or hypnotics. Generally, hypnotics are taken at bedtime to help you fall asleep. Sedatives can be taken during the day to help calm you and make you less nervous or excitable and at bedtime to help you fall asleep.

Barbiturates
(bar bi′ tyoo rates)

PRODUCT INFORMATION
Brand name for amobarbital (am oh bar′ bi tal): Amytal
Brand names for butabarbital (byoo ta bar′ bi tal): Buta-Kay, Butal, Buticaps, Butisol
Brand name for pentobarbital (pen toe bar′ bi tal): Nembutal
Brand names for phenobarbital (fee noe bar′ bi tal): Barbita, Barbipil, Luminal, Sherital, Solfoton
Brand name for secobarbital (see koe bar′ bi tal): Seconal
Brand name for a combination product containing amobarbital and secobarbital: Tuinal

USES
Barbiturates depress the central nervous system. They are used to help people fall asleep and stay asleep through the night. They also are prescribed to help relieve anxiety and tension. Some barbiturates are helpful in controlling epileptic seizures and convulsions caused by certain diseases.

Many of the barbiturates listed above are included in combination products with other drugs. A commonly prescribed combination containing amobarbital and secobarbital has the brand name Tuinal.

UNDESIRED EFFECTS
The drowsiness caused by barbiturates may persist until the next day, even though you take the medicine at bedtime. Even low doses taken during the day to control seizures may cause drowsiness. Do not drive a car, operate dangerous machinery or engage in any activity that requires mental alertness until you know how barbiturates will affect you.

Less often, barbiturates will cause diarrhea, headache, joint or muscle pain, nausea or vomiting and slurred speech. These effects may disappear as you continue to take the drug and as your body adjusts to it. If they continue or get worse, contact your doctor.

More serious side effects of barbiturates are allergic reactions, blood problems, liver problems and too much depression of the central nervous system. If any of these effects occur, they will require medical attention. Contact your doctor if you have mental confusion or depression; shortness of breath or difficulty breathing; skin rash or hives; sore throat and fever; swelling of the eyelids, face or lips; unusual bleeding or bruising; unusual excitement (more likely in children or older people); unusual tiredness or weakness; unusually slow heartbeat; wheezing or tightness in the chest; or yellowing of the eyes and skin.

When you stop taking a barbiturate, your body may need time to adjust, particularly if you have been taking it for a long time. During this adjustment period, be alert for symptoms of withdrawal. Contact your doctor if you have convulsions or seizures, faintness, hallucinations (seeing, hearing or feeling things that are not there), increased dreaming, nightmares, trembling, difficulty sleeping, unusual rest-lessness or unusual weakness.

PRECAUTIONS

If you ever had an unusual reaction to any barbiturate—the ones listed above or aprobarbital, hexobarbital, mephobarbital and talbutal—you should not take a bar-biturate. If you have any questions, check with your doctor or pharmacist.

Because barbiturates can make some medical conditions worse, tell your doctor if you have asthma (or a history of this problem), emphysema, any other chronic disease, hyperactivity (in children), kidney disease, liver disease, porphyria (or a history of it) or underactive adrenal glands.

Barbiturates taken with certain other medicines can increase the chance of and/or severity of side effects. These medicines include antihistamines, medicine for aller-gies or colds, narcotics, other barbiturates, prescription medicine for pain, sedatives, tranquilizers, medicine to help you sleep, medicine for seizures, medicine for depression, MAO inhibitors (isocarboxazid, pargyline, phenelzine or tranylcypro-mine), even if you stopped taking them within the past two weeks, anticoagulants (blood thinners), steroids, digitalis, digitoxin, doxycycline, griseofulvin and pheny-toin.

Tell your doctor what prescription or nonprescription medicines you are taking. If you do not know the names of the drugs or what they were prescribed for, bring them in their labeled containers to your doctor or pharmacist.

Do not drink alcoholic beverages while you are taking barbiturates. Do not start taking any of the drugs listed above unless you have your doctor's permission. You can avoid serious side effects this way.

Because barbiturates can be habit-forming, take them only as directed by your doctor. Do not take more of them, do not take them more often and do not take them for a longer time than your doctor has ordered.

If you accidentally take too much of a barbiturate, contact your doctor immedi-ately or go to the nearest hospital emergency room. Signs of overdosage are delirium, confusion, shortness of breath, difficult breathing, unusually slow or irregular heartbeat, deep sleep and coma. Overdosage can cause death.

Do not stop taking this medicine unless you first check with your doctor. Your doctor may want you to reduce the amount you take gradually before you stop completely. Be sure you have enough medicine to take all doses prescribed. Check your supply before vacations and holidays when it may be difficult for you to get more.

If you will be taking a barbiturate for a long period of time, your doctor will want to check your response to the drug at regular visits. *Be sure to keep all appointments with your doctor.*

To help your doctor select the best treatment for you and your baby, be sure to tell your doctor if you are pregnant or are breast-feeding a baby. If you become pregnant while taking a barbiturate, notify your doctor at once.

DOSAGE

Your doctor will determine how often you should take a barbiturate and how much you should take at each dose. When this medicine is prescribed to help control seizures and convulsions, it must be taken on a regular schedule to be effective. If you are taking a barbiturate to relieve anxiety and restlessness, your doctor may want you to take it at evenly spaced intervals during the day or, to help you sleep, at bedtime. Carefully follow the instructions on your prescription label, and ask your doctor or pharmacist to explain any part of the instructions you do not understand.

Barbiturates come in extended-release capsules, tablets and liquid form to be taken orally and in rectal suppositories. Do not break, crush or chew the capsules or tablets. They are to be swallowed whole.

The liquid form comes with a dropper for measuring the correct dose. Be sure you know how to use the dropper. If you have questions, ask your doctor or pharmacist. Each dose may be taken straight or mixed with water, milk or fruit juice. Do not use the liquid if it has become cloudy.

The rectal suppository should be removed from the foil wrapper and the tip moistened with water. Then lie on your side, bring your top knee up to your chest, insert the suppository well into your rectum with your finger and hold it there for a few moments. Try not to have a bowel movement for at least an hour after inserting the suppository.

If you forget to take a dose of this medicine, take it as soon as you remember and take the remaining doses for that day at evenly spaced intervals. However, if you do not remember a missed dose until it is almost time to take another, omit the missed dose entirely and take only the regularly scheduled dose. *Do not take two doses to make up for a missed dose.*

STORAGE
Keep this medicine in the container it came in. Keep it out of the reach of children, because an overdose is especially dangerous in children. Do not allow anyone else to take your barbiturates.

Chloral Hydrate
(klor al hey' drate)

PRODUCT INFORMATION
Brand names: Aquachloral, Cohidrate, Kessodrate, Noctec and others

USES
Chloral hydrate is a sedative and hypnotic drug used to treat sleeplessness or insomnia. It helps people fall asleep and stay asleep through the night. Usually it begins to work in 30 to 60 minutes. It also is used to help calm or relax people who are anxious, tense or nervous.

UNDESIRED EFFECTS
The most common side effects of chloral hydrate are indigestion, nausea, stomach

pain and vomiting. To lessen stomach upset, take this medicine with water, milk, fruit juice or ginger ale.

Chloral hydrate makes some people drowsy, dizzy, lightheaded, clumsy or unsteady on their feet. Do not drive a car or operate dangerous machinery until you know how this medicine will affect you. These effects tend to lessen or disappear as you continue to take chloral hydrate and as your body adjusts to it. If they continue or they bother you, contact your doctor.

More serious side effects do not occur very often but will need medical attention if they do occur. Contact your doctor if you have an allergic reaction (skin rash or hives), hallucinations (seeing, hearing or feeling things that are not there), mental confusion or unusual excitement.

After you stop taking chloral hydrate, your body may need time to adjust. For a few weeks after you stop taking this medicine, be alert for withdrawal problems. Contact your doctor if you have hallucinations, mental confusion, nausea, nervousness, restlessness, stomach pain, trembling, unusual excitement or vomiting.

PRECAUTIONS

Before you start to take chloral hydrate, tell your doctor if you have heart disease, kidney disease or liver disease. This medicine may make these conditions worse.

Tell your doctor what prescription or nonprescription drugs you are taking, including antihistamines, medicine for allergies or colds, barbiturates, narcotics, other sedatives, tranquilizers, other medicine to help you sleep, prescription medicine for pain, medicine for seizures, medicine for depression, anticoagulants (blood thinners) or MAO inhibitors (isocarboxazid, pargyline, phenelzine or tranylcypromine), even if you stopped taking them within the past two weeks. If you do not know the names of the drugs or what they were prescribed for, bring them in their labeled containers to your doctor or pharmacist.

Do not drink alcoholic beverages while you are taking chloral hydrate. Do not start taking any of the drugs listed above without your doctor's permission. All of them can increase the chance of and/or severity of side effects.

Because this medicine can be habit-forming and is potentially dangerous taken in large amounts or continually over a long time, be sure to take chloral hydrate exactly as prescribed by your doctor. Do not take more of it, do not take it more often and do not take it for a longer period than your doctor has prescribed.

If you accidentally take too much chloral hydrate, contact your doctor immediately or go to the nearest hospital emergency room. Signs of overdose are delirium, confusion, shortness of breath, difficult breathing, unusually slow or irregular heartbeat, deep sleep and coma.

Do not stop taking chloral hydrate without first checking with your doctor. Your doctor may want you to reduce the amount you are taking gradually before you stop completely.

If you will be taking chloral hydrate over a long period of time, your doctor will want to check your response to this medicine. *Be sure to keep all appointments with your doctor.*

Before you start to take chloral hydrate, tell your doctor if you are pregnant or are breast-feeding a baby. Safe use of this drug during pregnancy and while breast-feeding has not been established. If you become pregnant while taking this medicine, stop taking the drug immediately and contact your doctor.

DOSAGE

Your doctor will determine how often you should take chloral hydrate and how much you should take at each dose. Carefully follow the instructions on your prescription label, and ask your doctor or pharmacist to explain any part of the instructions you do not understand.

Chloral hydrate comes in capsules, tablets and liquid form to be taken orally and in rectal suppositories. The capsules and tablets should be taken with a full eight-ounce glass of water, milk, fruit juice or ginger ale to lessen the chance of upset stomach. Do not take any of the oral forms with solid food.

If you are taking the liquid form of chloral hydrate, it can be mixed with one-half glass (four ounces) of water or fruit juice.

To use the suppository, remove the foil wrapper and moisten the tip of the suppository with water. Then lie on your side, bring the knee of your top leg up to your chest, insert the suppository well into the rectum and hold it there for a few moments. Try not to have a bowel movement for at least an hour after inserting the suppository. If the suppository is too soft to insert, leave the wrapper on and put the wrapped suppository in the refrigerator for 30 minutes, or run cold water over it.

Chloral hydrate is prescribed to help you sleep. If you do not feel you need help in falling asleep on a certain night, you may omit the dose that night.

STORAGE

Keep chloral hydrate in the container it came in, and keep it out of the reach of children. Do not allow anyone else to take your chloral hydrate.

Flurazepam
(flure az' e pam)

PRODUCT INFORMATION
Brand name: Dalmane

USES

Flurazepam is one of the "benzodiazepine" group or family of drugs that is used as a sedative and hypnotic. It is used to treat sleeplessness or insomnia and helps people fall asleep and then remain asleep through the night. It seems to help restore normal sleep patterns with fewer problems than other drugs used to treat sleeplessness. Usually, flurazepam begins to work in 30 to 60 minutes.

UNDESIRED EFFECTS

The most common effects of flurazepam are clumsiness or unsteadiness, dizziness or lightheadedness and daytime drowsiness or "hangover," even though the medicine is taken at night. Do not drive a car, operate machinery or do anything that requires mental and/or physical alertness until you know how this medicine will affect you.

Less often, flurazepam will cause constipation, diarrhea, headache, heartburn, nausea or vomiting, slurred speech, stomach pain or unusual weakness or tiredness. These effects may disappear as you continue to take flurazepam and your body adjusts to it. If they continue or bother you, contact your doctor.

Rarely, flurazepam will cause more serious side effects, requiring medical attention. Contact your doctor if you experience hallucinations (seeing, hearing or feeling things that are not there), mental confusion or depression, skin rash or itching (signs of allergic reaction), unusual excitement, nervousness or irritability or yellowing of the skin and eyes (signs of a liver problem). If you take flurazepam for a long time, your doctor will probably ask you to have some laboratory tests, such as blood counts and tests for your liver and kidney functions.

After you stop taking flurazepam, your body may need time to adjust, particularly if you have been taking large doses or have been taking flurazepam for a long time. For at least two weeks after you stop taking this medicine, be alert for signs of withdrawal problems. Contact your doctor if you have convulsions or seizures, mental confusion, muscle cramps, nausea or vomiting, stomach cramps, trembling, unusual irritability or sweating.

PRECAUTIONS

If you ever had an unusual reaction to any medicine similar to flurazepam (alprazolam, chlordiazepoxide, clonazepam, clorazepate, diazepam, lorazepam, oxazepam, prazepam, temazepam or triazolam), you should not take flurazepam because you are likely to have a bad reaction to it. If you have any questions, check with your doctor or pharmacist.

Before you start to take flurazepam, tell your doctor if you have emphysema, asthma, chronic bronchitis or any other chronic lung disease, kidney disease, liver disease, epilepsy, porphyria or mental depression. Flurazepam may make these conditions worse.

Tell your doctor what other prescription or nonprescription drugs you are taking, including barbiturates, narcotics, other sedatives, tranquilizers, other medicine to help you sleep, antihistamines, medicine for allergies or colds, prescription medicine for pain, medicine for seizures, medicine for depression or MAO inhibitors (isocarboxazid, pargyline, phenelzine or tranylcypromine), even if you stopped taking them within the past two weeks. If you do not know the names of the drugs or what they were prescribed for, bring them in their labeled containers to your doctor or pharmacist.

Do not drink alcoholic beverages while you are taking flurazepam. Do not start to take any of the drugs listed above without first checking with your doctor or pharmacist. All of them can increase the chance of and/or severity of side effects.

Because flurazepam can be habit-forming and potentially dangerous when taken in very large amounts or continually for a long time, take this medicine exactly as prescribed by your doctor. Do not take more of it, do not take it more often and do not take it for a longer period than your doctor has prescribed.

If you accidentally take too much flurazepam, contact your doctor immediately or go to the nearest hospital emergency room. Signs of an overdose include deep sleep or coma, confusion, delirium, unusually slow heartbeat, shortness of breath and difficult breathing.

If you have been taking large doses of flurazepam for a long time, do not stop taking this medicine without your doctor's permission. Your doctor may want you to reduce the amount you are taking gradually before you stop completely.

Children under the age of 15 years should not take flurazepam. Safe use of this medicine in this age group has not been established.

Before you start to take flurazepam, be sure to tell your doctor if you are pregnant or are nursing a baby. The effects of flurazepam on an unborn child or a breast-fed baby are not known.

DOSAGE
Your doctor will determine how much flurazepam you should take. Carefully follow the instructions on your prescription label, and ask your doctor or pharmacist to explain any part of the instructions you do not understand.

Flurazepam comes in capsules, which are taken at bedtime. Because this medicine can lose its effectiveness after several weeks of regular use, take it only when you cannot sleep. You do not need to follow a regular schedule.

You may have to take flurazepam for two or three nights before your sleeping problem improves. It will take this long for the medicine to reach its full effect.

STORAGE
Keep flurazepam in the container it came in, and keep it out of the reach of children. Do not allow anyone else to take your flurazepam.

Meprobamate
(me proe ba' mate)

PRODUCT INFORMATION
Brand names: Bamate, Bamo, Corpobate, Equanil, Kesso-Bamate, Mepriam, Meprospan, Miltown, SK-Bamate, Tranmep and others

Brand names of some products containing meprobamate in combination with other drugs: Deprol, Equagesic, Meprogesic, Mepro-Hex, Meprotrate, Milpath, Milprem, Miltrate, Pathibamate

USES
Meprobamate is a sedative used to help people fall asleep, particularly people who are anxious or tense. Usually it begins to work within two hours. It also is used to calm and relax people who are nervous, anxious or tense.

UNDESIRED EFFECTS
The most common side effects of meprobamate are clumsiness, unsteadiness and drowsiness. Even when you take this medicine at bedtime, you still may be drowsy

and less alert than normal on the next day. Do not drive a car or operate dangerous machinery until you know how this medicine will affect you.

Less often, meprobamate will cause blurred vision, a change in near or distant vision, diarrhea, dizziness or lightheadedness, headache, nausea or vomiting, slurred speech or unusual weakness or tiredness. These effects may disappear as you continue to take meprobamate and as your body adjusts to it. Contact your doctor if they continue or bother you.

More serious side effects do not occur often, but they may require medical attention if they do occur. Contact your doctor if you experience skin rash, itching or hives (signs of allergic reaction); unusual excitement; mental confusion; sore throat and fever; unusual bleeding or bruising (signs of blood problems); or unusually fast, pounding or irregular heartbeat. If you take this drug for a long time, your doctor probably will order laboratory tests, including a blood count.

When you stop taking meprobamate, your body may need time to adjust. For the next few days, contact your doctor if you have convulsions or seizures, hallucinations (seeing, hearing or feeling things that are not there), increased dreaming, muscle twitching, nausea or vomiting, nightmares, trembling, difficulty sleeping or unusual nervousness or restlessness.

PRECAUTIONS

You should not take meprobamate if you ever had an unusual reaction to similar medicines such as carbromal, carisoprodol, mebutamate and tybamate. If you have questions, check with your doctor or pharmacist.

Because meprobamate can make some medical conditions worse, tell your doctor if you have epilepsy, kidney or liver disease, impaired kidney or liver function or porphyria.

Tell your doctor what prescription or nonprescription drugs you are taking, including antihistamines, medicine for allergies or colds, barbiturates, narcotics, other sedatives, tranquilizers, other medicine to help you sleep, prescription medicine for pain, medicine for seizures, medicine for depression and MAO inhibitors (isocarboxazid, pargyline, phenelzine or tranylcypromine), even if you stopped taking them within the past two weeks.

Do not drink alcoholic beverages while you are taking meprobamate. Do not start taking any of the drugs listed above unless you first check with your doctor. All of them can increase the chance of and/or severity of side effects.

Meprobamate can be habit-forming. It is important that you take it exactly as prescribed by your doctor. Do not take more of it, do not take it more often and do not take it for a longer time than directed by your doctor.

If you accidentally take too much meprobamate, contact your doctor immediately or go to the nearest hospital emergency room. Signs of overdose are slurred speech, staggering, unusually slow heartbeat, wheezing, shortness of breath or difficult breathing, deep sleep and coma.

If you take meprobamate in large doses or over a long period, do not stop taking it until your doctor tells you that you may. Your doctor may want you to reduce the amount you are taking gradually before stopping completely.

If you will be taking meprobamate for a long time, your doctor will want to check your response to this medicine regularly. *Be sure to keep all your appointments with your doctor.* Check with your doctor at least every four months to be sure you need to continue taking meprobamate.

Before you start to take meprobamate, tell your doctor if you are pregnant or think you may be or if you are nursing a baby. The effects of this drug on an unborn child or a breast-fed baby are not known.

DOSAGE
Your doctor will determine how often you should take meprobamate and how much you should take at each dose. Carefully follow the instructions on your prescription label, and ask your doctor or pharmacist to explain any part of the instructions you do not understand. Meprobamate comes in capsules and tablets.

If you forget to take a dose, *do not* take the missed dose when you remember it. Omit it and take the next dose at the regularly scheduled time. *Do not take a double dose.*

STORAGE
Keep meprobamate in the container it came in, and keep it out of the reach of children. Do not allow anyone else to take your meprobamate.

Temazepam
(te maz′ e pam)

PRODUCT INFORMATION
Brand name: Restoril

USES
Temazepam is used to help people fall asleep and stay asleep during the night.

UNDESIRED EFFECTS
Temazepam causes drowsiness and may affect your coordination and ability to exercise judgment, even on the morning following the dose. Do not drive a car, operate dangerous machinery or do anything that requires mental and physical alertness after you have taken a dose. Other side effects that are less common are tiredness, confusion, weakness, loss of appetite and diarrhea.

After you stop taking temazepam, your body may need time to adjust, particularly if you have been taking large doses or have been taking temazepam for a long time. For at least two weeks after you stop taking this medicine, be alert for signs of withdrawal problems. Contact your doctor if you have convulsions or seizures, mental confusion, muscle cramps, nausea or vomiting, stomach cramps, trembling, unusual irritability or sweating.

PRECAUTIONS
If you ever had an unusual reaction to any medicine similar to temazepam

(alprazolam, chlordiazepoxide, clonazepam, clorazepate, diazepam, flurazepam, lorazepam, oxazepam, prazepam or triazolam), you should not take temazepam because you are likely to have a bad reaction to it. If you have any questions, check with your doctor or pharmacist.

Before you start to take temazepam, tell your doctor if you have kidney disease, liver disease, epilepsy or mental depression. Temazepam may make these conditions worse.

Tell your doctor what other prescription or nonprescription drugs you are taking, including barbiturates, narcotics, other sedatives, tranquilizers, other medicine to help you sleep, antihistamines, medicine for allergies or colds, prescription medicine for pain, medicine for seizures or medicine for depression. If you do not know the names of the drugs or what they were prescribed for, bring them in their labeled containers to your doctor or pharmacist.

Do not drink alcoholic beverages while you are taking temazepam. Do not start taking any of the drugs listed above without first checking with your doctor or pharmacist. All of them can increase the chance of and/or severity of side effects.

Because temazepam can be habit-forming and potentially dangerous when taken in very large amounts or continually for a long period, take this medicine exactly as prescribed by your doctor. Do not take more of it, do not take it more often and do not take it for a longer time than your doctor has prescribed.

If you accidentally take too much temazepam, contact your doctor immediately or go to the nearest hospital emergency room. Signs of an overdose include deep sleep or coma, confusion, delirium, unusually slow heartbeat, shortness of breath and difficult breathing.

If you have been taking large doses of temazepam for a long time, do not stop taking this medicine without your doctor's permission. Your doctor may want you to reduce the amount you are taking gradually before you stop completely.

Children should not take temazepam. Safe use of this medicine in children under 18 has not been established.

Before you start to take temazepam, be sure to tell your doctor if you are pregnant or are nursing a baby. The effects of temazepam on an unborn child or a breast-fed baby are not known.

DOSAGE

Temazepam comes in capsules to be taken by mouth. Your doctor will determine how much temazepam you should take. Carefully follow the instructions on your prescription label, and ask your doctor or pharmacist to explain any part of the instructions you do not understand. Because this drug may lose its effectiveness after several weeks of use, take it only when you cannot sleep.

STORAGE

Keep this medication in the container it came in and out of the reach of children.

Triazolam
(trye ay′ zoe lam)

PRODUCT INFORMATION
Brand name: Halcion

USES
Triazolam is one of the group of drugs known as benzodiazepines. It is used to treat sleeplessness or insomnia.

UNDESIRED EFFECTS
Common effects during the first few days of therapy are drowsiness, dizziness and weakness. Do not drive a car or operate dangerous machinery until you know how triazolam will affect you. If fatigue continues past the first few days, contact your doctor.

If this medicine makes your mouth dry, suck hard candies or chew gum. Headache and slurring of speech may occur when you start to take triazolam and then disappear as your body adjusts to it.

More serious side effects, which will require medical attention, include allergic reactions, blood problems, liver problems and signs that your body is not tolerating the drug well. Contact your doctor if you have mental confusion, depression, skin rash or itching, trouble sleeping, unusual nervousness or irritability, unusually slow heartbeat, shortness of breath, difficulty breathing, continuing ulcers or sores in the mouth or throat or yellowing of the eyes or skin.

If you have taken triazolam for a long time, you may have withdrawal symptoms when you stop taking this medicine. Contact your doctor if you experience mental confusion, muscle cramps, nausea or vomiting, stomach cramps, trembling, unusual sweating or seizures.

PRECAUTIONS
Before you start taking this medicine, tell your doctor if you ever had an unusual reaction to any of the benzodiazepines (alprazolam, chlordiazepoxide, clonazepam, clorazepate, diazepam, flurazepam, lorazepam, oxazepam, prazepam and temazepam). You are more likely to have a bad reaction to triazolam if you have reacted badly to any of these other drugs.

Tell your doctor if you have any of these medical problems: asthma, emphysema, bronchitis or other chronic lung disease, glaucoma, kidney disease, liver disease, mental depression, myasthenia gravis, severe mental illness or hyperactivity (in children). Triazolam may make these conditions worse.

Certain medication may increase the possibility or severity of side effects when taken with triazolam. Tell your doctor what prescription or nonprescription drugs you are taking, including antihistamines or medicine for hay fever, other allergies or colds; barbiturates, narcotics or other sedatives; tranquilizers or medicine to help you sleep; prescription medicine for pain; medicine for depression; or MAO inhibitors (isocarboxazid, pargyline, phenelzine or tranylcypromine), even if you have not taken them for two weeks. If you do not know the names of the drugs you are taking, check with your doctor or pharmacist before taking triazolam because serious side effects can result from certain combinations. Do not start taking any of the drugs listed above without checking first with your doctor or pharmacist.

Take this medication exactly as directed by your doctor. Do not take more of it, do not take it more often and do not take it for a longer period than your doctor has ordered. This medicine can be habit-forming if you take it too often. Keep all appointments with your doctor.

Before you start to take triazolam, tell your doctor if you are pregnant, if you intend to become pregnant while taking this medicine or if you are nursing a baby. If you become pregnant while taking triazolam, stop taking the drug and contact your doctor.

DOSAGE
Triazolam comes in tablets to be taken by mouth at bedtime. Your doctor will determine how much triazolam you should take. Carefully follow the instructions on your prescription label, and ask your doctor or pharmacist to explain any part of the instructions you do not understand.

STORAGE
Keep this medicine in the container it came in and out of the reach of children.

Psychiatric Problems

DRUGS USED TO TREAT
PSYCHIATRIC PROBLEMS

Anxiety

A feeling of anxiety or fear in the face of danger is a normal reaction that is part of the body's "fight or flight" response. When the threat is real, fear is an appropriate response that is essential to survival. However, if the threat is nonexistent or trivial or if the level of anxiety greatly exceeds that indicated by the situation, the anxiety is considered inappropriate.

Anxiety may be manifested in different ways. Many patients never experience feelings of anxiety but have symptoms such as chest pain, palpitations, breathlessness and fatigue. Often, anxiety is found to be the cause of these symptoms after a thorough evaluation rules out other disease.

Treatment of anxiety relies on both psychotherapy and drugs. Because the nature of the problem varies greatly among individuals, treatment is tailored to each individual.

Alprazolam
(al pray' zoe lam)

PRODUCT INFORMATION
Brand name: Xanax

USES
Alprazolam is one of the group of drugs known as benzodiazepines. It is used to treat anxiety disorders and for anxiety associated with depression.

UNDESIRED EFFECTS
Common effects during the first few days of therapy are drowsiness, dizziness and lightheadedness. Do not drive a car or operate dangerous machinery until you know how alprazolam will affect you. If fatigue continues past the first few days, contact your doctor.

If this medicine makes your mouth dry, suck hard candies or chew gum. Headache, confusion and constipation may occur when you start to take alprazolam and then disappear as your body adjusts to it.

More serious side effects, which will require medical attention if they occur, include allergic reactions, blood problems, liver problems and signs that your body is not tolerating alprazolam well. Contact your doctor if you have mental confusion, depression, skin rash or itching, trouble sleeping, unusual nervousness or irritability, unusually slow heartbeat, shortness of breath, difficulty breathing, continuing ulcers or sores in the mouth or throat or yellowing of the eyes or skin.

If you have taken large doses of alprazolam for a long time, you may have withdrawal symptoms when you stop taking this medicine. Contact your doctor if you experience mental confusion, muscle cramps, nausea or vomiting, stomach cramps, trembling, unusual sweating or seizures.

PRECAUTIONS

Before you start to take alprazolam, tell your doctor if you ever had an unusual reaction to this medicine or to any other benzodiazepine (chlordiazepoxide, clonazepam, clorazepate, diazepam, flurazepam, lorazepam, oxazepam, prazepam, temazepam and triazolam). You are likely to have a bad reaction to alprazolam if you have reacted badly to these other drugs.

Alprazolam may make some medical conditions worse. Tell your doctor if you have a history of seizures, glaucoma, kidney or liver disease, asthma, emphysema, bronchitis or other chronic lung disease, mental depression or severe mental illness, myasthenia gravis or hyperactivity (in children).

Certain medication, when taken with alprazolam, may increase the possibility or severity of side effects. Tell your doctor what prescription or nonprescription drugs you are taking, including antihistamines or medicine for hay fever, other allergies or colds; barbiturates; narcotics; sedatives; tranquilizers; medicine for pain; medicine to help you sleep; medicine for depression; or MAO inhibitors (isocarboxazid, pargyline, phenelzine or tranylcypromine) even if you have not taken them for two weeks. If you do not know the names of the medicines you are taking or what they were prescribed for, check with your doctor or pharmacist before taking alprazolam. Serious side effects can result from certain combinations. Do not start taking any of the drugs listed above without checking first with your doctor or pharmacist.

Drinking alcoholic beverages can increase the drowsiness caused by alprazolam. Ask your doctor if you have any questions about alcohol consumption.

Take alprazolam exactly as directed by your doctor. Do not take more of it, do not take it more often and do not take it for a longer period than your doctor has ordered. This medicine can be habit-forming if you take it too often.

Do not stop taking alprazolam without consulting your doctor, particularly if you have been taking it for a long time or have been taking large doses. You may suffer withdrawal symptoms if you stop this medicine abruptly. If you have a history of seizures, it may be dangerous to stop taking this medication suddenly. If you want to stop taking alprazolam, contact your doctor.

If you will be taking alprazolam for a long time, *keep all appointments with your doctor* so that your responses to this medicine can be checked. Your doctor also will want to determine whether you need to continue to take this medicine.

Children under 18 years of age should not take this medicine. Safe use of alprazolam in this age group has not been established.

Before you start to take alprazolam, tell your doctor if you are pregnant, if you intend to become pregnant while taking this medicine or if you are nursing a baby. If you become pregnant while taking alprazolam, contact your doctor. Alprazolam is passed from a mother to her unborn baby and to a breast-fed baby through the milk and can have bad effects on the baby.

DOSAGE
Your doctor will determine how often you should take alprazolam tablets and how many you should take at each dose. Carefully follow the instructions on your prescription label, and ask your doctor or pharmacist to explain any part of the instructions you do not understand.

If you forget to take a dose, *do not* take it when you remember. Omit the missed dose completely, and take the next dose at the regularly scheduled time.

STORAGE
Keep this medicine in the container it came in, and store it out of the reach of children.

Chlordiazepoxide
(klor dye az e pox′ ide)

PRODUCT INFORMATION
Brand names: A-Poxide, Libritabs, Librium, Sereen, SK-Lygen

USES
Chlordiazepoxide is one of a group of drugs known as benzodiazepines. Chlordiazepoxide is a tranquilizer used to calm people who are anxious or tense. It may be prescribed for a wide variety of medical problems that cause anxiety. It also is used to calm people before an operation and to treat the symptoms of alcohol withdrawal.

UNDESIRED EFFECTS
During the first few days of chlordiazepoxide therapy, drowsiness, dizziness and weakness are common. Even if you take this medicine at bedtime, you may notice these effects when you get up in the morning. Do not drive a car or operate dangerous machinery until you know how this medicine will affect you.

Chlordiazepoxide may make your mouth dry. Suck hard candies or chew gum to relieve the dryness. Nausea and constipation may occur when you start to take this medicine and then decrease or disappear as your body adjusts to it. If these effects continue or are severe, contact your doctor. Your doctor may want to adjust your dose.

More serious side effects include allergic reactions, blood problems, liver problems and signs that your body is not tolerating this medicine well. Contact your doctor if your have mental confusion, depression, skin rash or itching (allergic problems), trouble sleeping, unusual nervousness or irritability, unusually slow heartbeat, shortness of breath, difficulty breathing, continuing ulcers or sores in the mouth or throat or yellowing of the eyes or skin.

When you stop taking this medicine, you may experience withdrawal symptoms, especially if you have taken large doses for a long time. Contact your doctor if you notice mental confusion, muscle cramps, nausea or vomiting, stomach cramps, trembling, unusual sweating or seizures.

PRECAUTIONS

Before you start to take chlordiazepoxide, tell your doctor if you ever had an unusual reaction to this medicine or to any other benzodiazepine (alprazolam, clonazepam, clorazepate, diazepam, flurazepam, lorazepam, oxazepam, prazepam, temazepam or triazolam). You are likely to have a bad reaction to chlordiazepoxide if you have had an unusual reaction to any of these other drugs.

Chlordiazepoxide can make certain medical conditions worse. Tell your doctor if you have asthma, emphysema, bronchitis or other chronic lung disease, glaucoma, kidney disease, liver disease, mental depression, myasthenia gravis, severe mental illness or hyperactivity (in children).

Tell your doctor what prescription or nonprescription drugs you are taking, including antihistamines or medicine for hay fever, other allergies or colds; barbiturates; narcotics; sedatives; tranquilizers or sleeping medicine; prescription medicine for pain; medicine for depression; or MAO inhibitors (isocarboxazid, pargyline, phenelzine or tranylcypromine) even if you have not taken them for two weeks. If you do not know the names of the drugs or what they were prescribed for, bring them in their labeled containers to your doctor or pharmacist.

Do not drink alcoholic beverages while you are taking chlordiazepoxide because serious effects may result. Do not start taking any of the drugs listed above without first checking with your doctor or pharmacist.

Because chlordiazepoxide can be habit-forming, you should take it exactly as directed by your doctor. Do not take more of it, do not take it more often and do not take it for a longer time than your doctor has ordered.

If you have been taking chlordiazepoxide in large doses or for a long period, do not stop taking it without your doctor's permission. To avoid withdrawal problems, your doctor may want you to reduce the amount you are taking gradually before you stop completely.

Your doctor will want to check your response to chlordiazepoxide if you are going to be taking it for a long time. Your doctor may want to check you at least every four months to determine whether you still need it. *Be sure to keep all appointments with your doctor.*

Chlordiazepoxide is passed from a mother to her unborn child and to a nursing baby. Be sure to tell your doctor if you are pregnant or plan to get pregnant while you are taking this medicine and if you are nursing a baby. If you become pregnant while taking this medicine, contact your doctor.

DOSAGE

Chlordiazepoxide comes in capsules and tablets. Your doctor will determine how often you should take this medicine and how much you should take at each dose. Carefully follow the instructions on your prescription label, and ask your doctor or pharmacist to explain any part of the instructions you do not understand.

If you forget to take a dose, *do not* take it when you remember. Omit the missed dose completely, and take the next dose at the regularly scheduled time.

STORAGE
Keep this medicine in the container it came in. Keep chlordiazepoxide out of the reach of children. Do not allow anyone else to take your chlordiazepoxide.

Clorazepate
(klor az′ e pate)

PRODUCT INFORMATION
Brand name: Tranxene

USES
Clorazepate is one of the benzodiazepine tranquilizers. Clorazepate is used to calm people who are anxious or tense. It may be prescribed for a wide variety of medical problems, including relief of the symptoms of alcohol withdrawal. Clorazepate also has been used investigationally for the treatment of epilepsy.

UNDESIRED EFFECTS
The most common side effect of clorazepate is drowsiness. Do not drive a car or operate dangerous machinery until you know what effect this medicine will have on you.

Less frequently, clorazepate will cause dizziness, stomach upset or nausea, nervousness, blurred vision, dry mouth, headache or mental confusion. If these effects bother you, contact your doctor.

More serious side effects will require medical attention if they occur. Contact your doctor if you experience difficulty sleeping, skin rash, tiredness, clumsiness or unsteadiness, irritability, double vision, depression or slurred speech. Your doctor may want to adjust your dosage or change your medication if you have any of these side effects.

When you stop taking clorazepate, it may take your body as long as two weeks to adjust. Be alert for symptoms of withdrawal; contact your doctor if you experience convulsions or seizures, mental confusion, muscle cramps, nausea or vomiting, stomach cramps, trembling, unusual irritability or unusual sweating.

PRECAUTIONS
Before you start to take clorazepate, tell your doctor if you ever had an unusual reaction to this medicine or to any other benzodiazepine (alprazolam, chlordiazepoxide, clonazepam, diazepam, flurazepam, lorazepam, oxazepam, prazepam, temazepam or triazolam). You may be sensitive to this whole group of drugs.

Clorazepate may make certain medical conditions worse. Be sure to tell your doctor if you have emphysema, asthma, bronchitis or other chronic lung disease, glaucoma, kidney disease, liver disease, mental depression, myasthenia gravis or severe mental illness.

Tell your doctor what prescription or nonprescription drugs you are taking. Certain medications, when taken with clorazepate, can increase the possibility or severity of side effects. These drugs include antihistamines or medicine for hay fever, other allergies or colds; barbiturates, narcotics and prescription medicine for pain; sedatives, tranquilizers or other medicine to help you sleep; medicine for seizures; medicine for depression; and MAO inhibitors (isocarboxazid, pargyline, phenelzine or tranylcypromine) even if you stopped taking them within the past two weeks. If you do not know the names of the drugs you are taking or what they were prescribed for, bring them in their labeled containers to your doctor or pharmacist.

Do not drink alcoholic beverages while you are taking clorazepate because you can experience side effects. Do not start taking any of the drugs listed above unless you have your doctor's permission. If you have any questions, check with your doctor or pharmacist.

Because clorazepate can be habit-forming, do not take more of this medicine than your doctor has directed and do not take it more often or for a longer period than directed.

Do not stop taking clorazepate without your doctor's permission, particularly if you have been taking it for a long time or have been taking large doses. You may suffer withdrawal symptoms if you stop this medicine abruptly. If you want to stop taking clorazepate, contact your doctor.

If you will be taking clorazepate for a long period, *keep all appointments with your doctor* so that your response to this medicine can be checked. Your doctor also will want to determine whether you need to continue to take this medicine.

Before you start to take clorazepate, tell your doctor if you are pregnant, if you intend to become pregnant while taking this medicine or if you are nursing a baby. If you become pregnant while taking clorazepate, contact your doctor. Clorazepate is passed from a mother to her unborn baby and to a breast-fed baby through the milk and can have bad effects on the baby.

DOSAGE

Your doctor will determine how often you should take clorazepate capsules and how many you should take at each dose. Carefully follow the instructions on your prescription label, and ask your doctor or pharmacist to explain any part of the instructions you do not understand.

If you forget to take a dose, *do not* take it when you remember. Omit the missed dose completely, and take the next dose at the regularly scheduled time.

STORAGE

Keep this medicine in the container it came in. Keep clorazepate out of the reach of children. Do not allow anyone else to take your clorazepate.

Diazepam
(dye az′ e pam)

PRODUCT INFORMATION
Brand name: Valium

USES
Diazepam is one of the group of drugs known as benzodiazepines. Diazepam acts on the brain to relieve anxiety and tension and to relax muscles. Diazepam is used to treat muscle spasm and cerebral palsy as well as to calm people who are anxious or tense.

UNDESIRED EFFECTS
Common effects during the first few days of therapy are drowsiness, dizziness and weakness. Even if you take diazepam at bedtime, you may notice these effects when you get up the next morning. Do not drive a car or operate dangerous machinery until you know how diazepam will affect you. If fatigue continues past the first few days, contact your doctor.

If this medicine makes your mouth dry, suck hard candies or chew gum. Headache and slurring of speech may occur when you start to take diazepam and then disappear as your body adjusts to it.

More serious side effects, which will need medical treatment if they occur, include allergic reactions, blood problems, liver problems and signs that your body is not tolerating diazepam well. Contact your doctor if you have mental confusion, depression, skin rash or itching, trouble sleeping, unusual nervousness or irritability, unusually slow heartbeat, shortness of breath, difficulty breathing, continuing ulcers or sores in the mouth or throat or yellowing of the eyes or skin.

If you have taken large doses of diazepam for a long time, you may have withdrawal symptoms when you stop taking this medicine. Contact your doctor if you experience mental confusion, muscle cramps, nausea or vomiting, stomach cramps, trembling, unusual sweating or seizures.

PRECAUTIONS
Before you start to take diazepam, tell your doctor if you ever had an unusual reaction to this medicine or to any other benzodiazepine (alprazolam, chlordiazepoxide, clonazepam, clorazepate, flurazepam, lorazepam, oxazepam, prazepam, temazepam or triazolam). You are likely to have a bad reaction to diazepam if you have reacted badly to any of these other drugs.

Tell your doctor if you have any of these medical problems: asthma, emphysema, bronchitis or other chronic lung disease, glaucoma, kidney disease, liver disease, mental depression, myasthenia gravis, severe mental illness or hyperactivity (in children). Diazepam may make these conditions worse.

Certain medication, when taken with diazepam, may increase the possibility or severity of side effects. Tell your doctor what prescription or nonprescription drugs you are taking, including antihistamines or medicine for hay fever, other allergies or colds; barbiturates, narcotics or other sedatives; tranquilizers or medicine to help you sleep; prescription medicine for pain; medicine for depression; or MAO inhibitors (isocarboxazid, pargyline, phenelzine or tranylcypromine) even if you have not taken them for two weeks. If you do not know the names of the drugs you are taking, check with your doctor or pharmacist before taking diazepam because serious side effects can result from certain combinations. Do not start taking any of the drugs listed above without checking first with your doctor or pharmacist.

Avoid drinking alcoholic beverages because they add to the drowsiness caused by diazepam.

Take diazepam exactly as directed by your doctor. Do not take more of it, do not take it more often and do not take it for a longer time than your doctor has ordered. This medicine can be habit-forming if you take it too often.

Do not stop taking diazepam without your doctor's permission, particularly if you have been taking it for a long period or have been taking large doses. You may suffer withdrawal symptoms if you stop this medicine abruptly. If you want to stop taking diazepam, contact your doctor.

If you will be taking diazepam for a long time, *keep all appointments with your doctor* so that your response to this medicine can be checked. Your doctor also will want to determine whether you need to continue to take this medicine.

Before you start to take diazepam, tell your doctor if you are pregnant, if you intend to become pregnant while taking this medicine or if you are nursing a baby. If you become pregnant while taking diazepam, contact your doctor. Diazepam is passed from a mother to her unborn baby and to a breast-fed baby through the milk and can have bad effects on the baby.

DOSAGE
Your doctor will determine how often you should take diazepam tablets and how many you should take at each dose. Carefully follow the instructions on your prescription label, and ask your doctor or pharmacist to explain any part of the instructions you do not understand.

If you forget to take a dose, *do not* take it when you remember. Omit the missed dose completely, and take the next dose at the regularly scheduled time.

STORAGE
Keep this medicine in the container it came in. Keep diazepam out of the reach of children. Do not allow anyone else to take your diazepam.

Hydroxyzine
(hye drox′ i zeen)

PRODUCT INFORMATION
Brand names: Atarax, Hy-Pam, Sedaril, Vistaril
Brand names of preparations containing hydroxyzine: Catarax, Enarax, Marax, Theophedrizine, Vistrax

USES

Hydroxyzine is a tranquilizer used to calm people who are tense or anxious because of a nervous or emotional condition. Because this medicine also acts as an antihistamine, it is used to help relieve the itching of allergies and the symptoms of hay fever.

The injectable form of hydroxyzine is used to control nausea and vomiting and to relieve anxiety before dental procedures, minor surgery and childbirth.

UNDESIRED EFFECTS

With usual doses of hydroxyzine, there are few side effects. This medicine can cause some people to be drowsy or less alert than they normally are. Do not drive a car or operate dangerous machinery until you know how this medicine will affect you. Drowsiness tends to disappear as your body adjusts to hydroxyzine.

If hydroxyzine gives you a dry mouth, chew gum or suck hard candies or bits of ice to relieve the dryness.

Large doses of this medicine can cause a skin rash or shakiness. If you experience these effects, contact your doctor.

PRECAUTIONS

Do not take hydroxyzine if you ever had an unusual reaction to this medicine in the past.

Before you start to take hydroxyzine, tell your doctor what prescription or nonprescription drugs you are taking, including antihistamines or medicine for hay fever, other allergies or colds (check the labels of nonprescription drugs); barbiturates, narcotics or prescription medicine for pain; medicine for seizures; sedatives, tranquilizers or sleeping medicine; and medicine for depression.

If you do not know the names of the drugs you are taking or what they were prescribed for, bring them in their labeled containers to your doctor or pharmacist.

Do not drink alcoholic beverages while you are taking this medicine. Alcohol will add to the drowsiness caused by hydroxyzine. Do not start taking any of the drugs listed above unless you have permission from your doctor. They may increase the possibility and severity of side effects.

Do not take more of this medicine and do not take it more often than directed by your doctor.

Because hydroxyzine may affect an unborn child if taken early during pregnancy, tell your doctor if you are pregnant or think you may be. Also tell your doctor if you are breast-feeding a baby.

DOSAGE

Your doctor will determine how often you should take hydroxyzine and how much you should take at each dose. Carefully follow the instructions on your prescription label, and ask your doctor or pharmacist to explain any part of the instructions you do not understand.

Hydroxyzine comes in capsules, tablets and liquid form. Your doctor will choose the form best for you. If you are taking hydroxyzine liquid, shake it well before use to distribute the medication evenly.

If you forget to take a dose of hydroxyzine, *do not* take the missed dose when you remember it. Take the next dose at the regularly scheduled time.

STORAGE
Keep hydroxyzine in the container it came in, and keep it out of the reach of children. Do not allow anyone else to take your hydroxyzine.

Lorazepam
(lor az′ e pam)

PRODUCT INFORMATION
Brand name: Ativan

USES
Lorazepam is one of the group of drugs known as benzodiazepines. Lorazepam acts on the brain to relieve anxiety and tension. It is also used to treat insomnia.

UNDESIRED EFFECTS
Common effects during the first few days of therapy are drowsiness, dizziness and weakness. Even if you take lorazepam at bedtime, you may notice these effects when you get up the next morning. Lorazepam may also cause loss of memory. Do not drive a car or operate dangerous machinery until you know how lorazepam will affect you. If fatigue continues past the first few days, contact your doctor.

If this medicine makes your mouth dry, suck hard candies or chew gum. Headache and slurring of speech may occur when you start to take lorazepam and then disappear as your body adjusts to it.

More serious side effects, which will need medical treatment if they occur, include allergic reactions, blood problems, liver problems and signs that your body is not tolerating lorazepam well. Contact your doctor if you have mental confusion, depression, skin rash or itching, trouble sleeping, unusual nervousness or irritability, unusually slow heartbeat, shortness of breath, difficulty breathing, continuing ulcers or sores in the mouth or throat or yellowing of the eyes or skin.

If you have taken large doses of lorazepam for a long time, you may have withdrawal symptoms when you stop taking this medicine. Contact your doctor if you experience mental confusion, muscle cramps, nausea or vomiting, stomach cramps, trembling, unusual sweating or seizures.

PRECAUTIONS
Before you start to take lorazepam, tell your doctor if you ever had an unusual reaction to this medicine or to any other benzodiazepine (alprazolam, chlordiazepoxide, clonazepam, clorazepate, diazepam, flurazepam, oxazepam, prazepam,

temazepam or triazolam). You are likely to have a bad reaction to lorazepam if you have reacted badly to any of these other drugs.

Tell your doctor if you have any of these medical problems: asthma, emphysema, bronchitis or other chronic lung disease, epilepsy, glaucoma, kidney disease, liver disease, mental depression, myasthenia gravis, blood disorders, severe mental illness or hyperactivity (in children). Lorazepam may make these conditions worse.

Certain medication, when taken with lorazepam, may increase the possibility or severity of side effects. Tell your doctor what prescription or nonprescription drugs you are taking, including antihistamines or medicine for hay fever, other allergies or colds; barbiturates, narcotics or other sedatives; tranquilizers or medicine to help you sleep; prescription medicine for pain; medicine for depression; and MAO inhibitors (isocarboxazid, pargyline, phenelzine or tranylcypromine) even if you have not taken them for two weeks.

If you do not know the names of the drugs you are taking, check with your doctor or pharmacist before taking lorazepam because serious side effects can result from certain combinations. Do not start taking any of the drugs listed above without checking first with your doctor or pharmacist. Alcohol and other depressants will increase the drowsiness caused by lorazepam.

Take lorazepam exactly as directed by your doctor. Do not take more of it, do not take it more often and do not take it for a longer time than your doctor has ordered. This medicine can be habit-forming if you take it too often.

Do not stop taking lorazepam without your doctor's permission, particularly if you have been taking it for a long period or have been taking large doses. You may suffer withdrawal symptoms if you stop this medicine abruptly. If you want to stop taking lorazepam, contact your doctor.

If you will be taking lorazepam for a long time, *keep all appointments with your doctor* so that your response to this medicine can be checked. Your doctor also will want to determine whether you need to continue to take this medicine.

Before you start to take lorazepam, tell your doctor if you are pregnant, if you intend to become pregnant while taking this medicine or if you are nursing a baby. If you become pregnant while taking lorazepam, contact your doctor. Lorazepam is passed from a mother to her unborn baby and to a breast-fed baby through the milk and can have bad effects on the baby.

DOSAGE
Your doctor will determine how often you should take lorazepam tablets and how much you should take at each dose. Carefully follow the instructions on your prescription label, and ask your doctor or pharmacist to explain any part of the instructions you do not understand.

If you forget to take a dose, *do not* take it when you remember. Omit the missed dose completely, and take the next dose at the regularly scheduled time.

STORAGE
Keep this medicine in the container it came in. Keep lorazepam out of the reach of children. Do not allow anyone else to take your lorazepam.

Oxazepam

(ox aze′ e pam)

PRODUCT INFORMATION
Brand name: Serax

USES
Oxazepam is one of the benzodiazepine tranquilizers. Oxazepam is used to treat the anxiety, tension, restlessness and irritability caused by a wide variety of medical problems, including alcohol withdrawal.

UNDESIRED EFFECTS
Transient, mild drowsiness is common during the first days of therapy. Do not drive a car or operate dangerous machinery until you know how oxazepam will affect you or until the drowsiness disappears. If the drowsiness continues, contact your doctor. Your doctor may want to adjust the dose.

Unsteadiness, dizziness or headache can occur with or without drowsiness. These effects tend to decrease as you continue to take oxazepam and as your body adjusts to it. If they are persistent or severe, contact your doctor. Less often this medicine will cause blurred vision, nausea, slurred speech or unusual weakness or tiredness. Contact your doctor if these effects continue or are severe.

More serious effects, although they do not occur often, will require medical attention. Contact your doctor if you experience mental confusion (a sign that you are not tolerating this medicine), skin rash or itching (signs of allergic reaction), trouble sleeping or unusual nervousness and irritability (signs of a reaction opposite to the desired one), unusually slow heartbeat or difficulty breathing (signs of slowed function of the central nervous system), sore throat and fever (signs of blood problems) or yellowing of the eyes or skin (signs of a liver problem).

When you stop taking oxazepam, it may take your body up to two weeks to adjust. Be alert for withdrawal symptoms; contact your doctor if you experience convulsions or seizures, mental confusion, muscle cramps, nausea or vomiting, stomach cramps, trembling, unusual irritability or unusual sweating.

PRECAUTIONS
Anyone who has had an unusual reaction to any other benzodiazepine is likely to react badly to oxazepam. Tell your doctor if you ever had an unusual reaction to alprazolam, chlordiazepoxide, clonazepam, clorazepate, diazepam, flurazepam, lorazepam, prazepam, temazepam or triazolam.

Tell your doctor if you have asthma, emphysema, bronchitis or other chronic lung disease, glaucoma, kidney disease, liver disease, mental depression, myasthenia gravis, severe mental illness or hyperactivity (in children). Oxazepam can make these conditions worse.

Certain medications, when taken with oxazepam, can increase the possibility or severity of side effects. Tell your doctor what prescription or nonprescription medicines you are taking, including antihistamines or medicine for hay fever, other allergies or colds; barbiturates, narcotics or other sedatives; tranquilizers or medicine to help you sleep; prescription medicine for pain; medicine for depression; or MAO inhibitors (isocarboxazid, pargyline, phenelzine or tranylcypromine) even if you have not taken them for two weeks. If you do not know the names of the drugs you are taking or what they were prescribed for, bring them in their labeled containers to your doctor or pharmacist.

Do not drink alcoholic beverages while you are taking oxazepam because serious side effects may result. Do not start taking any of the drugs listed above unless you have permission from your doctor. If you have any questions, check with your doctor or pharmacist.

Take oxazepam exactly as directed by your doctor. Do not take more of it, do not take it more often and do not take it longer than your doctor has ordered. This medicine can be habit-forming if you take it too often.

Your doctor will want to check your response to oxazepam if you are going to be taking it for a long time. Your doctor will check at least every four months to determine if you need to continue taking this medicine. *Be sure to keep all appointments with your doctor.*

If you have been taking oxazepam in large doses or for a long time, do not stop taking it without your doctor's permission. To avoid withdrawal problems, your doctor may want you to reduce the amount you are taking gradually before you stop completely.

Before you start to take oxazepam, tell your doctor if you are pregnant, if you plan to become pregnant while taking this medicine or if you are breast-feeding a baby. This drug can be passed from a mother to her unborn child and to a nursing baby through the milk. It can create problems for the baby. If you become pregnant while taking this medicine, contact your doctor.

DOSAGE

Your doctor will determine how often you should take oxazepam capsules and how much you should take at each dose. Carefully follow the instructions on your prescription label, and ask your doctor or pharmacist to explain any part of the instructions you do not understand.

If you forget to take a dose, *do not* take it when you remember. Omit the missed dose completely, and take only the next dose at the regularly scheduled time.

STORAGE

Keep oxazepam in the container it came in. Keep it out of the reach of children. Do not allow anyone else to take your oxazepam.

Prazepam
(pra′ ze pam)

PRODUCT INFORMATION
Brand name: Centrax

USES
Prazepam is a tranquilizer used to calm people who are anxious or tense. It may be prescribed for a variety of medical problems.

UNDESIRED EFFECTS
Common effects during the first few days of therapy are drowsiness, dizziness and weakness. Do not drive a car or operate dangerous machinery until you know how prazepam will affect you. If fatigue continues past the first few days, contact your doctor.

If this medicine makes your mouth dry, suck hard candies or chew gum. Other side effects that may occur include nausea, vomiting, constipation, restlessness, insomnia and skin rash. Contact your doctor if they persist.

More serious side effects, which will require medical attention, include allergic reactions, shortness of breath, difficulty breathing, mental confusion, hallucinations (seeing, hearing or feeling things that are not there), unusually slow heartbeat, continuing ulcers or sores in the mouth or throat or yellowing of the eyes or skin.

If you have taken large doses of prazepam for a long time, you may have withdrawal symptoms when you stop taking this medicine. Contact your doctor if you experience mental confusion, muscle cramps, nausea or vomiting, stomach cramps, trembling, unusual sweating or seizures.

PRECAUTIONS
Before you start to take prazepam, tell your doctor if you ever had an unusual reaction to any other benzodiazepine (alprazolam, chlordiazepoxide, clonazepam, clorazepate, diazepam, flurazepam, lorazepam, oxazepam, temazepam or triazolam). You are likely to have a bad reaction to prazepam if you have reacted badly to any of these other drugs.

Tell your doctor if you have glaucoma, lung disease, myasthenia gravis or hyperactivity (in children). Prazepam may make these conditions worse.

Certain medications, when taken with prazepam, increase the possibility or severity of side effects. Tell your doctor what prescription or nonprescription drugs you are taking, including antihistamines or medicine for hay fever, other allergies or colds; barbiturates, narcotics or other sedatives; tranquilizers or medicine to help you sleep; prescription medicine for pain; medicine for depression; or MAO inhibitors (isocarboxazid, pargyline, phenelzine or tranylcypromine) even if you have not taken them for two weeks.

If you do not know the names of the drugs you are taking, check with your doctor or pharmacist before taking prazepam because serious side effects can result from certain combinations. Do not start taking any of the drugs listed above without checking with your doctor or pharmacist.

Take prazepam exactly as directed by your doctor. Do not take more of it, do not take it more often and do not take it for a longer time than your doctor has ordered. This medicine can be habit-forming if you take it too often.

Do not drink alcoholic beverages while taking this drug.

Do not stop taking prazepam without your doctor's permission, particularly if you have been taking it for a long period or have been taking large doses. You may suffer withdrawal symptoms if you stop this medicine abruptly. If you want to stop taking prazepam, contact your doctor.

Before you start to take prazepam, tell your doctor if you are pregnant, if you intend to become pregnant while taking this medicine or if you are nursing a baby. If you become pregnant while taking prazepam, contact your doctor. Prazepam is passed from a mother to her unborn baby and to a breast-fed baby through the milk and can have bad effects on the baby.

DOSAGE

Your doctor will determine how often you should take prazepam capsules or tablets and how much you should take at each dose. Carefully follow the instructions on your prescription label, and ask your doctor or pharmacist to explain any part of the instructions you do not understand.

If you forget to take a dose, *do not* take it when you remember. Omit the missed dose completely, and take the next dose at the regularly scheduled time. Do not take a double dose.

STORAGE

Keep this medicine in the container it came in. Keep prazepam out of the reach of children. Do not allow anyone else to take your prazepam.

Depression

Grief is the normal response to loss of a loved one, illness, failure or frustration. Depression is a state of continual feelings of demoralization, unhappiness and pessimism that is not related to a specific event or situation. In bipolar depression, periods of elation alternate with depression.

Depression causes many different symptoms, depending on the exact nature and severity of the disease. Weight loss, insomnia and "agitated" behavior such as hand wringing or pacing are common. Anxiety and depression often appear together, making diagnosis of the underlying problem difficult even for professionals.

The treatment of depression may involve electroconvulsive therapy, psychotherapy or antidepressant drugs. Often these treatments are used together.

Amitriptyline
(a mee trip′ ti leen)

PRODUCT INFORMATION
Brand names: Amitid, Amitril, Elavil, Endep, SK-Amitriptyline
Brand names of preparations containing amitriptyline: Etrafon (with perphenazine), Limbitrol (with chlordiazepoxide), Triavil (with perphenazine)

USES
Amitriptyline is one of the group of drugs called antidepressants or mood elevators. It is used to treat mental depression and the depression that can occur with anxiety.

UNDESIRED EFFECTS
The most common side effects of amitriptyline are dry mouth (suck hard candy or chew gum to relieve the dryness), headache, increased appetite for sweets, tiredness and weakness. Less often, this medicine will cause diarrhea, excessive sweating, heartburn, sleeping difficulty or vomiting. These effects tend to decrease and may disappear as your body adjusts to the medicine. If they continue or are severe, contact your doctor.

Amitriptyline makes some people drowsy or dizzy, particularly when they first begin to take it. Do not drive a car or operate dangerous machinery until you know how this medicine will affect you.

If this medicine makes you dizzy, lightheaded or faint when you get up from a lying or sitting position, try getting up slowly. Contact your doctor if this problem continues or gets worse.

Although more serious side effects do not occur often, they will require medical attention. Contact your doctor if you have blurred vision, constipation, irregular heartbeat, difficulty urinating, eye pain, hallucinations (seeing, hearing or feeling things that are not there), shakiness, unusually slow pulse, skin rash and itching, sore throat and fever or yellowing of the eyes or skin.

PRECAUTIONS

If you ever had an allergic reaction to any tricyclic antidepressant (desipramine, doxepin, imipramine, nortriptyline or protriptyline), you are likely to have a bad reaction to amitriptyline. Talk this problem over with your doctor.

Amitriptyline can make some medical conditions worse. Be sure to tell your doctor if you have a history of asthma, alcoholism, difficult urination, enlarged prostate, glaucoma, heart disease, high blood pressure, liver disease, overactive thyroid or stomach or bowel problems.

Tell your doctor what prescription or nonprescription drugs you are taking, particularly anticoagulants (blood thinners), antihistamines, allergy medicine, barbiturates, medicine for blood pressure, cold remedies, medicine for hay fever, narcotics, other medicine for depression, medicine for pain, sedatives, medicine for seizures, medicine to help you sleep, tranquilizers and MAO inhibitors (isocarboxazid, pargyline, phenelzine or tranylcypromine) even if you stopped taking them within the past two weeks. If you do not know the names of the drugs or what they were prescribed for, bring them in their labeled containers to your doctor or pharmacist.

Do not drink alcoholic beverages while you are taking amitriptyline. Do not start to take any of the drugs listed above without your doctor's permission. All of them can increase the possibility or severity of side effects.

You may have to take amitriptyline for several weeks before you begin to feel better. Do not stop taking amitriptyline unless your doctor tells you to. Your doctor may want you to decrease the amount you are taking gradually before you stop completely.

Before you have any kind of surgery (including dental surgery) or emergency treatment, tell the doctor or dentist in charge that you are taking amitriptyline.

Children under 12 years of age should not take this medicine. Safe use of amitriptyline in this age group has not been established.

Before beginning to take amitriptyline, tell your doctor if you are pregnant or are breast-feeding. If you become pregnant while taking this medicine, contact your doctor at once.

DOSAGE

Your doctor will determine how often you should take amitriptyline and how much you should take at each dose. Carefully follow the instructions on your prescription label, and ask your doctor or pharmacist to explain any part of the instructions you do not understand.

Amitriptyline comes in tablets. They may be taken with food to decrease the chance of an upset stomach, unless your doctor has told you to take them on an empty stomach.

If you forget to take a dose of this medicine, take it as soon as you remember it and take any remaining doses for that day at evenly spaced intervals. If you remember a missed dose when it is almost time for you take another one, take only the regularly scheduled dose. Omit the missed dose completely. *Do not take a double dose.*

STORAGE

Keep this medicine in the container it came in. Keep amitriptyline out of the reach of children, because an overdose can be especially dangerous to young children. Do not allow anyone else to take your amitriptyline.

Amoxapine

(a mox′ a peen)

PRODUCT INFORMATION

Brand name: Asendin

USES

Amoxapine is used to treat anxiety and depression.

UNDESIRED EFFECTS

The most common side effects of amoxapine are drowsiness, dry mouth (suck hard candy or chew gum to relieve the dryness), constipation and blurred vision. Less often, this medicine will cause difficulty sleeping, nervousness, anxiety, nightmares, nausea, dizziness and headache. These effects tend to decrease and may disappear as your body adjusts to the medicine. If they continue or are severe, contact your doctor.

Amoxapine may make you drowsy or dizzy. Do not drive a car or operate dangerous machinery until you know how this medicine will affect you.

Although more serious side effects do not occur often, they will require medical attention. Contact your doctor if you have blurred vision, constipation, irregular heartbeat, eye pain, hallucinations (seeing, hearing or feeling things that are not there), shakiness, unusually slow pulse, skin rash and itching, sore throat and fever or yellowing of the eyes or skin.

PRECAUTIONS

If you ever had a bad reaction to loxapine or any tricyclic antidepressant (amitriptyline, desipramine, doxepin, imipramine, nortriptyline or protriptyline), you are likely to have a bad reaction to amoxapine. Talk this problem over with your doctor.

This medicine can make some medical conditions worse. Be sure to tell your doctor if you have a history of glaucoma, urinary retention, seizures, heart disease (especially a recent heart attack), asthma, alcoholism, enlarged prostate, difficult urination, high blood pressure, liver disease, overactive thyroid or stomach or bowel problems.

Tell your doctor what prescription and nonprescription drugs you are taking, particularly MAO inhibitors (isocarboxazid, pargyline, phenelzine or tranylcypromine) even if you stopped taking them within the past two weeks, barbiturates, sedatives, medicine to help you sleep, tranquilizers, medicine for pain, other medicine for depression, narcotics, cold and allergy medicines, antihistamines and anticoagulants (blood thinners). If you do not know the names of the drugs or what they were prescribed for, bring them in their labeled containers to your doctor or pharmacist.

Do not drink alcoholic beverages while taking amoxapine. Alcohol can increase the possibility or severity of side effects.

Before you have any kind of surgery (including dental surgery) or emergency treatment, tell the doctor or dentist in charge that you are taking amoxapine.

Children under 16 years of age should not take this medicine. Safe use of amoxapine in this age group has not been established.

Before beginning to take amoxapine, tell your doctor if you are pregnant or are breast-feeding. If you become pregnant while taking this medicine, contact your doctor at once.

DOSAGE

Your doctor will determine how often you should take amoxapine and how much you should take at each dose. Carefully follow the instructions on your prescription label, and ask your doctor or pharmacist to explain any part of the instructions you do not understand.

Amoxapine comes in tablets. They may be taken with food to decrease the chance of stomach upset, unless your doctor has told you to take them on an empty stomach.

If you forget to take a dose of this medicine, take it as soon as you remember it and take any remaining doses for that day at evenly spaced intervals. If you remember a missed dose when it is almost time for you to take another one, take only the regularly scheduled dose. Omit the missed dose completely. *Do not take a double dose.*

STORAGE

Keep this medicine in the container it came in, and store it out of the reach of children.

Desipramine
(dess ip' ra meen)

PRODUCT INFORMATION
Brand names: Norpramin, Pertofrane

USES

Desipramine is one of the group of drugs called antidepressants or mood elevators. Desipramine is used to treat anxiety and depression, particularly when these conditions exist together.

UNDESIRED EFFECTS

Desipramine often causes dry mouth (suck hard candy or chew gum to relieve the dryness), headache, increased appetite for sweets, tiredness or weakness. Less common effects are diarrhea, excessive sweating, heartburn, difficulty sleeping and vomiting. All of these effects tend to decrease or disappear as your body adjusts to desipramine. If they continue or get worse, contact your doctor.

Some people become drowsy when they start to take desipramine. Do not drive a car or operate dangerous machinery until you know what effect this medicine will have on you.

Desipramine can make you dizzy, lightheaded or faint when you get up from a sitting or lying position. Getting up slowly may help to relieve this problem. Contact your doctor if this problem continues or gets worse.

Although more serious side effects do not occur often, they will require medical attention. Contact your doctor if you have blurred vision, constipation, irregular heartbeat, difficulty urinating, eye pain, hallucinations (seeing, hearing or feeling things that are not there), shakiness, unusually slow pulse, skin rash and itching, sore throat and fever or yellowing of the eyes or skin.

PRECAUTIONS

Before you start to take desipramine, tell your doctor if you ever had an unusual reaction to any tricyclic antidepressant (amitriptyline, doxepin, imipramine, nortriptyline or protriptyline). If you have had a bad reaction to any of these drugs, you might have a bad reaction to desipramine and should not take it.

Because desipramine can make certain medical conditions worse, tell your doctor if you have a history of asthma, alcoholism, difficult urination, enlarged prostate, glaucoma, heart disease, high blood pressure, liver disease, overactive thyroid or stomach or bowel problems.

Tell your doctor what prescription or nonprescription drugs you are taking, including antihistamines, medicine for allergy, barbiturates, medicine for high blood pressure, cold remedies, medicine for hay fever, narcotics, other medicine for depression, medicine for pain, tranquilizers, sedatives, medicine for seizures, medicine to help you sleep and MAO inhibitors (isocarboxazid, pargyline, phenelzine or tranylcypromine) even if you stopped taking them within the past two weeks. If you do not know the names of the drugs you are taking or what they were prescribed for, bring them in their labeled containers to your doctor or pharmacist.

Do not drink alcoholic beverages while you are taking desipramine. Do not start taking any of the drugs listed above without your doctor's permission. All of them can increase the possibility and severity of side effects.

It may take several weeks before you notice the full effects of desipramine. Do not stop taking this medicine without your doctor's permission. Your doctor probably will want you to reduce the amount you take gradually before you stop taking this medicine completely.

Before you have emergency treatment or any kind of surgery, including dental surgery, tell the doctor or dentist in charge that you are taking desipramine.

Children under 12 years of age should not take this medicine. Safe use of desipramine in this age group has not been established.

Before you start to take this medicine, tell your doctor if you are pregnant or are breast-feeding. If you become pregnant while taking desipramine, contact your doctor at once.

DOSAGE
Your doctor will determine how often you should take desipramine and how much you should take at each dose. Carefully follow the instructions on your prescription label, and ask your doctor or pharmacist to explain any part of the instructions you do not understand.

Desipramine comes in tablets and capsules. Unless your doctor instructs you otherwise, you may take it with food if desipramine upsets your stomach.

If you forget to take a dose of desipramine, take it as soon as you remember and take any remaining doses for that day at evenly spaced intervals. If you do not remember a missed dose until it is almost time for you to take another, take only the regularly scheduled dose. Omit the missed dose completely. *Do not take a double dose to make up for a missed one.*

STORAGE
Keep desipramine in the container it came in. Keep this medicine out of the reach of children. An overdose of desipramine may be particularly dangerous for young children. Do not allow anyone else to take your desipramine.

Doxepin
(dox′ e pin)

PRODUCT INFORMATION
Brand names: Adapin, Sinequan

USES
Doxepin is one of the antidepressant or mood-elevating drugs. Doxepin is used to treat anxiety and depression, particularly when these conditions exist together. It also is used to treat alcoholism.

UNDESIRED EFFECTS
Drowsiness and dizziness are common side effects during the first few weeks of therapy. Do not drive a car or operate dangerous machinery until you know how doxepin will affect you. These effects tend to decrease or disappear as your body adjusts to doxepin. If they continue, contact your doctor.

Other common effects are dry mouth (suck hard candy or chew gum to relieve the dryness), headache, increased appetite for sweets, nausea and tiredness or weakness. Less often, doxepin will cause diarrhea, excessive sweating, heartburn, sleeping difficulty or vomiting. Contact your doctor if these effects continue or are severe.

More serious side effects, which require medical attention, do not occur often. However, you should contact your doctor if you have blurred vision, constipation, irregular heartbeat, problems urinating, eye pain, fainting, hallucinations (seeing, hearing or feeling things that are not there), shakiness, unusually slow pulse, skin rash and itching, sore throat and fever or yellowing of the eyes or skin.

PRECAUTIONS

Before you start to take doxepin, tell your doctor if you ever had an unusual reaction to any tricyclic antidepressant (amitriptyline, desipramine, imipramine, nortriptyline or protriptyline). If you have had a bad reaction to any of these drugs, you are likely to have a bad reaction to doxepin.

Because doxepin can make certain medical conditions worse, tell your doctor if you have any of the following: alcoholism, history of asthma, difficulty urinating, enlarged prostate, glaucoma, heart disease, high blood pressure, liver disease, overactive thyroid or stomach or bowel problems.

Tell your doctor what prescription or nonprescription drugs you are taking, particularly medicine for allergy, antihistamines, medicine for high blood pressure, cold remedies, medicine for hay fever, narcotics, other medicine for depression, medicine for pain, sedatives, medicine for seizures, medicine to help you sleep, tranquilizers and MAO inhibitors (isocarboxazid, pargyline, phenelzine or tranyl-cypromine) even if you stopped taking them within the past two weeks. If you do not know the names of the drugs or what they were prescribed for, bring them in their labeled containers to your doctor or pharmacist.

Do not drink alcoholic beverages while you are taking doxepin. Do not start taking any of the drugs listed above without your doctor's permission. All of them can increase the chance and severity of side effects.

Take doxepin only as directed, and *keep all appointments with your doctor* so your doctor can determine how you are responding to this medicine.

Sometimes doxepin must be taken for several weeks before you begin to feel better. Do not stop taking this medicine without your doctor's permission. Your doctor may want you to reduce the amount you are taking gradually before you stop taking this medicine completely.

If you need emergency treatment or surgery, including dental surgery, tell the doctor or dentist in charge that you are taking doxepin.

Children under the age of 12 years should not take doxepin. Safe use of this medicine in this age group has not been established.

Before you start to take doxepin, tell your doctor if you are pregnant or are breast-feeding. If you become pregnant while taking this medicine, contact your doctor at once.

DOSAGE

Your doctor will determine how often you should take doxepin and how much you should take at each dose. Carefully follow the instructions on your prescription label, and ask your doctor or pharmacist to explain any part of the instructions you do not understand.

Doxepin comes in capsules and liquid form to be taken orally. You may take this medicine with food to decrease stomach upset, unless your doctor has told you to take it on an empty stomach.

If you are taking the liquid form, be sure that you know how to measure the proper dose with the enclosed dropper. The liquid must be diluted. Just before you take this medicine, place the dose in at least half a glass of water, milk or juice (except grape). Do not mix this medicine with grape juice or carbonated beverages because they may reduce doxepin's effectiveness.

If you forget to take a dose of doxepin, take it as soon as you remember and take any remaining doses for that day at evenly spaced intervals. If you remember a missed dose when it is almost time for you to take another, omit the missed dose completely and take only the regularly scheduled dose. *Do not take a double dose to make up for a missed one.*

STORAGE

Keep doxepin in the container it came in. Keep this medicine out of the reach of children. Overdose is especially dangerous for young children. Do not allow anyone else to take your doxepin.

Imipramine
(im ip' ra meen)

PRODUCT INFORMATION
Brand names: Imavate, Janimine, Presamine, SK-Pramine, Tofranil

USES

Imipramine is one of the antidepressant or mood-elevating drugs. Imipramine is used to treat depression in adults and bed-wetting in children.

UNDESIRED EFFECTS

Imipramine makes some people drowsy or dizzy, especially during the first few weeks of treatment. Do not drive a car or operate dangerous machinery until you know how this drug will affect you.

If imipramine makes your mouth dry, suck hard candy or chew gum to relieve the dryness. Imipramine may cause nausea, vomiting or diarrhea. Taking this medicine with food or a light snack may help prevent stomach upset. Contact your doctor if these effects continue in spite of your precautions.

Other effects, which may occur early in treatment and then disappear as your body adjusts to the medicine, are headache, increased appetite for sweets, tiredness or weakness, excessive sweating, heartburn and difficulty sleeping. If these effects continue or bother you, contact your doctor.

Although more serious effects do not occur often, they may require medical attention. Contact your doctor if you have blurred vision, constipation, irregular heartbeat, difficulty urinating, eye pain, fainting, hallucinations (seeing, hearing or feeling things that are not there), shakiness, unusually slow pulse, skin rash and itching, sore throat and fever or yellowing of the eyes or skin.

The most common side effects in children taking imipramine for bed-wetting are nervousness, sleeping problems, tiredness and mild stomach upset. Although these effects usually disappear as the child continues to take the medicine, contact your doctor if they continue.

PRECAUTIONS

If you ever had an unusual reaction to any tricyclic antidepressant (amitriptyline, desipramine, doxepin, nortriptyline or protriptyline), you are likely to have a bad reaction to imipramine. Tell your doctor if you have had problems with these drugs.

Imipramine can make certain medical conditions worse. Tell your doctor if you have a history of asthma, alcoholism, difficult urination, enlarged prostate, glaucoma, heart disease, high blood pressure, liver disease, overactive thyroid or stomach or bowel problems.

Tell your doctor what prescription or nonprescription drugs you are taking, particularly medicine for allergy, antihistamines, barbiturates, medicine for high blood pressure, cold remedies, medicine for hay fever, narcotics, other medicine for depression, medicine for pain, sedatives, medicine for seizures, medicine to help you sleep, tranquilizers and MAO inhibitors (isocarboxazid, pargyline, phenelzine or tranylcypromine) even if you stopped taking them within the past two weeks. If you do not know the names of the drugs or what they were prescribed for, bring them in their labeled containers to your doctor or pharmacist.

Do not drink alcoholic beverages while you are taking imipramine. Do not start taking any of the drugs listed above without your doctor's permission. All of them can increase the chance and severity of side effects.

Take imipramine exactly as directed by your doctor, and *keep all appointments with your doctor* so your response to this medicine can be checked.

You may have to take imipramine for several weeks before you begin to feel better. Do not stop taking this medicine without your doctor's permission. Your doctor may want you to decrease the amount you are taking gradually before you stop taking imipramine completely.

If you have to have emergency treatment or any kind of surgery, including dental surgery, be sure to tell the doctor or dentist in charge that you are taking imipramine.

Before you start to take imipramine, tell your doctor if you are pregnant or are breast-feeding. If you become pregnant while you are taking this medicine, contact your doctor at once.

DOSAGE

Your doctor will determine how often you should take imipramine and how much you should take at each dose. Carefully follow the instructions on your prescription label, and ask your doctor or pharmacist to explain any part of the instructions you do not understand.

Imipramine comes in tablets and capsules. If this medicine upsets your stomach, take it with food or a light snack.

If you forget to take a dose of imipramine, take it as soon as you remember and take any remaining doses for the day at evenly spaced intervals. If you remember a missed dose when it is almost time for you to take another, omit the missed dose entirely and take only the regularly scheduled dose. *Do not take a double dose to make up for a missed one.*

STORAGE

Keep imipramine in the container it came in. Keep this medicine out of the reach of children. An overdose of imipramine is especially dangerous for young children. Do not let anyone else take your imipramine.

Maprotiline
(ma proe' ti leen)

PRODUCT INFORMATION
Brand name: Ludiomil

USES

Maprotiline is a member of the class of drugs known as antidepressants or mood elevators. It is used to treat depression and the anxiety associated with it.

UNDESIRED EFFECTS

Maprotiline may cause dizziness, lightheadedness or faintness. Do not drive a car or operate dangerous machinery until you know how this medicine will affect you. If you become lightheaded when you get up from a lying or sitting position, try getting up slowly. Contact your doctor if this problem continues or gets worse.

Some common side effects of maprotiline include nausea, vomiting, seizures, difficult urination and constipation. Although more serious side effects do not occur often, they will require medical attention. Contact your doctor if you have blurred vision, irregular heartbeat, eye pain, hallucinations (seeing, hearing or feeling things that are not there), shakiness, unusually slow pulse, skin rash and itching, sore throat and fever or yellowing of the eyes or skin.

PRECAUTIONS

This medicine can make some medical conditions worse. Tell your doctor if you have a history of seizures, asthma, alcoholism, difficult urination, enlarged prostate, glaucoma, heart disease, high blood pressure, liver disease, overactive thyroid or stomach or bowel problems.

If you ever had an unusual reaction to any tricyclic antidepressant (amitriptyline, desipramine, doxepin, imipramine, nortriptyline or protriptyline), you are likely to have a bad reaction to maprotiline. Talk this problem over with your doctor.

Tell your doctor what prescription or nonprescription drugs you are taking, particularly anticoagulants (blood thinners), antihistamines, allergy medicine, barbiturates, medicine for blood pressure, cold remedies, medicine for hay fever, narcotics, other medicine for depression, medicine for pain, sedatives, medicine for seizures, medicine to help you sleep, tranquilizers and MAO inhibitors (isocarboxazid, pargyline, phenelzine or tranylcypromine) even if you stopped taking them within the past two weeks. If you do not know the names of the drugs or what they were prescribed for, bring them in their labeled containers to your doctor or pharmacist.

Do not drink alcoholic beverages while taking maprotiline. Alcohol may increase the possibility and severity of side effects.

You may have to take maprotiline for two to three weeks before you begin to feel better. Do not stop taking maprotiline without your doctor's permission. Your doctor may want you to decrease the amount you are taking gradually before you stop completely.

Before you have any kind of surgery (including dental surgery) or emergency treatment, tell the doctor or dentist in charge that you are taking maprotiline.

Children under 18 years of age should not take this medicine. Safe use of maprotiline in this age group has not been established.

Before beginning to take maprotiline, tell your doctor if you are pregnant or are breast-feeding. If you become pregnant while taking this medicine, contact your doctor at once.

DOSAGE
Maprotiline comes in tablets to be taken by mouth. Your prescription label tells you how much maprotiline to take at each dose. Your doctor has determined how often you should take this medication. Maprotiline must be taken on a regular schedule to be effective, so be sure to follow the dosage schedule prescribed by your doctor. Follow the instructions on your prescription label carefully, and ask your doctor or pharmacist to explain any part you do not understand. Do not skip a dose, even though you may not feel that you need to take the drug at the time you are scheduled to take it.

If you are on a once a day at bedtime dosage schedule and forget to take a dose, do not take the drug until the next evening unless you check with your doctor first. If you are on a more than once daily dosage schedule, take the missed dose as soon as you remember it. Take the remaining doses for that day at evenly spaced intervals. However, if you remember a missed dose near the time you are scheduled to take the next dose, take only one dose. *Do not take a double dose to make up for the missed one.*

STORAGE
Keep this medicine in the container it came in, and store it out of the reach of children.

Nortriptyline
(nor trip′ ti leen)

PRODUCT INFORMATION
Brand names: Aventyl Hydrochloride, Pamelor

USES
Nortriptyline belongs to the group of drugs known as antidepressants or mood elevators. Nortriptyline is used to relieve mental depression and anxiety, particularly when these conditions exist together.

UNDESIRED EFFECTS
The most common side effects of nortriptyline are dry mouth (suck hard candy or chew gum to relieve the dryness), headache, increased appetite for sweets, tiredness and weakness. Less often, this medicine will cause diarrhea, excessive sweating, heartburn, sleeping difficulty or vomiting. These effects tend to decrease and may disappear as your body adjusts to nortriptyline. If they continue or bother you, contact your doctor.

Some people become drowsy or dizzy when they begin to take nortriptyline. Do not drive a car or operate dangerous machinery until you know how this medicine will affect you.

Nortriptyline may make you dizzy, lightheaded or faint when you get up from a lying or sitting position. Getting up slowly may help. If this problem continues or gets worse, contact your doctor.

Although more serious side effects do not occur often, they will require medical attention. Contact your doctor if you have blurred vision, constipation, irregular heartbeat, difficulty urinating, eye pain, hallucinations (seeing, hearing or feeling things that are not there), shakiness, unusually slow pulse, skin rash and itching, sore throat and fever or yellowing of the eyes or skin.

PRECAUTIONS
If you ever had an unusual reaction to any tricyclic antidepressant (amitriptyline, desipramine, doxepin, imipramine or protriptyline), you are likely to have a bad reaction to nortriptyline and should not take it. If you have any questions about this problem, ask your doctor.

Because nortriptyline can make some medical conditions worse, tell your doctor if you have a history of asthma, alcoholism, difficult urination, enlarged prostate, glaucoma, heart disease, high blood pressure, liver disease, overactive thyroid or stomach or bowel problems.

Tell your doctor what prescription or nonprescription drugs you are taking, particularly antihistamines, medicine for allergy, barbiturates, medicine for high blood pressure, cold remedies, medicine for hay fever, narcotics, other medicine for depression, medicine for pain, sedatives, medicine for seizures, medicine to help you sleep, tranquilizers and MAO inhibitors (isocarboxazid, pargyline, phenelzine or tranylcypromine) even if you stopped taking them within the past two weeks. If you do not know the names of the drugs or what they were prescribed for, bring them in their labeled containers to your doctor or pharmacist.

Do not drink alcoholic beverages while you are taking nortriptyline. Do not start taking any of the drugs listed above without your doctor's permission. All of the them can increase the chance and severity of side effects.

You may have to take this medicine for several weeks before you begin to feel better. Do not stop taking nortriptyline without your doctor's permission. Your doctor may want you to decrease the amount you are taking gradually before you stop taking nortriptyline completely.

Before you have emergency treatment or surgery, including dental surgery, tell the doctor or dentist in charge that you are taking nortriptyline.

Children under 12 years of age should not take this medicine. Safe use of nortriptyline in this age group has not been established.

Before beginning to take nortriptyline, tell your doctor if you are pregnant or are breast-feeding. If you become pregnant while taking this medicine, contact your doctor at once.

DOSAGE

Your doctor will determine how often you should take nortriptyline and how much you should take at each dose. Carefully follow the instructions on your prescription label, and ask your doctor or pharmacist to explain any part of the instructions you do not understand.

Nortriptyline comes in capsules and liquid form. It may be taken with food or a light snack to decrease the chance of an upset stomach, unless your doctor has told you to take it on an empty stomach.

Measure the liquid form in a specially marked measuring spoon to be sure of an accurate dose. The liquid must be diluted. Just before you take this medicine, place the dose in at least half a glass of water, milk or juice (except grape). Do not mix this medicine with grape juice or carbonated beverages because they may decrease the effectiveness of nortriptyline.

If you forget to take a dose of this medicine, take it as soon as you remember it and take any remaining doses for that day at evenly spaced intervals. If you remember a missed dose when it is almost time for you to take another, take only the regularly scheduled dose. Omit the missed dose completely. *Do not take a double dose.*

STORAGE

Keep nortriptyline in the container it came in. Keep this medicine out of the reach of children. An overdose of nortriptyline can be especially dangerous to young children. Do not allow anyone else to take your nortriptyline.

Trazodone
(traz′ oh done)

PRODUCT INFORMATION
Brand name: Desyrel

USES
Trazodone is an antidepressant drug that is used to treat depression and anxiety. It has been shown to produce improvements in anxiety, irritability, fatigue and sleep disturbances.

Trazodone also has been used investigationally in the treatment of shakiness, anxiety and depression associated with alcoholism.

Trazodone may be preferred over some other antidepressant drugs because it causes a lower incidence of certain side effects. These effects include dry mouth, blurred vision, constipation, difficulty urinating and heart problems.

UNDESIRED EFFECTS
Side effects from trazodone are usually mild and will go away after you take the drug for a few weeks. Contact your doctor if they persist because it may be necessary to reduce your dosage.

The most common side effect of trazodone is drowsiness. Do not drive a car or operate dangerous machinery until you know how this drug will affect you.

If this medicine makes you dizzy, lightheaded or faint when you get up from a lying or sitting position, try getting up slowly. Contact your doctor if this problem continues or gets worse.

Other side effects include dry mouth (suck hard candies or chew gum to relieve the dryness), muscle aches and nausea.

Although it is uncommon, contact your doctor if you develop a fever or sore throat while taking trazodone.

PRECAUTIONS
Trazodone may cause abnormal heartbeats (palpitations, fast heartbeats or skipped heartbeats) in people with heart disease or who have had a recent heart attack. Tell your doctor if you have a history of heart disease. Contact your doctor immediately if you experience abnormal heartbeats.

Tell your doctor what prescription or nonprescription drugs you are taking, particularly antihistamines, medicine for allergies or colds, sedatives, tranquilizers, barbiturates, narcotics, medicine for depression, pain relievers, sleeping aids, medicine for blood pressure, digoxin, phenytoin and MAO inhibitors (isocarboxazid, pargyline, phenelzine or tranylcypromine) even if you have stopped taking them in the last two weeks.

If you do not know the names of the medicines that you are taking or what they were prescribed for, bring them in their labeled containers to your doctor or pharmacist.

Drinking alcoholic beverages can add to the drowsiness caused by trazodone. Ask your doctor how much alcohol is safe to drink.

It is not known if trazodone is safe for children younger than 18 years of age.

Tell your doctor if you are pregnant, plan to become pregnant or are breast-feeding a baby. It is not known whether trazodone will harm the baby.

If you need surgery with a general anesthetic, including dental surgery, be sure the doctor or dentist knows that you are taking trazodone.

Do not stop taking trazodone without consulting your doctor. It may take up to four weeks to feel the full effect of the medication.

DOSAGE

Trazodone comes in tablets. It should be taken after a meal or light snack to decrease the chance of dizziness or lightheadedness.

Your doctor will decide when you should take trazodone and how much you should take at each dose. Follow the directions on your prescription label, and ask your doctor or pharmacist to explain any part you do not understand.

If you forget to take a dose of trazodone, take it as soon as you remember unless it is time for the next dose. Take any remaining doses for that day at evenly spaced intervals. *Do not take a double dose to make up for a missed dose.*

STORAGE

Keep your trazodone in the container it came in and away from light, heat and moisture. Do not let anyone else take this medication.

Schizophrenia

Schizophrenia is a serious mental illness characterized by delusions, hallucinations and changes in behavior. Often, schizophrenics have delusions about body control. They feel that they are under the control of an outside force or power and are forced to speak a certain way or perform certain actions. In many cases, expression of emotions is disturbed and inappropriate. For example, the schizophrenic may laugh while describing a sad event.

The causes of schizophrenia are controversial. Although the disease appears to be hereditary, heredity may only make a person susceptible to schizophrenia, but other contributing factors may have to be present for a person to develop the disease. Environment and life experiences are major factors. Current investigations suggest that chemical imbalances may also play a part in the development of the disease.

Treatment of schizophrenia usually involves a period of hospitalization followed by psychotherapy, drug treatment and social planning.

Chlorpromazine
(klor proe' ma zeen)

PRODUCT INFORMATION
Brand name: Thorazine

USES
Chlorpromazine is a tranquilizer used to treat patients who are anxious, tense, apprehensive or overexcited. Sometimes it is prescribed to control nausea, vomiting and severe hiccups.

UNDESIRED EFFECTS
During the first few weeks in which you are taking chlorpromazine, it may make you drowsy or less alert than normal. Do not drive a car or operate dangerous machinery until you know how this medicine will affect you. The drowsiness usually will disappear after a time, but contact your doctor if it continues to trouble you.

Chlorpromazine can cause dry mouth. Suck hard candy or chew gum to relieve this dryness. Other side effects, which may go away as your body adjusts to chlorpromazine, include blurred vision, constipation, decreased sweating, dizziness, nasal congestion, unusually fast heartbeat, changes in menstrual period, decreased sexual ability, difficult urination and swelling of the breast. If these effects continue or are severe, contact your doctor.

If your doctor increases your dosage of chlorpromazine, you may experience other effects. Contact your doctor if you have muscle spasm in the neck or back; restlessness; shuffling walk; jerky movements of the head, neck, face and mouth; or trembling and shaking of the hands and fingers.

Other side effects, which may require medical attention, are fainting; fine, worm-like movements of the tongue; skin rash; eye problems; sore throat and fever; and yellowing of the eyes or skin. Contact your doctor if you have any of these effects.

Chlorpromazine may turn your urine red or brown. This effect is harmless.

PRECAUTIONS
If you ever had an unusual reaction to any phenothiazine (chlorpromazine, flu-phenazine, perphenazine, prochlorperazine, promazine, thioridazine or trifluopera-zine), you should not take chlorpromazine. If you have questions about this problem, check with your doctor or pharmacist.

Before you start to take chlorpromazine, tell your doctor if you have any of the following medical problems: alcoholism, blood disease, glaucoma, heart or blood vessel disease, liver disease, lung disease, Parkinson's disease, enlarged prostate, stomach ulcers or urination problems. Chlorpromazine may make these conditions worse.

Tell your doctor what prescription or nonprescription drugs you are taking, because certain medications can increase the possibility and severity of side effects. These drugs include amphetamines, medicine for seizures, medicine for asthma, epinephrine, guanethidine (medicine for high blood pressure), levodopa and medi-cine for ulcers. If you do not know the names of the drugs or what they were prescribed for, bring them in their labeled containers to your doctor or pharmacist.

Other medicines that can influence the effect of chlorpromazine are antihista-mines or medicine for hay fever, other allergies or colds; barbiturates, narcotics or prescription medicine for pain; sedatives, tranquilizers or medicine to help you sleep; medicine for depression; and MAO inhibitors (isocarboxazid, pargyline, phenelzine or tranylcypromine) even if you stopped taking them within the past two weeks. Tell your doctor if you are taking any of these medicines.

Take chlorpromazine exactly as prescribed by your doctor. Do not take more of it or take it more often than your doctor has ordered. This precaution is particularly important when you give this medicine to children, since they may react very strongly to its effects.

It may take several weeks before you notice the full effects of this medicine. Do not stop taking chlorpromazine without your doctor's permission. Your doctor may want you to reduce the amount you take gradually before you stop taking it complete-ly.

Do not drink alcoholic beverages while you are taking chlorpromazine. Alcohol can make the side effects more severe. Do not start taking any other medicine while you are taking chlorpromazine unless you first check with your doctor or pharmacist.

Chlorpromazine may make you sweat less than normal and your body temperature will increase. Be careful to avoid situations in which you might become overheated (such as exercise and hot weather) while taking this medicine.

When taking chlorpromazine, some people are more sensitive to sunlight. Stay out of sunlight or use a sunscreen preparation until you know how this medicine will affect you. If you sunburn more easily while taking chlorpromazine, contact your doctor.

Before you start to take chlorpromazine, tell your doctor if you are pregnant, if you plan to become pregnant or if you are nursing a baby. Chlorpromazine is passed to an unborn baby or to a breast-feeding baby and can have bad effects on it. If you become pregnant while taking chlorpromazine, contact your doctor at once.

DOSAGE

Your doctor will determine how often you should take chlorpromazine and how much you should take at each dose. Carefully follow the instructions on your prescription label, and ask your doctor or pharmacist to explain any part of the instructions you do not understand.

Chlorpromazine comes in extended-release capsules, tablets and liquid form to be taken orally, and in rectal suppositories. The tablets and capsules should be taken with a full eight-ounce glass of water or milk to avoid stomach irritation. The extended-release capsules should be swallowed whole. Do not break, crush or chew them before swallowing them.

If you are taking the liquid form, you may take it in water, milk, a soft drink, coffee, tea or tomato or fruit juice. Try to avoid getting this medicine on your skin or clothing. It may cause a skin rash.

To use the rectal suppository, remove the foil wrapper and dip the tip of the suppository in water. Lie on your side, and bring the knee of your top leg up to your chest. Then insert the suppository well into your rectum and hold it there for a few minutes. Try to avoid having a bowel movement for at least an hour after inserting the suppository.

If the suppository is too soft to insert because it was stored in a warm place, leave the foil wrapper on and refrigerate the suppository for 30 minutes or run cold water over it.

If you forget to take a dose of chlorpromazine, take it as soon as you remember and take any remaining doses for that day at evenly spaced intervals. If you do not remember the missed dose until it is almost time to take another one, omit the missed dose completely and take only the regularly scheduled dose. *Do not take a double dose.*

STORAGE

Keep chlorpromazine in the container it came in, and keep it out of the reach of children. Do not allow anyone else to take your chlorpromazine.

Haloperidol
(ha loe per' i dole)

PRODUCT INFORMATION
Brand name: Haldol

USES
Haloperidol is a tranquilizer used to treat emotional and mental conditions. It also is used to control nausea and vomiting; muscular tics of the face, neck, hands and shoulders; and severe behavior problems in children.

UNDESIRED EFFECTS
The most common side effects are dry mouth (suck hard candies or chew gum to relieve it), constipation and blurred vision. Less often, haloperidol will cause nausea or vomiting and decreased sexual ability. These side effects tend to decrease or disappear as your body adjusts to the medicine. If they continue or are severe, contact your doctor.

Haloperidol causes some people to become drowsy or less alert than normal. Do not drive a car or operate dangerous machinery until you know how haloperidol will affect you.

Larger doses of haloperidol can cause shuffling walk; stiffness of the arms and legs; jerky movements of the head, face, mouth and neck; or trembling and shaking of the hands and fingers. If you experience any of these effects, contact your doctor. Your doctor may want to adjust your dose or prescribe another drug that will control these effects.

Other effects, which may require medical attention, include difficult urination, dizziness, lightheadedness, fainting, worm-like movements of the tongue, skin rash, sore throat and fever and yellowing of the eyes or skin. Contact your doctor if you have any of these effects.

PRECAUTIONS
Because haloperidol can make certain medical conditions worse, tell your doctor if you have blood disease, alcoholism, epilepsy, glaucoma, heart or blood vessel disease, kidney disease, liver disease, lung disease, overactive thyroid, Parkinson's disease, enlarged prostate, severe mental depression, stomach ulcers or problems urinating.

Tell your doctor what prescription or nonprescription drugs you are taking, including amphetamines, medicine for seizures, medicine for high blood pressure, medicine for asthma, epinephrine, medicine for ulcers, antihistamines, medicine for allergies or colds, barbiturates, narcotics, prescription medicine for pain, sedatives, tranquilizers, medicine to help you sleep, medicine for depression and MAO inhibitors (isocarboxazid, pargyline, phenelzine or tranylcypromine) even if you stopped taking them within the past two weeks. If you do not know the names of the drugs or what they were prescribed for, bring them in their labeled containers to your doctor or pharmacist.

Do not drink alcoholic beverages while you are taking haloperidol. Do not start to take any of the drugs listed above without your doctor's permission. All of them can increase the possibility and severity of side effects.

Take haloperidol exactly as directed by your doctor. Do not take more of it, do not take it more often and do not take it for a longer time than your doctor has instructed.

Do not stop taking haloperidol without your doctor's permission. Your doctor may want you to cut down on the amount you take gradually before you stop taking it completely.

To help your doctor select the best treatment for you and your baby, tell your doctor if you are pregnant or are breast-feeding. If you become pregnant while taking haloperidol, contact your doctor at once.

DOSAGE

Your doctor will determine how often you should take haloperidol and how much you should take at each dose. Carefully follow the instructions on your prescription label, and ask your doctor or pharmacist to explain any part of the instructions you do not understand.

Haloperidol comes in tablets and liquid form. If this medicine upsets your stomach, the tablets may be taken with solid food or milk.

The liquid comes in a container with a dropper to be used in measuring the proper dose. Be sure you understand how much to take and how to measure it. If you have any questions, check with your doctor or pharmacist.

The liquid should be taken with a four-ounce glass of milk, water, soft drink or juice. Put the medicine in the beverage just before you take it. If you get any of the beverage on the dropper, rinse it with tap water before you put it back into the container.

Try not to get any liquid haloperidol on your skin or clothing. Liquid haloperidol may cause a skin rash.

If you forget to take a dose of haloperidol, take it as soon as you remember and take any remaining doses for the day at evenly spaced intervals. If you remember a missed dose when it is almost time to take another one, omit the missed dose completely and take only the regularly scheduled dose. *Do not take more than one dose at a time.*

STORAGE

Keep haloperidol in the container it came in, and store it away from heat and out of direct sunlight. Keep this medicine out of the reach of children. Do not allow anyone else to take your haloperidol.

Lithium
(li′ thee um)

PRODUCT INFORMATION
Brand names: Eskalith, Lithane, Lithionate

USES
Lithium works on the nervous system to stabilize the mood of people with manic-depressive illness.

UNDESIRED EFFECTS
When you begin to take lithium, you may have shaking of the hands and fingers, thirst, frequent urination or brief episodes of nausea and diarrhea. Usually, these effects disappear as your body adjusts to the medicine. If they do not stop, contact your doctor.

Lithium also can decrease the function of the thyroid gland. Symptoms of this problem include coldness of the fingers and toes, constipation, dry and puffy skin, headache, menstrual changes, muscle aches, sleepiness, tiredness and unusual weight gain. Contact your doctor if you experience any of these effects. Your doctor may want to prescribe a thyroid supplement for you.

The most serious side effect of this medicine is lithium poisoning. Stop taking lithium and contact your doctor if you experience nausea and vomiting, shakiness, drowsiness, mental confusion, slurred speech, ringing in the ears, weakness, blurred vision or jerking of the arms and legs. Also contact your doctor if you have pains in the lower stomach (a sign of stomach irritation) or swelling of the feet and lower legs (a sign that your body is retaining water).

PRECAUTIONS
Because lithium can make some medical conditions worse, tell your doctor if you have heart disease, kidney disease, Parkinson's disease, any kind of severe infection or thyroid disease.

Tell your doctor what prescription or nonprescription drugs you are taking, including medicine for asthma; caffeine (a common ingredient of many colas and nonprescription medicines for pain); chlorpromazine; diuretics (water pills), especially the thiazide type; haloperidol; potassium iodide; and sodium bicarbonate (baking soda). If you do not know the names of the drugs or what they were prescribed for, bring them in their labeled containers to your doctor or pharmacist.

While you are taking lithium, drink two or three quarts of water or other fluids each day and use a normal amount of salt in your food. If you are on a low-salt diet, discuss this with your doctor.

Lithium may cause some people to become drowsy or less alert than they normally are. Do not drive a car or operate machinery until you know how lithium will affect you.

Be careful to avoid situations in which you will sweat heavily (such as hot weather, strenuous exercise and hot or sauna baths). The loss of too much water and salt from your body may lead to serious side effects from taking lithium.

Do not drink large amounts of beverages that contain caffeine (such as coffee, tea or cola) while you are taking lithium. Lithium is excreted from the body in the urine, and the increased flow of urine caused by caffeine may decrease the effect of lithium.

While you are taking lithium, your doctor will want to monitor the amount of drug in your blood to make sure you do not have serious side effects. *Be sure to keep all appointments with your doctor for blood tests.*

Usually, lithium must be taken for seven to 10 days before you begin to feel better. Do not take more of this medicine, do not take it more often and do not take it for a longer time than your doctor has ordered.

Do not drink alcoholic beverages or take any other drugs while you are taking lithium without your doctor's permission.

Lithium should not be given to children under 12 years of age. Safe use of lithium in this age group has not been established.

Be sure to tell your doctor if you are pregnant or think you may become pregnant. Also tell your doctor if you are breast-feeding. Lithium is passed from a mother to her unborn baby or to a nursing baby, and it may have bad effects on the baby. If you become pregnant while you are taking lithium, contact your doctor at once.

DOSAGE

Your doctor will determine how often you should take lithium and how much you should take at each dose. Carefully follow the instructions on your prescription label, and ask your doctor or pharmacist to explain any part of the instructions you do not understand.

Lithium comes in tablets and capsules. If this medicine upsets your stomach, take it immediately after meals or with solid food or milk. If you have any questions, check with your doctor or pharmacist.

If you forget to take a dose of lithium, *do not* take it when you remember. Omit the missed dose and take the next dose at the regularly scheduled time. *Do not take a double dose to make up for a missed dose.*

STORAGE

Keep lithium in the container it came in, and store the container out of direct sunlight. Keep this medicine out of the reach of children. Do not allow anyone else to take your lithium.

Loxapine
(lox′ a peen)

PRODUCT INFORMATION
Brand name: Loxitane

USES
Loxapine is a tranquilizer used to treat emotional and mental conditions. It is useful for controlling symptoms such as disorientation, hallucinations and hostility.

UNDESIRED EFFECTS
The most common side effect of loxapine is drowsiness. This effect may disappear as you continue to take the medication and as your body adjusts to it. Do not drive a car or operate dangerous machinery until you know how this medicine will affect you.

Other side effects that may occur include dry mouth (suck hard candies or chew gum to relieve it), constipation, fast heartbeat and weakness.

When first taking loxapine, you may experience dizziness when you stand. If you become dizzy, move slowly from a sitting to a standing position. This problem should go away as you continue to take loxapine.

Large doses of loxapine may cause stiffness of the arms and legs; jerky movement of the head, face, mouth and neck; or trembling and shaking of the hands and fingers. Contact your doctor if you experience any of these effects. It may be necessary to adjust your dose or prescribe another drug that will control these symptoms.

You should also seek medical attention if you experience worm-like movements of the tongue or have eye problems or difficulty breathing.

PRECAUTIONS
Because loxapine can make certain medical conditions worse, tell your doctor if you have a history of alcoholism; seizures or epilepsy; problems urinating; glaucoma; severe mental depression; Parkinson's disease; or heart, lung, liver or kidney disease.

Certain medications, when taken with loxapine, can increase the possibility and severity of side effects. Tell your doctor what prescription and nonprescription drugs you are taking, including medicine for allergies or colds; antihistamines; barbiturates; narcotics; pain relievers; sedatives; tranquilizers; sleeping medication; medicine for depression; MAO inhibitors (isocarboxazid, pargyline, phenelzine or tranylcypromine) even if you stopped taking them in the past two weeks; epinephrine; medicine for ulcers, asthma, seizures or Parkinson's disease; guanethidine (medicine for high blood pressure); and amphetamines.

If you do not know the names of the drugs you are taking or what they were prescribed for, take them in their labeled containers to your doctor or pharmacist.

Drinking alcoholic beverages may add to the drowsiness caused by loxapine. Discuss with your doctor how much alcohol is safe to drink.

Before you start to take loxapine, tell your doctor if you are pregnant, if you plan to become pregnant or if you are breast-feeding a baby. This drug can be passed from a mother to her unborn child and to a nursing baby through the milk. It is not known whether this exposure will have a harmful effect on the baby. Contact your doctor if you become pregnant while taking loxapine.

Loxapine should not be taken by children under the age of 16 years. It is not known whether this drug is safe for this age group.

DOSAGE

Your doctor will determine how often you should take loxapine and how much you should take at each dose. Follow the instructions on your prescription label, and ask your doctor or pharmacist to explain any part you do not understand.

Loxapine comes in capsules and liquid to be taken by mouth and in a liquid form for injection. If you are taking the oral liquid form, carefully measure the proper dose with the dropper provided and place it in orange or grapefruit juice before taking it. The liquid should be diluted.

If you forget to take a dose, take it as soon as you remember and take any remaining doses for that day at evenly spaced intervals. If you remember a missed dose when it is almost time for you to take another one, omit the missed dose completely and take only the regularly scheduled dose. *Do not take a double dose to make up for a missed one.*

STORAGE

Keep this medication in the container it came in, and keep it out of the reach of children. Do not allow anyone else to take it.

Perphenazine
(per fen′ a zeen)

PRODUCT INFORMATION
Brand name: Trilafon

USES

Perphenazine is a tranquilizer used to treat patients who are anxious, tense, apprehensive or overexcited. It also is prescribed to control severe nausea and vomiting and severe hiccups.

UNDESIRED EFFECTS

Perphenazine may make you drowsy, especially during the first few weeks you are taking it. Do not drive a car or operate dangerous machinery until you know how this medicine will affect you. If the drowsiness does not disappear or is severe, contact your doctor.

Other side effects, which tend to decrease or disappear as your body adjusts to perphenazine, include dry mouth (suck hard candy or chew gum to relieve the dryness), blurred vision, constipation, decreased sweating, dizziness, nasal congestion, unusually fast heartbeat, changes in menstrual period, decreased sexual ability, difficult urination and swelling of the breasts. Contact your doctor if these effects continue or are severe.

An increase in dosage can cause muscle spasm in the neck or back; restlessness; shuffling walk; jerky movements of the head, neck, face and mouth; or trembling and shaking of the hands and fingers. Contact your doctor if any of these effects occur.

Side effects that may require medical attention include fainting, worm-like movements of the tongue, skin rash, eye problems, sore throat and fever and yellowing of the skin or eyes. If any of these effects occur, contact your doctor.

This medicine may color your urine red or brown. This effect is harmless.

PRECAUTIONS

Tell your doctor if you ever had an unusual reaction to any phenothiazine (chlorpromazine, fluphenazine, perphenazine, prochlorperazine, promazine, thioridazine or trifluoperazine). If so, you are likely to have a bad reaction to perphenazine.

Perphenazine can make some medical problems worse. Before you start to take this medicine, tell your doctor if you have blood disease, alcoholism, glaucoma, heart or blood vessel disease, liver disease, lung disease, Parkinson's disease, enlarged prostate, stomach ulcers or urination problems.

Certain medications, when taken with perphenazine, can increase the possibility and severity of side effects. Tell your doctor what prescription or nonprescription drugs you are taking, including amphetamines, medicine for seizures, medicine for asthma, epinephrine, guanethidine (medicine for high blood pressure), levodopa, medicine for ulcers, antihistamines, medicine for allergies or colds, barbiturates, narcotics, prescription medicine for pain, sedatives, tranquilizers, medicine to help you sleep, medicine for depression and MAO inhibitors (isocarboxazid, pargyline, phenelzine or tranylcypromine) even if you stopped taking them within the past two weeks.

If you do not know the names of the drugs or what they were prescribed for, bring them in their labeled containers to your doctor or pharmacist.

Do not drink alcoholic beverages while you are taking perphenazine. Do not start to take any of the drugs listed above without your doctor's permission. All of them can increase the severity of side effects.

Take perphenazine exactly as prescribed by your doctor. Do not take more of it and do not take it more often than ordered by your doctor. This is particularly important if you are giving perphenazine to a child. Children may react strongly to this medicine's effects.

It may take several weeks for you to notice the full effects of perphenazine. Do not stop taking it without first checking with your doctor. Your doctor may want you to reduce the amount you are taking gradually before you stop taking it completely.

Avoid situations in which you may become overheated while you are taking perphenazine. This medicine can cause you to sweat less and, as a result, your body temperature will increase. Strenuous exercise and hot weather can create problems in this regard.

Some people become more sensitive to sunlight when they are taking perphenazine. Limit the amount of time you spend in sunlight until you know what effect this medicine will have on you. If this medicine causes you to sunburn easily, contact your doctor.

Perphenazine is passed by a mother to her unborn child or to a breast-feeding baby. Be sure to tell your doctor if you are nursing a baby, if you are pregnant or if you plan to become pregnant. If you become pregnant while taking this medicine, contact your doctor at once.

DOSAGE

Your doctor will determine how often you should take perphenazine and how much you should take at each dose. Carefully follow the instructions on your prescription label, and ask your doctor or pharmacist to explain any part of the instructions you do not understand.

Perphenazine comes in extended-release tablets, regular tablets and concentrated liquid form. The regular tablets should be taken with a full eight-ounce glass of water or milk to avoid stomach irritation. The extended-release tablets should be swallowed whole. Do not break, crush or chew them before swallowing them.

The concentrated liquid form must be diluted. Just before taking it, measure the correct dose and put it in half a glass (four ounces) of tomato or fruit juice, water, soup, coffee, tea or a soft drink. Try to avoid getting liquid perphenazine on your skin or clothing. Liquid perphenazine may cause a skin rash.

If you forget to take a dose of perphenazine, take it as soon as you remember and take any remaining doses for that day at evenly spaced intervals. If you do not remember a missed dose until it is almost time to take another one, omit the missed dose completely and take only the regularly scheduled dose. *Do not take a double dose.*

STORAGE

Keep this medicine in the container it came in, and keep it out of the reach of children. Do not allow anyone else to take your perphenazine.

Prochlorperazine
(pro klor peer' a zeen)

PRODUCT INFORMATION
Brand name: Compazine

USES
Prochlorperazine is a tranquilizer used to treat emotional and mental conditions. It also is prescribed to control anxiety, nausea and vomiting and severe hiccups.

UNDESIRED EFFECTS

During the first few weeks in which you are taking prochlorperazine, it may make you drowsy or less alert than normal. Do not drive a car or operate dangerous machinery until you know how this medicine will affect you. The drowsiness should disappear. If it does not, contact your doctor.

If prochlorperazine makes your mouth dry, suck hard candies or chew gum to relieve the dryness. Other side effects include blurred vision, unusually fast heartbeat, constipation, decreased sweating, dizziness, nasal congestion, changes in menstrual period, decreased sexual ability, difficult urination and swelling of the breasts. These effects tend to decrease as your body adjusts to prochlorperazine. If they continue or are severe, contact your doctor.

If your dosage of prochlorperazine is increased, you may experience muscle spasm in the neck or back; restlessness; shuffling walk; jerky movements of the head, neck, face and mouth; or trembling and shaking of the hands and fingers. Contact your doctor.

Side effects that may require medical attention include fainting, worm-like movements of the tongue, skin rash, eye problems, sore throat and fever and yellowing of the skin or eyes. Contact your doctor if these problems occur.

Prochlorperazine may change the color of your urine to red or brown. This effect is harmless.

PRECAUTIONS

If you ever had an unusual reaction to prochlorperazine or any other phenothiazine (chlorpromazine, fluphenazine, perphenazine, promazine, thioridazine or trifluoperazine), you should not take prochlorperazine. If you have any questions, ask your doctor or pharmacist.

Before you start to take prochlorperazine, tell your doctor if you have any of the following medical conditions: blood disease, alcoholism, glaucoma, heart or blood vessel disease, liver disease, lung disease, Parkinson's disease, enlarged prostate, stomach ulcers or urination problems. This medicine may make these conditions worse.

Certain medication can increase or decrease the effects of prochlorperazine. Tell your doctor if you are taking amphetamines, medicine for seizures, medicine for asthma, epinephrine, guanethidine (medicine for high blood pressure), levodopa, medicine for ulcers, antihistamines, medicine for allergies or colds, barbiturates, narcotics, prescription medicine for pain, sedatives, tranquilizers, medicine to help you sleep, medicine for depression and MAO inhibitors (isocarboxazid, pargyline, phenelzine or tranylcypromine) even if you stopped taking them within the past two weeks.

If you do not know the names of the drugs you are taking or what they were prescribed for, bring them in their labeled containers to your doctor or pharmacist.

Do not drink alcoholic beverages while you are taking prochlorperazine. Do not start taking any of the drugs listed above without your doctor's permission. All of them can increase the possibility and severity of side effects.

Take this medicine exactly as prescribed by your doctor. Do not take more of it and do not take it more often than instructed. This precaution is particularly important if you are giving prochlorperazine to a child. Children may react strongly to this medicine's effects.

You may not notice the full effects of this medicine until you have taken it for several weeks. Do not stop taking prochlorperazine without your doctor's permission. Your doctor may want you to reduce the amount you are taking gradually before you stop taking it completely.

This medicine can cause you to sweat less and, as a result, your body temperature will increase. Be careful to avoid situations (such as strenuous exercise and hot weather) in which you may become overheated while taking prochlorperazine.

Because prochlorperazine makes some people more sensitive to sunlight than they normally are, limit the amount of time you spend in the sunlight until you know what effect this medicine will have on you. If you sunburn easily while taking prochlorperazine, contact your doctor.

Prochlorperazine should not be taken by pregnant women or by women who are breast-feeding. Be sure to tell your doctor if you are pregnant or are nursing a baby. If you become pregnant while you are taking this medicine, contact your doctor at once.

DOSAGE
Your doctor will determine how often you should take prochlorperazine and how much you should take at each dose. Carefully follow the instructions on your prescription label, and ask your doctor or pharmacist to explain any part of the instructions you do not understand.

Prochlorperazine comes in extended-release capsules, tablets and liquid to be taken orally and in rectal suppositories. The tablets should be taken with a full eight-ounce glass of water or milk to avoid stomach upset. The extended-release capsules should be swallowed whole. Do not break, crush or chew them before swallowing them.

If you are taking the liquid form of prochlorperazine, try to avoid getting it on your skin or clothing. Liquid prochlorperazine may cause a skin rash. The liquid may be taken in juice, water, soup, coffee, tea or a soft drink.

To use the rectal suppositories, remove the foil wrapper and dip the tip of the suppository in water. Then lie on your side, bring the knee of your top leg up to your chest, insert the suppository well into your rectum and hold it there for a few moments. Try not to have a bowel movement for at least an hour after inserting the suppository. If the suppository has been stored in a warm place and is too soft to insert easily, leave the wrapper on and refrigerate the suppository for 30 minutes or run cold water over it.

If you forget to take a dose of prochlorperazine, take it as soon as you remember and take any remaining doses for that day at evenly spaced intervals. If you do not remember a missed dose until it is almost time for another one, omit the missed dose completely and take only the regularly scheduled dose. *Do not take a double dose to make up for a missed dose.*

STORAGE

Keep this medicine in the container it came in. Keep it out of the reach of children. Do not allow anyone else to take your prochlorperazine.

Thioridazine
(the oh rid′ a zeen)

PRODUCT INFORMATION
Brand name: Mellaril

USES

Thioridazine is one of the phenothiazine tranquilizers used to treat mental depression and the depression often associated with anxiety. Thioridazine also is used to treat children with severe behavioral problems and children who are hyperactive.

UNDESIRED EFFECTS

Some common side effects of thioridazine are dry mouth (suck hard candy or chew gum to relieve it), blurred vision, constipation, decreased sweating, dizziness, nasal congestion and unusually fast heartbeat. Less often, thioridazine can cause difficulty urinating, changes in menstrual period, decreased sexual ability or swelling of the breasts. These effects usually disappear as your body adjusts to the medicine. Let your doctor know if they continue or are severe.

Some people become drowsy or less alert than normal when they take thioridazine. Do not drive a car or operate dangerous machinery until you know how this medicine will affect you. Usually the drowsiness will disappear after a few weeks. Contact your doctor if it does not.

If thioridazine makes you dizzy, lightheaded or faint when you get up from a sitting or lying position, try to get up slowly. If this problem continues, contact your doctor.

More serious side effects do not occur often, but they may require medical attention. Most often, these effects result from high doses or long-term therapy. Contact your doctor if you experience muscle spasm in the neck or back; restlessness; shuffling walk; jerky movements of the head, neck, face and mouth; trembling and shaking of the hands and fingers; fainting; worm-like movements of the tongue; skin rash; eye problems; sore throat and fever; or yellowing of the skin or eyes. Thioridazine may color your urine red or brown. This effect is harmless.

PRECAUTIONS

You should not take thioridazine if you ever had an unusual reaction to any phenothiazine (chlorpromazine, fluphenazine, perphenazine, prochlorperazine, promazine, thioridazine or trifluoperazine). If you have any questions, check with your doctor or pharmacist.

Because thioridazine can make some medical problems worse, tell your doctor if you have blood disease, alcoholism, glaucoma, heart or blood vessel disease, lung disease, Parkinson's disease, enlarged prostate, stomach ulcers or urination problems.

Tell your doctor what prescription or nonprescription drugs you are taking, including amphetamines, medicine for seizures, medicine for asthma, epinephrine, guanethidine (medicine for high blood pressure), levodopa, medicine for ulcers, antihistamines, medicine for allergies and colds, barbiturates, narcotics, prescription medicine for pain, sedatives, tranquilizers, medicine to help you sleep, medicine for depression and MAO inhibitors (isocarboxazid, pargyline, phenelzine or tranylcypromine) even if you stopped taking them within the past two weeks.

If you do not know the names of the drugs you are taking or what they were prescribed for, bring them in their labeled containers to your doctor or pharmacist.

Do not drink alcoholic beverages while you are taking thioridazine. Do not start taking any of the drugs listed above without your doctor's permission. All of them can increase the chance and severity of side effects.

Do not take more of this medicine or take it more often than instructed by your doctor. It is particularly important that thioridazine is given to a child exactly as prescribed. Children may react strongly to this medicine's effects.

You may have to take thioridazine for several weeks before you feel its full effects. Do not stop taking it without your doctor's permission. Your doctor may want you to reduce the amount you are taking gradually before you stop taking it completely.

Thioridazine can cause you to sweat less; as a result, your body temperature will rise. Avoid situations in which you may become overheated (such as strenuous exercise, hot weather and hot or sauna baths) while taking this medicine.

Thioridazine makes some people more susceptible to sunburn than they normally are. Avoid excessive exposure to sunlight or use a sunscreen preparation until you know whether this medicine will cause you to sunburn easily.

Pregnant women and women who are breast-feeding should not take this medicine because of possible bad effects on the baby. Before you start to take thioridazine, tell your doctor if you are pregnant or are nursing a baby. If you become pregnant while taking thioridazine, contact your doctor at once.

DOSAGE

Your doctor will determine how often you should take thioridazine and how much you should take at each dose. Carefully follow the instructions on your prescription label, and ask your doctor or pharmacist to explain any part of the instructions you do not understand.

Thioridazine comes in tablets and liquid form. It may be taken with food or with a full eight-ounce glass of water or milk to decrease stomach upset.

If you are taking the liquid form, use a specially marked measuring spoon to be sure you get an accurate dose. Some forms of the liquid must be diluted; be sure that you carefully follow the instructions for dilution on your prescription label. Try to avoid getting the liquid on your skin or clothing. Liquid thioridazine may cause a skin rash.

If you forget to take a dose of thioridazine, take it as soon as you remember and take any remaining doses for that day at evenly spaced intervals. If you do not remember a missed dose until it is almost time to take another one, omit the missed dose and take only the regularly scheduled dose. *Do not take a double dose.*

STORAGE
Keep this medicine in the container it came in, and store away from heat and direct sunlight. Keep it out of the reach of children. Do not allow anyone else to take your thioridazine.

Thiothixene
(thye oh thix' een)

PRODUCT INFORMATION
Brand name: Navane

USES
Thiothixene is a tranquilizer used to treat emotional and mental conditions. It may be particularly useful in treating people with chronic mental illness who have not responded to other drugs of this type.

UNDESIRED EFFECTS
During the first few weeks in which you take thiothixene, you may be drowsy or less alert than normal. Do not drive a car or operate dangerous machinery until you know how this medicine will affect you. The drowsiness should disappear as you continue to take this medicine. If it does not, contact your doctor.

You may become dizzy, lightheaded or faint when getting up from a sitting or lying position. Getting up slowly may help, but contact your doctor if these problems continue or get worse.

Other side effects that may occur are dry mouth (suck hard candy or chew gum to relieve it), blurred vision, constipation, decreased sweating, nasal congestion and unusually fast heartbeat. Less often, thiothixene can cause difficulty urinating, swelling of the breasts, changes in menstrual period and decreased sexual ability. If any of these effects bother you, contact your doctor.

If your doctor increases your dose of thiothixene, you may have muscle spasms of the neck or back; restlessness; shuffling walk; jerky movements of the head, face, mouth and neck; or trembling of the hands and fingers. Contact your doctor if these effects occur. It may be necessary to adjust your dose or prescribe another medicine to relieve these problems.

Other side effects require medical attention. Contact your doctor if you experience fainting, worm-like movements of the tongue, skin rash, eye problems, sore throat and fever or yellowing of the skin or eyes.

PRECAUTIONS
Before you start to take thiothixene, tell your doctor if you ever had an unusual

reaction to chlorprothixene or to any phenothiazine (chlorpromazine, fluphenazine, perphenazine, prochlorperazine, promazine, thioridazine or trifluoperazine). If so, you are likely to have a bad reaction to thiothixene.

Because thiothixene can make some medical conditions worse, tell your doctor if you have blood disease, alcoholism, glaucoma, heart or blood vessel disease, liver disease, lung disease, Parkinson's disease, enlarged prostate, stomach ulcers or urination problems.

Tell your doctor what prescription or nonprescription drugs you are taking, including amphetamines, medicine for seizures, medicine for asthma, epinephrine, guanethidine (medicine for high blood pressure), levodopa, medicine for ulcers, antihistamines, medicine for allergies and colds, barbiturates, narcotics, prescription medicine for pain, sedatives, tranquilizers, medicine to help you sleep, medicine for depression and MAO inhibitors (isocarboxazid, pargyline, phenelzine or tranylcypromine) even if you stopped taking them within the past two weeks. These drugs can influence the effects of thiothixene.

If you do not know the names of the drugs you are taking or what they were prescribed for, bring them in their labeled containers to your doctor or pharmacist.

Do not drink alcoholic beverages while you are taking this medicine. Do not start taking any of the drugs listed above without your doctor's permission. All of them can increase the possibility and severity of side effects.

Take thiothixene exactly as prescribed by your doctor. Do not take more of it and do not take it more often than instructed.

You may have to take thiothixene for several weeks before you feel its full effects. Do not stop taking this medicine without your doctor's permission. Your doctor may want you to reduce the amount you are taking gradually before you stop taking it completely.

Thiothixene can cause you to sweat less; as a result, your body temperature will rise. Be careful to avoid situations in which you may become overheated (such as strenuous exercise, hot weather and sauna baths) while taking this medicine.

Thiothixene may make some people more sensitive to sunlight than they normally are. Limit the amount of time you spend in sunlight until you know how this medicine will affect you. If you sunburn more easily while taking thiothixene, contact your doctor.

Do not take thiothixene within an hour of taking antacids or medicine for diarrhea. If these drugs are taken too close together, thiothixene may be less effective.

To help your doctor select the best treatment for you and your baby, tell your doctor if you are pregnant or are nursing a baby.

Thiothixene should not be given to children under 12 years of age. Its safe use in this age group has not been established.

DOSAGE

Your doctor will determine how often you should take thiothixene and how much you should take at each dose. Carefully follow the instructions on your prescription label, and ask your doctor or pharmacist to explain any part of the instructions you do not understand.

Thiothixene comes in capsules and concentrated liquid. The capsules should be taken with a full eight-ounce glass of water or milk to avoid stomach upset.

Thiothixene liquid comes in a container with a measuring dropper. If you are taking this form, be sure you understand how much to take and how to measure it with the dropper. Just before you take the liquid, measure the proper amount into a half glass (four ounces) of juice, water, soup, coffee, tea, milk or a soft drink. If any of the liquid with which you are diluting the medicine gets on the dropper, rinse the dropper with tap water before putting it back in the container.

Avoid getting liquid thiothixene on your skin or clothing. Liquid thiothixene may cause a skin rash.

If you forget to take a dose of thiothixene, take it as soon as you remember and take any remaining doses for that day at evenly spaced intervals. If you do not remember a missed dose until it is almost time to take another one, omit the missed dose completely and take only the regularly scheduled dose. *Do not take a double dose.*

STORAGE
Keep thiothixene in the container it came in, and store it away from heat and direct sunlight. Keep it out of the reach of children. Do not allow anyone else to take your thiothixene.

Trifluoperazine
(trye floo oh peer' a zeen)

PRODUCT INFORMATION
Brand name: Stelazine

USES
Trifluoperazine is a tranquilizer used to treat emotional and mental conditions. It also is prescribed to control anxiety, nausea and vomiting and severe hiccups.

UNDESIRED EFFECTS
When you start to take trifluoperazine, you may be drowsy or less alert than normal. Do not drive a car or operate dangerous machinery until you know how this medicine will affect you. The drowsiness should disappear after a few weeks. If it does not, contact your doctor.

Some common effects of this medicine are dry mouth (suck hard candy or chew gum to relieve it), blurred vision, constipation, decreased sweating, dizziness, nasal congestion and unusually fast heartbeat. Less often, trifluoperazine can cause difficulty urinating, changes in menstrual period, decreased sexual ability and swelling of the breasts. Tell your doctor if these effects bother you.

If your doctor increases the amount of trifluoperazine you take, you may experience muscle spasm in the neck or back; restlessness; shuffling walk; jerky movements of the head, neck, face and mouth; or trembling and shaking of the hands and fingers. Contact your doctor if you have any of these problems.

Other side effects, which may require medical attention, are fainting, worm-like movements of the tongue, skin rash, eye problems, sore throat and fever and yellowing of the skin or eyes. If any of these problems occur, contact your doctor.

You may notice a change in the color of your urine to red or brown. This effect is harmless.

PRECAUTIONS

If you ever had an unusual reaction to any phenothiazine (chlorpromazine, fluphenazine, perphenazine, prochlorperazine, promazine, thioridazine or trifluoperazine), you are likely to have a bad reaction to trifluoperazine and should not take it. If you have any questions, check with your doctor or pharmacist.

Before you start to take trifluoperazine, tell your doctor if you have blood disease, alcoholism, glaucoma, heart or blood vessel disease, liver disease, lung disease, Parkinson's disease, enlarged prostate, stomach ulcers or urination problems. This medicine may make these problems worse.

Tell your doctor what prescription or nonprescription drugs you are taking, including amphetamines, medicines for seizures, medicine for asthma, epinephrine, guanethidine (medicine for high blood pressure), levodopa, medicine for ulcers, antihistamines, medicine for allergies and colds, barbiturates, narcotics, prescription medicine for pain, sedatives, tranquilizers, medicine to help you sleep, medicine for depression and MAO inhibitors (isocarboxazid, pargyline, phenelzine or tranylcypromine) even if you stopped taking them within the past two weeks. These drugs can influence the effect of trifluoperazine.

If you do not know the names of the drugs you are taking or what they were prescribed for, bring them in their labeled containers to your doctor or pharmacist.

Do not drink alcoholic beverages while you are taking trifluoperazine. Do not start taking any of the drugs listed above without your doctor's permission. All of them can increase the possibility and severity of side effects.

Do not take more of this medicine or take it more often than instructed by your doctor. It is particularly important that trifluoperazine is given to a child exactly as prescribed. Children may react strongly to this medicine's effects.

You may have to take trifluoperazine for several weeks before you feel its full effects. Do not stop taking this medicine without first checking with your doctor. Your doctor may want you to reduce the amount you are taking gradually before you stop taking it completely.

Trifluoperazine can cause you to sweat less; as a result, your body temperature will rise. Be careful to avoid situations in which you may become overheated (such as strenuous exercise or hot weather) while taking this medicine.

Some people become more sensitive to sunlight while they are taking trifluoperazine. Limit the amount of time you spend in sunlight until you know how this medicine will affect you. If you sunburn easily while taking trifluoperazine, contact your doctor.

Pregnant women and women who are breast-feeding should not take trifluoperazine because of possible bad effects on the baby. Before you start to take this medicine, tell your doctor if you are pregnant or are nursing a baby. If you become pregnant while taking trifluoperazine, contact your doctor at once.

DOSAGE

Your doctor will determine how often you should take trifluoperazine and how much you should take at each dose. Carefully follow the instructions on your prescription label, and ask your doctor or pharmacist to explain any part of the instructions you do not understand.

Trifluoperazine comes in tablets and in concentrated liquid form to be taken orally. The tablets should be taken with a full eight-ounce glass of water or milk to avoid stomach upset.

Trifluoperazine liquid comes in a container with a measuring dropper. If you are taking this form, be sure you understand how much to take and how to measure it with the dropper. Just before you take the liquid, measure the proper amount into one-half glass (four ounces) of juice, water, soup, coffee, tea, milk or a soft drink. If any of the liquid with which you are diluting the medicine gets on the dropper, rinse the dropper with tap water before putting it back in the container.

Avoid getting liquid trifluoperazine on your skin or clothing. Liquid trifluoperazine may cause a skin rash.

If you forget to take a dose of trifluoperazine, take it as soon as you remember and take any remaining doses for that day at evenly spaced intervals. If you do not remember a missed dose until it is almost time to take another one, omit the missed dose completely and take only the regularly scheduled dose. *Do not take a double dose.*

STORAGE

Keep trifluoperazine in the container it came in, and store it away from heat and direct sunlight. Keep it out of the reach of children. Do not allow anyone else to take your trifluoperazine.

Miscellaneous
Drugs

MISCELLANEOUS DRUGS

Estrogen
(ess' tro jen)

PRODUCT INFORMATION
Brand name: Premarin
Brand name of a combination product containing meprobamate: Milprem

USES
Estrogen is a hormone produced by the body that is needed by women to bear children and for other natural functions. Additional estrogen is prescribed for women to relieve certain symptoms of menopause, such as "hot flashes," sweating, irritability, anxiety, depression and other discomforts.

Estrogen also is used to help promote normal physical growth in young women who are not maturing at the usual rate. Certain types of cancer, including cancer of the breast and prostate, are treated with estrogen.

UNDESIRED EFFECTS
Nausea is the most frequent side effect of estrogen. If you take this medicine with milk or a light snack, you may avoid this problem. The nausea should disappear as your body adjusts to estrogen. If it does not, contact your doctor. You may notice tenderness and fullness of the breast while you are taking estrogen. This side effect is harmless and will disappear when you stop taking estrogen.

More serious side effects will require medical attention. Contact your doctor if you have puffiness of the hands or ankles, weight gain, leg cramps, bleeding or discharge from the vagina or pain and tenderness of the calf or groin.

PRECAUTIONS
If you or any member of your family ever had lumps in the breast or breast cancer, you should not take estrogen. Tell your doctor about this problem and any other medical condition that may be made worse by estrogen such as diabetes, asthma, epilepsy, migraine headaches, heart or kidney disease, bone disease, liver disease or an underactive or overactive thyroid.

Estrogen may affect the way your body responds to any other medicine. Before you begin to take estrogen, tell your doctor what prescription or nonprescription drugs you are taking. If you do not know the names of the drugs or what they were prescribed for, bring them in their labeled containers to your doctor or pharmacist.

It is important that your doctor check the way you are responding to estrogen. *Be sure to keep all your appointments for checkups.* You may have to take estrogen for several weeks before its full effects can be determined.

Do not stop taking estrogen unless your doctor specifically tells you to do so. Before you have any laboratory test, tell the doctor in charge that you are taking estrogen.

To help your doctor select the best treatment for you and your baby, tell your doctor if you are pregnant or are breast-feeding. If you become pregnant while taking this medicine, contact your doctor.

DOSAGE

Your doctor will determine how much estrogen you should take and how often you should take it. Carefully follow the instructions on your prescription label, and ask your doctor or pharmacist to explain any part of the instructions you do not understand.

Estrogen comes in tablets to be taken orally and as a cream to be inserted in the vagina. If you are to use the estrogen cream, your doctor or pharmacist will tell you how to insert it. You may wish to wear a sanitary napkin after inserting the cream to avoid staining your clothes.

If you forget to take a tablet, take it as soon as you remember it. If you remember a missed dose when it is time for you to take another, omit the missed dose entirely and take only the regularly scheduled dose. *Do not take a double dose to make up for a missed dose.*

STORAGE

Keep estrogen in the container it came in, and keep it out of the reach of children. Do not allow anyone else to take your estrogen.

Estrogen and Progestogen Combinations
(ess′ tro jen) (proe jes′ to jen)

PRODUCT INFORMATION

Brand names: Brevicon, Demulen, Enovid, Loestrin, Lo-Ovral, Modicon, Nordette, Norinyl, Norlestrin, Ortho-Novum, Ovcon, Ovral, Ovulen, Tri-Norinyl, Triphasil

USES

Birth-control pills contain estrogen and progestogen, two female hormones. During pregnancy, your body manufactures these two hormones to prevent your ovaries from releasing eggs. Therefore, when you take these hormones regularly, they will keep you from getting pregnant by preventing the release of eggs from your ovaries.

Attempts to improve the effectiveness and decrease the side effects of birth-control pills have led to two variations on the original combination birth-control pills. These new products are the ''low dose'' pills (contain less than 50 micrograms of estrogen and 1.5 milligrams of progestogen) and biphasic and triphasic pills. Biphasic (Ortho-Novum 10/11) or triphasic (Ortho-Novum 7/7/7, Tri-Norinyl and Triphasil) pills containing varying amounts of the estrogen and progestogen components are used during different days of the menstrual cycle. To be effective, these pills must be taken in the proper sequence.

UNDESIRED EFFECTS

The most common side effects of birth-control pills are similar to those experienced during early pregnancy such as tenderness of the breasts, weight gain or loss, nausea and vomiting and spotted darkening of the skin. These effects usually are mild but should be reported to your doctor if they are bothersome.

Spotting or bleeding between menstrual periods is not uncommon during the first two months of taking birth-control pills. However, you should contact your doctor if such bleeding continues after the second month. You may need a change in your medication.

While serious side effects such as blood clots, stroke and liver problems are rare, be on the alert for symptoms of these problems. Contact your doctor if you develop a sharp pain in the chest or shortness of breath or cough up blood (symptoms of blood clots in the lungs); crushing pain or heaviness in the chest (possibly a heart attack); pain in the calf of the leg (possibly a blood clot); sudden severe headache or vomiting, dizziness or fainting, disturbance of vision or speech or weakness or numbness in an arm or a leg (symptoms of a stroke); sudden partial or complete loss of vision (possibly a blood clot in the eye); severe pain in the abdomen or yellowing of the skin (symptoms of liver problems); breast lumps; or severe depression.

PRECAUTIONS
Carefully read the package insert that comes with your birth-control pills. Ask your doctor or pharmacist for a copy if you do not have one. You should not take birth-control pills if you ever had blood clots in the legs or lungs; a stroke, heart attack or angina pectoris (heart pain); known or suspected cancer of the breast or sex organs; or unusual vaginal bleeding that has not been diagnosed.

To make taking birth-control pills as safe as possible, tell your doctor if you have breast nodules or cysts, diabetes, high blood pressure, high cholesterol level, migraine headaches, heart or kidney disease, epilepsy, mental depression, fibroid tumors of the uterus, gallbladder disease or a family history of breast cancer. Also tell your doctor if you smoke cigarettes. You should not smoke while taking this medication because smoking increases the risk of serious side effects.

Before you start to take birth-control pills, tell your doctor what prescription or nonprescription drugs you are taking including ampicillin, anticoagulants (blood thinners), barbiturates, medicine for depression or seizures, phenylbutazone, phenytoin, rifampin and tetracycline.

Oral contraceptives must be taken daily for at least two weeks before they can be considered fully effective in preventing pregnancy. To prevent pregnancy during these first two weeks, use some other form of birth control as well.

See your doctor regularly (every six to 12 months) for a complete physical examination, particularly breast and pelvic examinations and a Pap smear. Follow your doctor's instructions for examining your own breasts between checkups. Before having any surgery, including dental surgery, tell your doctor or dentist that you are taking birth-control pills.

Before you start to take birth-control pills, tell your doctor if you think you may be pregnant. Birth-control pills can harm your developing child. If you miss one menstrual period and have been taking your tablets as directed, continue taking them. However, if you miss one period and have not taken your tablets as directed or if you miss two menstrual periods and have taken the tablets as directed, notify your doctor and use another method of birth control until you can determine if you are pregnant. If you wish to stop taking birth-control pills and become pregnant, use another form of birth control for three months to be sure that the medication will not affect the baby. Tell your doctor if you are breast-feeding a baby. It is not known whether this medication is harmful to a breast-fed baby.

DOSAGE
Oral contraceptives come in tablets. They are available in packets of 21 or 28 tablets. In the 28-tablet packet, the last seven tablets are a different color. These tablets are not birth-control pills; they contain either iron (ferrous fumarate) or an inactive ingredient. Your menstrual period should begin while you are taking the last seven tablets of a 28-tablet packet. If you are using the 21-tablet packet, your menstrual period should begin after you take the last tablet.

Counting the first day of your period as day one, oral contraceptives are taken from day five through 25 of your menstrual cycle. Be sure you carefully follow your doctor's instructions. Always have your prescription refilled often enough so that you have another packet ready when you finish a packet of tablets.

Be sure to take one tablet regularly each day. It is a good idea to take a tablet at the same time every day and at a time when you do something else each day, such as brushing your teeth in the morning or eating dinner in the evening. If you have tablets of more than one color, be sure to take them in the proper sequence. Different colored tablets contain different ingredients and are not interchangeable.

If you forget to take one tablet at the scheduled time, take it as soon as you remember it. Take the next one at the regular time, even though you may be taking two tablets in one day. If you miss two tablets, take two tablets a day for the next two days. Also, use another method of birth control until you have taken one tablet each day for seven consecutive days.

If you miss three tablets, do not take them when you remember. Contact your doctor or pharmacist for instructions. Use another method of birth control.

STORAGE
Keep this medicine out of the reach of children.

Ferrous Sulfate
(fer′ us sul′ fate)

PRODUCT INFORMATION
Brand names: Feosol, Fer-in-Sol, Fero-Gradumet, Ferolix, Ferralyn, Ferospace, Fesotyme, Mol-Iron and others

USES
Ferrous sulfate provides the body with the extra amounts of iron needed to produce red blood cells. It is used to treat iron-deficiency anemia, a condition that

occurs when the body has too few red blood cells. Iron-deficiency anemia is usually the result of poor diet, excess bleeding or certain medical problems.

UNDESIRED EFFECTS

Stomach upset, nausea and vomiting are common side effects of taking ferrous sulfate. If you experience these effects, disregard instructions to take this medicine on an empty stomach and take it with meals or a snack.

If this medicine makes you constipated, drink extra fluids and add foods such as bran and prunes to your diet. If you have questions about foods that can help prevent constipation, check with your doctor or pharmacist.

Ferrous sulfate can cause darkening of the stools. This side effect is harmless. It also can darken the teeth of children. This effect is harmless, but the child's teeth can be cleaned once a week with tooth powder or baking soda.

PRECAUTIONS

Because ferrous sulfate can make some medical conditions worse, tell your doctor if you have hemochromatosis (anemia caused by something other than iron deficiency), stomach ulcer or inflammation or ulcerative disease of the bowel.

Before you start to take ferrous sulfate, tell your doctor what prescription or nonprescription drugs you are taking, particularly antacids, tetracycline, chloramphenicol and pencillamine (medicine for rheumatoid arthritis). If you do not know the names of the drugs or what they were prescribed for, bring them in their labeled containers to your doctor or pharmacist.

Take ferrous sulfate exactly as your doctor has prescribed. It may take several days or weeks before you begin to feel the full benefit of this medicine. Be sure to take ferrous sulfate as long as your doctor tells you to. Your doctor may want to perform blood tests to determine if this medication is working. *Be sure to keep all appointments for checkups.*

DOSAGE

Your doctor will determine how much ferrous sulfate you should take and how often you should take it. Carefully follow the instructions on your prescription label, and ask your doctor or pharmacist to explain any part of the instructions you do not understand.

Ferrous sulfate comes in tablets and in liquid form to be taken orally and in drops for small children. This medicine should be taken on an empty stomach (at least two hours after meals), unless it upsets your stomach; then it may be taken with meals or a snack.

Over time, liquid ferrous sulfate may change color from pale green-blue to light yellow. This change does not affect the strength of the drug, and you may continue to take it if this change occurs.

If you are giving drops to a child, you may place the drops directly into the child's mouth or mix them into water or fruit juice. Be sure to measure the drops carefully, and give your child only the amount the doctor has prescribed.

If you forget to take a dose of this medicine, take it as soon as you remember it. If you do not remember a missed dose until it is time for your next dose, omit the missed dose entirely and take only the regularly scheduled dose. *Do not take a double dose.*

STORAGE
Keep ferrous sulfate in the container it came in, and keep it out of the reach of children. This precaution is very important, because an overdose of ferrous sulfate can be fatal to a small child. Do not let anyone else take your ferrous sulfate.

Nicotine
(nick' o teen)

PRODUCT INFORMATION
Brand name: Nicorette

USES
Nicotine is a natural substance present in tobacco leaves. It is difficult for many people to stop smoking because nicotine is habit-forming.

Nicotine chewing gum is used in behavior modification programs (including counseling and education) to help people stop smoking. It is most successful when individuals have a strong motivation to stop smoking.

Chewing gum acts as a substitute oral activity and provides a source of nicotine that reduces the withdrawal symptoms experienced when smoking is stopped.

UNDESIRED EFFECTS
Side effects caused by nicotine are usually mild and disappear after using the gum for a few days. These effects include irritation or a tingling sensation of the tongue, mouth and throat; mouth ulcers; and jaw ache. Contact your doctor if these problems persist.

Indigestion and nausea may occur during the first week, particularly if you chew the gum too fast or vigorously (the nicotine is released too quickly). It may help to chew the gum more slowly.

Other side effects of nicotine include dizziness, headache, insomnia, irritability and hiccups. These symptoms should decrease as you follow your doctor's instructions to decrease the number of pieces of gum chewed per day. Contact your doctor if these side effects persist or are bothersome.

Nicotine chewing gum has a tobacco-like, slightly peppery taste and contains a sweetener (sorbitol). Most people find the taste somewhat unpleasant.

PRECAUTIONS
Because nicotine may make some medical conditions worse, tell your doctor if you have heart disease, particularly a history of heart attack, angina (heart pain) or irregular heartbeat (arrhythmia); high blood pressure; overactive thyroid gland (hy-

perthyroidism); pheochromocytoma (a disease of the adrenal gland); type I (insulin dependent) diabetes; or ulcers.

Tell your doctor what prescription and nonprescription drugs you are taking, particularly albuterol, beta blockers (atenolol, metoprolol, nadolol, pindolol, propranolol and timolol), furosemide, imipramine, metaproterenol, pentazocine, phenylephrine, phenylpropanolamine, propoxyphene, pseudoephedrine, theophylline and terbutaline. Stopping smoking may affect the way your body responds to these drugs. If you do not know the names of the drugs you are taking or what they were prescribed for, take them in their labeled containers to your doctor or pharmacist.

Follow your doctor's instructions for use of the chewing gum. Do not use more of it or use it more often than instructed. Do not smoke cigarettes while using nicotine chewing gum because nicotine overdose may result. Signs of nicotine overdose include nausea, increased salivation, abdominal pain, vomiting, diarrhea, sweating, headache, dizziness, hearing and visual disturbances, mental confusion and weakness. If you accidentally use too much or if a child ingests the gum, call your doctor or poison center immediately. Swallowing the gum is not dangerous because nicotine is absorbed slowly in the stomach.

Do not stop using the gum unless your doctor tells you to or your craving for cigarettes is satisfied by one or two pieces of gum per day. Ask your doctor if you want to stop using the gum. You should gradually reduce the number of pieces of gum chewed per day to prevent withdrawal from occurring. Symptoms of nicotine withdrawal (which may result when either the gum or smoking is stopped) include craving for tobacco, irritability, anxiety, difficulty concentrating, restlessness, headache, drowsiness and stomach upset. These symptoms vary in severity and duration. They usually appear within 24 hours of stopping smoking or using nicotine gum and last for several days or weeks.

Tell your doctor if you are pregnant, plan to become pregnant or are breastfeeding a baby. Nicotine is passed from a mother to an unborn baby and a breast-fed baby. Babies born to women that smoke during pregnancy generally weigh less than babies born to nonsmoking women.

DOSAGE

Nicotine comes in a chewing gum. Ask your pharmacist or doctor for a copy of the package insert (manufacturer's detailed labeling and instructions for use included inside the package).

Follow the instructions on your prescription label and the package insert carefully, and ask your doctor or pharmacist to explain any part you do not understand.

Stop smoking cigarettes immediately. Nicotine chewing gum should be used as a temporary substitute for smoking. Chew one piece of gum whenever you have the urge to smoke a cigarette. Chew the gum slowly until you can taste the nicotine or feel a slight tingling in your mouth. Stop chewing. Once the tingling is almost gone (about one minute), start chewing and repeat this procedure for about 30 minutes. Do not chew the gum rapidly because side effects, such as nausea, may occur.

Chewing nicotine gum does not satisfy your craving for nicotine as quickly as smoking a cigarette.

Keep in touch with your doctor at least once a month so that your progress can be evaluated. You should be able to decrease the number of pieces of gum you use per day gradually. If you are using only one or two pieces of gum per day, follow your doctor's instructions for stopping the gum completely. Do not use more than 30 pieces of gum per day or use nicotine gum for longer than six months without consulting your doctor.

STORAGE

Keep nicotine gum out of the reach of children and protect it from light. Do not allow anyone else to use your gum unless they are under a doctor's supervision.

Appendix
Canadian Brand Names

Many brand names under which drugs are sold in Canada differ from those used in the United States. Canadian readers who do not know the generic names of the drugs that have been prescribed for them can refer to this Appendix; Canadian brand names are followed here by the names of the generic drugs to which they refer. The pages of this book on which these generic drugs are discussed are listed in the Index.

A

Accutane Roche—isotretinoin
Acetazolam—acetazolamide
Acetophen—aspirin
Achromycin—tetracycline hydrochloride
Achromycin V—tetracycline hydrochloride
Actidil—triprolidine hydrochloride
Adalat—nifedipine
Adrenalin—epinephrine
Aeroseb HC—hydrocortisone
Aldactone—spironolactone
Aldomet—methyldopa
Algoverine—phenylbutazone
Allerdryl—diphenhydramine hydrochloride
Alloprin—allopurinol
Alupent—metaproterenol sulfate
Alu-Tab—aluminum hydroxide
Amcill—ampicillin
Amersol—ibuprofen
Amoxil—amoxicillin
Amphojel—aluminum hydroxide
Ampicin—ampicillin
Ampilean—ampicillin
Amytal—amobarbital
Ancasal—aspirin
Antazone—sulfinpyrazone
Anturan—sulfinpyrazone
Aparkane—trihexyphenidyl hydrochloride
Apo-Acetaminophen—acetaminophen
Apo-Acetazolamide—acetazolamide
Apo-Allopurinol—allopurinol
Apo-Amitriptyline—amitriptyline
Apo-Asen—aspirin
Apo-Benztropine—benztropine mesylate
Apo-Carbamazepine—carbamazepine
Apo-Chlordiazepoxide—chlordiazepoxide
Apo-Chlorpromazine—chlorpromazine

Apo-Chlorpropamide—chlorpropamide
Apo-Chlorthalidone—chlorthalidone
Apo-Cimetidine—cimetidine
Apo-Diazepam—diazepam
Apo-Dipyridamole—dipyridamole
Apo-Erythro-S—erythromycin stearate
Apo-Ferrous Sulfate—ferrous sulfate
Apo-Flurazepam—flurazepam hydrochloride
Apo-Furosemide—furosemide
Apo-Guanethidine—guanethidine sulfate
Apo-Haloperidol—haloperidol
Apo-Hydro—hydrochlorothiazide
Apo-Imipramine—imipramine
Apo-ISDN—isosorbide dinitrate
Apo-K—potassium chloride
Apo-Meprobamate—meprobamate
Apo-Methyldopa—methyldopa
Apo-Metronidazole—metronidazole
Apo-Naproxen—naproxen
Apo-Nitrofurantoin—nitrofurantoin
Apo-Oxazepam—oxazepam
Apo-Oxtriphylline—oxtriphylline
Apo-Perphenazine—perphenazine
Apo-Phenylbutazone—phenylbutazone
Apo-Prednisone—prednisone
Apo-Primidone—primidone
Apo-Propranolol—propranolol hydrochloride
Apo-Quinidine—quinidine hydrochloride
Apo-Sulfamethoxazole—sulfamethoxazole
Apo-Sulfatrim—co-trimoxazole
Apo-Sulfinpyrazone—sulfinpyrazone
Apo-Sulfisoxazole—sulfisoxazole
Apo-Tetra—tetracycline hydrochloride
Apo-Thioridazine—thioridazine hydrochloride
Apo-Tolbutamide—tolbutamide
Apo-Trifluoperazine—trifluoperazine

Apo-Trihex—trihexyphenidyl
  hydrochloride
Apresoline—hydralazine
Aristocort—triamcinolone
Aristospan hexacetonide—triamcinolone
Artane—trihexyphenidyl hydrochloride
Asendin—amoxapine
Astrin—aspirin
Atarax—hydroxyzine hydrochloride
Atasol—acetaminophen
Atasol Forte—acetaminophen
Athrombin-K potassium—warfarin
Ativan—lorazepam
Aventyl—nortriptyline hydrochloride
Ayercillin—penicillin G

B

Baciguent—bacitracin
Bacitin—bacitracin
Bactopen—cloxacillin sodium
Bactrim—co-trimoxazole
Balminil D.M. Syrup—dextromethorphan
  hydrobromide
Balminil Expectorant—guaifenesin
Banlin—propantheline bromide
Barriere—simethicone
Barseb—hydrocortisone
Basaljel—aluminum hydroxide
Beben—betamethasone
Beclovent—beclomethasone dipropionate
Beconase—beclomethasone dipropionate
Benadryl—diphenhydramine
  hydrochloride
Benemid—probenecid
Bensylate—benztropine mesylate
Bentylol—dicyclomine hydrochloride
Benuryl—probenecid
Benzedrine—amphetamine sulfate
Betacort—betamethasone
Betaderm—betamethasone
Betaloc—metoprolol tartrate
Betnelan—betamethasone
Betnesol—betamethasone
Betnovate—betamethasone
Bicillin—penicillin G
Biquin Durules—quinidine bisulfate
Bleph-10—sulfacetamide
Blocadren—timolol maleate

Bonamine—meclizine hydrochloride
Brevicon—estrogen and progestogen
  combinations
Bricanyl—terbutaline sulfate
Broncho-Grippol-DM—dextromethorphan
  hydrobromide
Bronkaid Mistometer—epinephrine
Buffazone—phenylbutazone
Butazolidin—phenylbutazone
Butisol Sodium—butabarbital

C

Campain—acetaminophen
Capoten—captopril
Carbolith—lithium carbonate
Cardilate—erythrityl tetranitrate
Cardioquin—quinidine polygalacturonate
Cardizem—diltiazem hydrochloride
Catapres—clonidine hydrochloride
Ceclor—cefaclor
Cefracycline—tetracycline hydrochloride
Celestoderm—betamethasone
Celestone—betamethasone
Celontin—methsuximide
Ceporex—cephalexin monohydrate
Cetamide—sulfacetamide
Chloronase—chlorpropamide
Chloroptic—chloramphenicol
Chlorphen—chlorpheniramine
Chlor-Promanyl—chlorpromazine
Chlor-Tripolon—chlorpheniramine
  maleate
Climestrone Tablets—estrogens
Clinoril—sulindac
Cloxilean—cloxacillin sodium
Cogentin—benztropine mesylate
Colace—docusate sodium
Combantrin—pyrantel pamoate
Conjugated Estrogens—estrogens
Corgard—nadolol
Coronex—isosorbide dinitrate
Corophyllin—aminophylline
Cortamed—hydrocortisone
Cortate—hydrocortisone
Cort-Dome—hydrocortisone
Cortef—hydrocortisone
Cortenema—hydrocortisone
Corticreme—hydrocortisone

Cortifoam—hydrocortisone
Cortiment—hydrocortisone
Cortoderm—hydrocortisone
Cortril—hydrocortisone
Corutol DH—hydrocodone bitartrate
Corutol Expectorant—guaifenesin
Coryphen—aspirin
Coumadin sodium—warfarin
Cremocort—triamcinolone
Crystapen—penicillin G
Cytomel—liothyronine sodium

D

Dalmane—flurazepam hydrochloride
Darbid—isopropamide iodide
Darvon-N—propoxyphene napsylate
Day-Barb—butabarbital
Decadron—dexamethasone
Declomycin—demeclocycline
Delsym—dextromethorphan
    hydrobromide
Deltasone—prednisone
Demo-Cineol Antitussive
    Syrup—dextromethorphan
    hydrobromide
Demulen—estrogen and progestogen
    combinations
Dermalar—fluocinolone acetonide
Dermophyl—fluocinolone acetonide
Deronil—dexamethasone
Desyrel—trazodone
Detensol—propranolol hydrochloride
Dexasone—dexamethasone
Dexedrine—dexamphetamine
Diaβeta—glyburide
Diabinese—chlorpropamide
Diamox—acetazolamide
Dilantin—phenytoin
Dimelor—acetohexamide
Dimetane—brompheniramine maleate
Diprosone—betamethasone
Diuchlor H—hydrochlorothiazide
Diuril—chlorothiazide
Dixarit—clonidine hydrochloride
DM Syrup—dextromethorphan
    hydrobromide
Dolobid—diflunisal
Dopamet—methyldopa

Drenison—flurandrenolide
Duretic—methyclothiazide
Duricef—cefadroxil
Dynapen—dicloxacillin sodium
    monohydrate
Dyrenium—triamterene
Dysne-Inhal hydrochloride—epinephrine

E

Ecostatin—econazole nitrate
Ecotrin—aspirin
Edecrin—ethacrynic acid
EES-200—erythromycin
EES-400—erythromycin
Elavil—amitriptyline hydrochloride
Elixophyllin—theophylline
Eltor—pseudoephedrine hydrochloride
Eltroxin—levothyroxine sodium
Emo-Cort—hydrocortisone
E-Mycin—erythromycin
Enovid E—estrogen and progestogen
    combinations
Entrophen—aspirin
E-Pam—diazepam
Epifrin hydrochloride—epinephrine
Epitrate bitartrate—epinephrine
Equanil—meprobamate
Eryc—erythromycin base
Erythrocin ethyl succinate, stearate or
    lactobionate—erythromycin
Erythromid—erythromycin
Esidrix—hydrochlorothiazide
Estinyl—estrogens
Estrace—estrogens
Etibi—ethambutol hydrochloride
Exdol—acetaminophen

F

Feldene—piroxicam
Fenicol—chloramphenicol
Fer-In-Sol—ferrous sulfate
Fero-Grad—ferrous sulfate
Fesofor—ferrous sulfate
Fivent—cromolyn sodium
Flagyl—metronidazole
Flexeril—cyclobenzaprine hydrochloride

Fluoderm—fluocinolone acetonide
Fluolar—fluocinolone acetonide
Formulex—dicyclomine hydrochloride
Fulvicin P/G—griseofulvin
Fulvicin U/F—griseofulvin
Furacin—nitrofurazone
Furoside—furosemide

G

Gantanol—sulfamethoxazole
Gantrisin—sulfisoxazole
Garamycin—gentamicin sulfate
Gardenal—phenobarbital
gBh—lindane
Grisovin-FP—griseofulvin

H

Halcion—triazolam
Haldol—haloperidol
Halotex—haloprogin
Herplex—idoxuridine
Herplex-D Liquifilm—idoxuridine
Hexadrol—dexamethasone
Histantil—promethazine hydrochloride
Humulin-N—insulin (human biosynthetic)
Humulin-R—insulin (human biosynthetic)
Hycodan—hydrocodone bitartrate
Hyderm—hydrocortisone
Hydro-Cortilean—hydrocortisone
Hydrocortone—hydrocortisone
HydroDiuril—hydrochlorothiazide
Hygroton—chlorthalidone

I

Iletin Lente—insulin zinc suspension
Iletin II Pork Lente—insulin zinc
    suspension
Iletin Semilente—insulin zinc suspension
Iletin Ultralente—insulin zinc suspension
Ilosone estolate—erythromycin
Imodium—loperamide hydrochloride
Impril—imipramine hydrochloride
Inderal—propranolol hydrochloride
Inderal-LA—propranolol hydrochloride
Indocid—indomethacin

Insomnal—diphenhydramine
    hydrochloride
Insulin Lente—insulin zinc suspension
Insulin Semilente—insulin zinc
    suspension
Insulin Ultralente—insulin zinc
    suspension
Intal—cromolyn sodium
Intrabutazone—phenylbutazone
Ionamin ion-exchange resin
    complex—phentermine
Ismelin—guanethidine sulfate
Isobec base—amobarbital
Isoptin—verapamil hydrochloride
Isopto Carbachol—carbachol
Isopto Carpine
    hydrochloride—pilocarpine
Isopto Cetamide—sulfacetamide
Isopto Fenicol—chloramphenicol
Isordil—isosorbide dinitrate
Isotamine—isoniazid
Isuprel—isoproterenol

K

K-10—potassium chloride
Kalium Durules—potassium chloride
Kaochlor—potassium chloride
Kaochlor-20 Concentrate—potassium
    chloride
Kaon—potassium gluconate
Kay Ciel—potassium chloride
KCL 5%—potassium chloride
KCL 20%—potassium chloride
Keflex—cephalexin monohydrate
Kenacort—triamcinolone
Kenalog—triamcinolone
Kenalog-E acetonide—triamcinolone
K-Long—potassium chloride
K-Lor—potassium chloride
K-Lyte/Cl—potassium chloride
Koffex Syrup—dextromethorphan
    hydrobromide
Kwellada—lindane

L

Lanoxin—digoxin

Largactil—chlorpromazine
Larodopa—levodopa
Lasix—furosemide
Laxagel—docusate sodium
Ledercillin VK potassium—penicillin V
Lente Insulin—insulin zinc suspension
Levate—amitriptyline hydrochloride
Librium—chlordiazepoxide hydrochloride
Lidemol—fluocinonide
Lidex—fluocinonide
Lioresal—baclofen
Lithane—lithium carbonate
Lithizine—lithium carbonate
Loestrin—estrogen and progestogen
  combinations
Lomine—dicyclomine hydrochloride
Lomotil—diphenoxylate hydrochloride
Loniten—minoxidil
Lopresor—metoprolol tartrate
Lorelco—probucol
Loxapac—loxapine
Ludiomil—maprotiline hydrochloride
Luminal—phenobarbital
Lyderm Cream—fluocinonide

M

Macrodantin—nitrofurantoin
Mandelamine—methenamine mandelate
Maxidex—dexamethasone
Mazepine—carbamazepine
Medicycline—tetracycline hydrochloride
Medihaler-Epi bitartrate—epinephrine
Medihaler-Iso—isoproterenol
Medilium—chlordiazepoxide
  hydrochloride
Medimet-250—methyldopa
Meditran—meprobamate
Megacillin Suspension—penicillin G
Megacillin Tablets—penicillin G
Mellaril—thioridazine hydrochloride
Menrium—chlordiazepoxide and
  estrogens
Meprospan-400—meprobamate
Meravil—amitriptyline hydrochloride
Metaderm—betamethasone
Meval—diazepam
Micatin—miconazole nitrate
Microcort—hydrocortisone

Micro-K—potassium chloride
Micronor—progestogen
Midamor—amiloride
Miltown—meprobamate
Minestrin—estrogen and progestogen
  combinations
Minims—chloramphenicol, pilocarpine
  and sulfacetamide
Minipress—prazosin hydrochloride
Minocin—minocycline hydrochloride
Min-Ovral—estrogen and progestogen
  combinations
Miocarpine hydrochloride—pilocarpine
Miostat—carbachol
Mobenol—tolbutamide
Monistat—miconazole nitrate
Motrin—ibuprofen
Moxilean trihydrate—amoxicillin
Multipax—hydroxyzine hydrochloride
Myambutol—ethambutol hydrochloride
Mycifradin—neomycin sulfate
Myciguent—neomycin sulfate
Mycostatin—nystatin
Mydfrin—phenylephrine hydrochloride
Mysoline—primidone

N

Nadopen-V—penicillin V
Nadostine—nystatin
Nadozone—phenylbutazone
Nafrine—oxymetazoline hydrochloride
Nalcrom—cromolyn sodium
Nalfon calcium—fenoprofen
Naprosyn—naproxen
Natigoxine—digoxin
Natrimax—hydrochlorothiazide
Navane—thiothixene
Nefrol—hydrochlorothiazide
NegGram—nalidixic acid
Neo-Barb—butabarbital
Neo-Calme—diazepam
Neo-Codema—hydrochlorothiazide
Neo-DM—dextromethorphan
  hydrobromide
Neo-K—potassium bicarbonate and
  chloride
Neo-Renal—furosemide
Neo-Spec—guaifenesin

Neo-Synephrine—phenylephrine
hydrochloride
Neo-Tetrine—tetracycline hydrochloride
Neo-Tran—meprobamate
Neo-Tric—metronidazole
Neo-Zoline—phenylbutazone
Nephronex—nitrofurantoin
Nicorette—nicotine
Nifuran—nitrofurantoin
Nilstat—nystatin
Nitro-Bid—nitroglycerin
Nitrogard-SR—nitroglycerin
Nitrol—nitroglycerin
Nitrong SR—nitroglycerin
Nitrostabilin—nitroglycerin
Nitrostat—nitroglycerin
Noctec—chloral hydrate
Norinyl—estrogen and progestogen
combinations
Norlestrin—estrogen and progestogen
combinations
Norpace—disopyramide phosphate
Norpace CR—disopyramide phosphate
Norpramin—desipramine
Novamobarb—amobarbital
Novamoxin trihydrate—amoxicillin
Novasen—aspirin
Novo-Ampicillin—ampicillin
Novobetamet—betamethasone
Novobutamide—tolbutamide
Novobutazone—phenylbutazone
Novochlorhydrate—chloral hydrate
Novochlorpromazine—chlorpromazine
Novocimetidine—cimetidine
Novocloxin—cloxacillin sodium
Novocolchine—colchicine
Novodigoxin—digoxin
Novodipam—diazepam
Novoferrosulfa—ferrous sulfate
Novoflupam—flurazepam hydrochloride
Novoflurazine—trifluoperazine
Novofuran—nitrofurantoin
Novohexidyl—trihexyphenidyl
hydrochloride
Novohydrazide—hydrochlorothiazide
Novohydrocort—hydrocortisone
Novolente-K—potassium chloride
Novolexin—cephalexin monohydrate
Novomedopa—methyldopa

Novomepro—meprobamate
Novomethacin—indomethacin
Novonaprox—naproxen
Novoniacin—niacin
Novonidazol—metronidazole
Novopen-G—penicillin G
Novopen-VK—penicillin V
Novopheniram—chlorpheniramine
maleate
Novophenytoin—phenytoin
Novopoxide—chlordiazepoxide
hydrochloride
Novopramine—imipramine hydrochloride
Novopranol—propranolol hydrochloride
Novoprednisone—prednisone
Novopropamide—chlorpropamide
Novopropanthil—propantheline bromide
Novopropoxyn—propoxyphene
hydrochloride
Novopurol—allopurinol
Novopyrazone—sulfinpyrazone
Novoquinidin—quinidine
Novoquinine—quinine sulfate
Novoreserpine—reserpine
Novoridazine—thioridazine hydrochloride
Novorythro base, stearate or
estolate—erythromycin
Novosecobarb—secobarbital
Novosemide—furosemide
Novosorbide—isosorbide dinitrate
Novosoxazole—sulfisoxazole
Novotetra—tetracycline hydrochloride
Novothalidone—chlorthalidone
Novotrimel—cotrimoxazole
Novotriphyl—oxtriphylline
Novotriptyn—amitriptyline hydrochloride
Nyaderm—nystatin

O

Ocusert Pilo-20—pilocarpine
Ocusert Pilo-40—pilocarpine
Oestrilin—estrogens
Ogen Tablets—estrogens
Opticrom—cromolyn sodium
Orbenin—cloxacillin sodium
Orciprenaline sulfate—metaproterenol
sulfate
Orinase—tolbutamide

Ortho—estrogen and progestogen
　combinations
Ortho-Novum—estrogen and progestogen
　combinations
Ovol—simethicone
Ovral—estrogen and progestogen
　combinations
Ovulen—estrogen and progestogen
　combinations
Ox-Pam—oxazepam

P

P-50—penicillin G
Palaron—aminophylline
Pamovin—pyrvinium pamoate
Panadol—acetaminophen
Panectyl—trimeprazine tartrate
Panolol—propranolol hydrochloride
Paveral—codeine phosphate
Penbritin—ampicillin
Penioral 500—penicillin G
Pen-Vee K—penicillin V
Pen-Vee potassium or
　benzathine—penicillin V
Peptol—cimetidine
Periactin—cyproheptadine hydrochloride
Peridol—haloperidol
Peritrate—pentaerythritol tetranitrate
Persantine—dipyridamole
Pertofrane—desipramine
Phenazine—perphenazine
Phenazo—phenazopyridine hydrochloride
Phenbuff—phenylbutazone
Phenergan—promethazine hydrochloride
Phyllocontin—aminophylline
Pitrex—tolnaftate
PMS Dopazide—methyldopa
Polymox trihydrate—amoxicillin
Ponstan—mefenamic acid
Potassium-Rougier—potassium gluconate
Potassium-Sandoz—potassium
　bicarbonate and chloride
Premarin—estrogens
Pro-Banthine—propantheline bromide
Profedrine—pseudoephedrine
　hydrochloride
Program Tablets—estrogens
Proloid—thyroglobulin

Proloprim—trimethoprim
Pronestyl—procainamide hydrochloride
Propanthel—propantheline bromide
Propyl-Thyracil—propylthiouracil
Protophylline—dyphylline
Protrin—co-trimoxazole
Protylol—dicyclomine hydrochloride
Pseudofrin—pseudoephedrine
　hydrochloride
Pulmophylline—theophylline
Purinol—allopurinol
P.V. Carpine nitrate—pilocarpine
PVF benzathine—penicillin V
PVF K potassium—penicillin V
Pyribenzamine hydrochloride or
　citrate—tripelennamine
Pyridium—phenazopyridine
　hydrochloride
Pyronium—phenazopyridine
　hydrochloride

Q

Questran—cholestyramine resin
Quibron-T—theophylline
Quibron-T/SR—theophylline
Quinaglute—quinidine gluconate
Quinate—quinidine gluconate
Quinidex Extentabs—quinidine sulfate

R

Regulex—docusate sodium
Reserfia—reserpine
Respbid—theophylline
Restocort—hydrocortisone
Restoril—temazepam
Resyl—guaifenesin
Rifadin—rifampin
Rimactane—rifampin
Rimifon—isoniazid
Riphen-10—aspirin
Rival—diazepam
Robaxin—methocarbamol
Robidex—dextromethorphan
　hydrobromide
Robidone—hydrocodone bitartrate

Robidrine—pseudoephedrine hydrochloride
Robigesic—acetaminophen
Robitussin—guaifenesin
Rofact—rifampin
Roubac—co-trimoxazole
Roucol—allopurinol
Rounox—acetaminophen
Roychlor—potassium chloride
Royonate—potassium gluconate
Rynacrom—cromolyn sodium
Rythmodan—disopyramide

S

Sal-Adult—aspirin
Salazopyrin—sulfasalazine
Salbutamol—albuterol
Sal-Infant—aspirin
SAS-500—sulfasalazine
S-Cortilean—hydrocortisone
Secogen sodium—secobarbital
Seconal sodium—secobarbital
Sedatuss—dextromethorphan hydrobromide
Septra—cotrimoxazole
Serax—oxazepam
Serenack—diazepam
Serpasil—reserpine
Sertan—primidone
Sinequan—doxepin hydrochloride
642—propoxyphene hydrochloride
Slo-Pot—potassium chloride
Slow-Fe—ferrous sulfate
Slow-K—potassium chloride
Sodium Amytal—amobarbital
Sodium Sulamyd—sulfacetamide
Solazine—trifluoperazine
Solium—chlordiazepoxide hydrochloride
Solu-Cortef—hydrocortisone
Somophyllin-T—theophylline
Somophyllin-12—theophylline
Sopamycetin—chloramphenicol
Spasmoban—dicyclomine hydrochloride
Stabinol—chlorpropamide
Stelazine—trifluoperazine
Stemetil—prochlorperazine
Sterine—methenamine mandelate
StieVAA—tretinoin

Stoxil—idoxuridine
Stress-Pam—diazepam
Sudafed—pseudoephedrine hydrochloride
Sulcrate—sucralfate
Sulfex—sulfacetamide
Sulf-10—sulfacetamide
Supasa—aspirin
Supeudol—oxycodone
Surfak—docusate calcium
Sus-Phrine—epinephrine
Symmetrel—amantadine hydrochloride
Synalar—fluocinolone acetonide
Synamol—fluocinolone acetonide
Synthroid—levothyroxine sodium

T

Tagamet—cimetidine
Talwin—pentazocine
Tapazole—methimazole
Tegopen—cloxacillin sodium
Tegretol—carbamazepine
Tempra—acetaminophen
Tenormin—atenolol
Terfluzine—trifluoperazine
Terramycin—oxytetracycline
Tertroxin—liothyronine sodium
Tetracyn—tetracycline hydrochloride
Tetralean—tetracycline hydrochloride
Theo-Dur—theophylline
Theolair—theophylline
Thioril—thioridazine hydrochloride
Tigan—trimethobenzamide hydrochloride
Timoptic—timolol maleate
Tinactin—tolnaftate
Tofranil—imipramine hydrochloride
Tolectin—tolmetin sodium
Topsyn Gel—fluocinonide
Tranxene—clorazepate dipotassium
Triaderm—triamcinolone
Trialean acetonide—triamcinolone
Triamacort—triamcinolone
Triamalone—triamcinolone
Triaphen-10—aspirin
Tridil—nitroglycerin
Triflurin—trifluoperazine
Trilafon—perphenazine
Triphasil—estrogen and progestogen combinations

Turbinaire Decadron
    phosphate—dexamethasone
Tylenol—acetaminophen

U

Unicort—hydrocortisone
Uridon—chlorthalidone
Uritol—furosemide
Urozide—hydrochlorothiazide

V

Valisone Scalp Lotion—betamethasone
Valium—diazepam
Vancenase—beclomethasone dipropionate
Vanceril—beclomethasone dipropionate
Vanquin—pyrvinium pamoate
Vaponefrin—epinephrine
V-Cillin K potassium—penicillin V
VC-K 500 potassium—penicillin V
Velosef—cephradine
Ventolin—albuterol
Vibramycin—doxycycline
Vimicon—cyproheptadine hydrochloride
Vira-A—vidarabine

Viscerol—dicyclomine hydrochloride
Visken—pindolol
Vitamin A Acid—tretinoin
Vivol—diazepam

W

Warfilone sodium—warfarin
Warnerin sodium—warfarin
Wel-K—potassium tartrate
Westcort—hydrocortisone
Winpred—prednisone
Wycillin 300—penicillin G
Wycillin 600—penicillin G

X

Xanax—alprazolam

Z

Zantac—ranitidine hydrochloride
Zapex—oxazepam
Zarontin—ethosuximide
Zaroxolyn—metolazone
Zovirax—acyclovir
Zyloprim—allopurinol
Zynol—sulfinpyrazone

Index

Note: The page numbers listed in this Index refer to the pages of the book on which discussion of a given drug begins. Also, Canadian readers may need to refer first to the Appendix, page 499, where the generic drugs to which Canadian brand names apply are listed; they can then check the Index to find where in the book discussions of each generic drug can be found.

A

B

C

O

Q

T

U